NURSING CARE DURING THE LABOR PROCESS

Edition 3

Janet Swanson Malinowski, R.N., M.S.N.
Associate Professor
Mercy College of Detroit
Detroit, Michigan

with

Carolyn G. Pedigo, R.N., M.S.N.
Associate Professor
University of Southwestern Louisiana
Lafayette, Louisiana

Celeste R. Phillips, R.N., Ed.D.
President of Phillips & Fenwick
Women's Health Care Consulting Firm
Capitola, California

F. A. DAVIS COMPANY • Philadelphia

Printed in the United States of America

Last digit indicates print number: 10 9 8 7 6 5 4

NOTE: As new scientific information becomes available through basic and clinical research, recommended treatments and drug therapies undergo changes. The author(s) and publisher have done everything possible to make this book accurate, up-to-date, and in accord with accepted standards at the time of publication. However, the reader is advised always to check product information (package inserts) for changes and new information regarding dose and contraindications before administering any drug. Caution is especially urged when using new or infrequently ordered drugs.

Library of Congress Cataloging-in-Publication Data

Malinowski, Janet S.
Nursing care during the labor process.
Bibliography: p.
Includes index.
1. Obstetrical nursing. 2. Labor (Obstetrics)
I. Pedigo, Carolyn G. II. Phillips, Celeste R.,
III. Title.
RG951.M28 1989 610.73′678 88-30981
ISBN 0-8036-5803-6

PREFACE

This book provides current knowledge about the labor process and nursing interventions based on contemporary standards for nursing practice. The book is a foundational textbook for student or practicing nurses. It can serve as an introduction to, a reference for, or a review of nursing care during the labor process. It is useful for both classroom and independent study in schools of nursing and hospital inservice education programs. It is a useful tool when preparing for N-CLEX and certification exams.

The format of this third edition remains the same as that of the first and second editions. It is written in a clear, concise, and organized way, using a self-instructional approach. The objectives and self-test questions and answers in each chapter facilitate the reader's understanding of the subject matter.

The reader can use the contents of this book to develop individualized nursing care plans based on the nursing process. The authors assume that the reader has a working knowledge of the nursing process. Therefore, it is integrated throughout the book. The reader will note that the NANDA approved nursing diagnoses are highlighted. Since there are multiple classifications of nursing diagnoses, an effort is made to meet the needs of a wide variety of readers. Three appendices of nursing diagnoses are provided. Appendix A lists the nursing diagnoses in the order in which they appear in each chapter; Appendix B lists them according to Doenges' diagnostic divisions; and Appendix C lists them according to Gordon's functional health patterns.

This edition is purposefully more comprehensive than the previous editions. New chapters address contemporary approaches, selected maternal complications, fetal well-being, and legal considerations. Psychosocial aspects are included. Appendix D provides guidelines for working with AIDS patients. Content on fetal monitoring interpretation is expanded. These additions and numerous others update the book and make it more valuable to the student nurse, as well as the graduate nurse, who finds nursing knowledge and technology to be ever changing.

J.S.M.

ACKNOWLEDGMENTS

This book acknowledges those student and practicing nurses who used previous editions and encouraged us to write this one, and our immediate families who not only cooperated with our endeavors but provided us with support. These family members include:

my son, David, and husband (in memory), Michael;
Carolyn Pedigo's daughter, Claire Burdin, and son, J. J. Burdin, III;
and Celeste Phillips's husband, Roger.

I furthermore express appreciation to Mercy College of Detroit, which granted me a sabbatical leave providing me time to achieve this publishing project. On behalf of all the authors, I wish to acknowledge the help provided by the many reviewers listed in the Consultants list and the conscientious efforts of the publisher's Nursing Editor, Linda Nold.

J.S.M.

CONSULTANTS

Katherine Camacho Carr, R.N., C.N.M., Ph.C.
University of Washington
Seattle, Washington

Linda Chagnon, R.N.C., B.S.
Risk Management Consultant
Northwest Nursing Associates
Seattle, Washington

Bonnie Flood Chez, R.N.C., M.S.N.
Perinatal Clinical Specialist/Consultant
Nursing Education Resources, Inc.
Secaucus, New Jersey

Beverly Easterwood, R.N.C., B.S.N.
Risk Management Consultant
Northwest Nursing Associates
Seattle, Washington

Claire Grande, R.N.C., B.S.N.
Assistant Director
Maternal Child Nursing
Columbus Hospital
Newark, New Jersey

Ann Marie Rhodes, R.N., M.A., J.D.
University of Iowa
Iowa City, Iowa

Jean Tillman, R.N., B.S.N., M.S.N.
Professor of Nursing
Holyoke Community College
Holyoke, Massachusetts

Norman D. Tucker, J.D.
Sommers, Schwartz, Silver and Schwartz
Professional Corporation
Southfield, Michigan

Lois J. Vice, R.N.
Perinatal Consultant
The Woodlands Community Hospital
The Woodlands, Texas

Jean E. Walton, R.N., Ed.D.
Assistant Professor
North Carolina Central University
Durham, North Carolina

CONTENTS

1. ***AN OVERVIEW OF LABOR AND DELIVERY*** **1**
Carolyn G. Pedigo

The Labor and Delivery Process 2
Theories of Labor 2
Premonitory Signs of Labor 3
Stages of Labor 8
Fetal Relationship to Maternal Pelvis 10
Mechanisms of Labor 14
Nursing Care During the Labor and Delivery Process 16
Recognition of the Onset of Labor 16
Admission Assessment 17
Latent Phase of the First Stage of Labor 22
Emotional Fears Commonly Associated with Childbirth 22
Early Active Phase of the First Stage of Labor 27
Transition Phase of the First Stage of Labor 28
Second Stage of Labor 30
Third Stage of Labor 31
Fourth Stage of Labor 32
Immediate Care of the Newborn 35
Emergency Delivery—A Nursing Responsibility 37
Conclusion 39
References 41
Bibliography 41
Post-Test 43

2. ***MECHANISMS OF LABOR*** **53**
Janet S. Malinowski

The Normal Mechanisms of Labor Through a Gynecoid Pelvis 54

Adaptation by the Fetal Head 54
Pelvic Characteristics 57
The Pelvic Inlet 58
The Midpelvis 61
The Pelvic Outlet 63
Modified Mechanisms 64
Occipital Posterior Position 64
Breech Presentation 66
Conversion To Cephalic Presentation 68
Nursing Implications Related to the Mechanisms of Labor 69
Using Predictive Assessment Data 69
Nursing Interventions That Promote Descent 71
Nursing Interventions That Provide Changes in Fetal Position 75
Conclusion 76
References 76
Bibliography 77
Post-Test 79

3. MATERNAL-FETAL MONITORING 83
Janet S. Malinowski

Uterine Activity 84
Anatomy and Physiology of the Uterus During Labor 84
Terms Used to Describe Uterine Contractions 88
Uterine Contraction Assessment Methods 90
Abnormal Uterine Contraction Patterns 93
Assessing Pain of Uterine Contractions 97
Fetal Response 98
Intermittent Fetal Heart Rate Assessment 98
Continuous Fetal Heart Rate Assessment 103
Fetal Heart Rate Baseline 108
Recognizing Periodic Changes: Decelerations 110
Assessment and Intervention for FHR Decelerations 114
Recognizing Periodic Changes: Accelerations 115
Variability in Fetal Heart Rate 116
Conclusion 120
References 121
Bibliography 122
Post-Test 124

4. *GRAPHING LABOR CURVES* **129**
Janet S. Malinowski

Methodology of Graphing Stage 1 Labor Patterns 130
Phases of the S Curve in a Normal Cervical Dilatation Pattern 132
Abnormal Cervical Dilatation Patterns 134
Definitions, Associated Factors, and Interventions for Abnormal Dilatation Patterns 134
- Precipitous Labor 134
- Prolonged Labor 136
- Prolonged Labor: Active Phase 139

Descent Patterns 141
Care in the Presence of Prolonged Labor 145
Conclusion 147
Bibliography 147
Post-Test 149

5. *LABOR STIMULATION* **158**
Janet S. Malinowski

Labor Stimulants 158
- Ambulation 158
- Stripping Membranes 160
- Enema 161
- Nipple Stimulation 163

Induction—A Form of Labor Stimulation 165
- Surgical Induction of Labor with Rupture of Membranes 165
- Medical Induction 169
- Medical Induction of Labor with Oxytocin 171
- Medical Induction of Labor with Prostaglandin Gel 176

Conclusion 177
References 178
Bibliography 179
Post-Test 181

6. *MANAGEMENT OF PAIN WITH DRUGS* **185**
Carolyn G. Pedigo

Psycho-Physiologic Responses to Pain 186
- Pain as Stress 187

Pain as Distress 187
Cause of Pain in Labor 187
Nonpharmacologic Nursing Interventions for Pain Relief During Labor and Delivery 189
Analgesia and Anesthesia 191
Considerations that Influence the Decision to Use Drugs 193
The Action and Side Effects of Drugs Used During Labor 195
Narcotic Agonists 195
Narcotic Antagonists 198
Mixed Narcotic Agonists/Antagonists 200
Sedatives 202
Drug-Induced Anesthesia During Labor and Delivery 203
Regional Anesthesia During Labor and Delivery 204
Lumbar Epidural Block 209
Caudal Block 210
Saddle Block 210
Spinal Block 210
Paracervical Block 212
Pudendal Block 214
Local Perineal Infiltration 215
Emergency Nursing Measures for Complications Following Anesthetic Administration 216
General Anesthesia During Labor and Delivery 218
Inhalation Anesthesia 219
Intravenous Anesthesia 220
Conclusion 222
References 222
Bibliography 224
Post-Test 225

7. *CONTEMPORARY APPROACHES TO THE LABOR PROCESS* **232**
Celeste R. Phillips

Dynamic Maternity Care System 233
Health Care Trends in General 233
Family-Centered Maternity and Newborn Care 234
Historical Perspectives 234
Consumer Influence 235
Contemporary Maternity Care 236
Philosophic Foundation 236
Clinical Practice 237
VBAC (Vaginal Birth After Previous Cesarean) 237

Obstetrical Design Trends 240
Marketing and Education 241
Preparation for Birth 242
Self-Care Concepts 242
Prepared Childbirth Methods 243
Childbirth Education 243
Read Method: Childbirth Without Fear 243
Bradley Method 245
Lamaze Method (PPM) 246
Basic Breathing for Labor and Birth 249
Pushing 253
Exhalation Breathing 253
Other Nonpharmaceutical Methods 255
Other Options 256
Physical Means 256
Hydrotherapy 256
Therapeutic Touch 256
Acupressure 257
Acupuncture 257
Massage 257
Psychological Support 257
Biofeedback 258
Transcutaneous Electrical Nerve Stimulation (TENS) 258
Autogenic Training 258
Hypnosuggestion 258
Labor and Birth Support 260
Passage to Parenthood 260
Supportive Roles 260
Nursing Implications for Labor Support 261
Out-of-Hospital Options 261
Freestanding Birthing Centers 261
Home Birth 262
Conclusion 262
A Vision of the Future 263
References 264
Bibliography 265
Post-Test 266

8. *SELECTED MATERNAL COMPLICATIONS* **272**
Janet S. Malinowski

The Adolescent in Labor 273
The Older Woman in Labor 275

The Substance Abuser 277
Bleeding 280
Abruptio Placenta and Placenta Previa 282
Postpartum Hemorrhage 286
Pregnancy-Induced Hypertension 288
Pregnancy-Induced Hypertension Treatment 291
Cesarean Delivery 295
Emotional Aspects Prior to Cesarean Delivery 296
Confirming Diagnostic Procedures 297
Preparation Prior to Cesarean Delivery 298
Postoperative Care 300
Conclusion 301
References 302
Bibliography 303
Post-Test 305

9. FETAL WELL-BEING IN PRETERM AND POST-TERM GESTATION **309**
Janet S. Malinowski

Preterm Labor 310
Psychological Effects of Preterm Labor on the Mother 310
Physiologic Hindrances of the Preterm Infant 311
Methods of Determining Gestational Age 313
Interventions to Arrest Preterm Labor 318
Appropriate Nursing Measures When Preterm Delivery is Imminent 328
Variations in Physical Features of the Preterm Infant 329
Psychological Tasks for Mothers of Preterm Infants 331
Ways a Nurse Can Facilitate Parental-Infant Attachment 332
Death of a Preterm Infant 333
Post-Term Labor 333
Effects of Post-Term Labor on Mother and Infant 333
Assessment for Postmaturity and Fetal Well-Being 335
Nursing Measures During Post-Term Labor 341
Immediate Care of the Post-Term Infant 342
Conclusion 343
References 343
Bibliography 346
Post-Test 348

10. LEGAL CONSIDERATIONS **354**
Janet S. Malinowski

Overview of General Law Applied to Nursing 355
Negligence 358
Who is Liable? 358
Standard of Care 360
"Reasonable Nurse" Standard 361
Potential Liability in Each Step of the Nursing Process 363
Malpractice Insurance 367
Patient's Rights and Consent 368
Documentation: Strategies to Discourage Legal Actions 372
Components and Procedures of a Malpractice Lawsuit 375
Conclusion 377
References 377
Bibliography 378
Post-Test 380

APPENDIX:

A. LIST OF NURSING DIAGNOSES BY CHAPTERS **384**

B. LIST OF NURSING DIAGNOSES ACCORDING TO DOENGES' DIAGNOSTIC DIVISIONS **393**

C. LIST OF NURSING DIAGNOSES ACCORDING TO GORDON'S FUNCTIONAL HEALTH PATTERNS **400**

D. RECOMMENDATIONS FOR PREVENTION OF HIV TRANSMISSION IN HEALTH-CARE SETTINGS **407**

INDEX **415**

1 AN OVERVIEW OF LABOR AND DELIVERY

Carolyn G. Pedigo

OBJECTIVES

Upon completing this chapter, you will be able to:

- Briefly explain three theories regarding the cause of labor.
- Explain the significance of the following for a normal course of labor and delivery:
  a. premonitory signs of labor
  b. rupture of membranes
  c. physiologic/psychologic aspects of the four stages of labor
  d. fetal lie, attitude, presentation, position, and station
  e. mechanisms of labor
- Distinguish between false labor and true labor.
- Describe at least five physiologic/psychologic changes that the nurse should recognize as significant signs of progress in labor.
- Formulate nursing diagnoses based on the assessed data.
- Identify nursing measures that:
  a. assess maternal/fetal well-being
  b. provide comfort during labor
  c. promote parent-newborn attachment
- Describe nursing responsibilities related to:
  a. the four stages of labor
  b. immediate care of the newborn
  c. the unexpected, unattended birth

Labor generally begins at 38 to 42 weeks' gestation, when the fetus is mature enough to cope with extrauterine conditions. Even though the mother may have experienced the normal developmental stages of pregnancy, labor and delivery can be an acute developmental and situational crisis for her. With skillful intervention by the health care team, the negative impact of the experience can be significantly decreased. The birth experience can become a positive one. It can even foster stronger relationships among all family members.

This chapter is divided into two parts: The first part, the labor and delivery process, focuses on essential terminology that is fundamental to nursing care; the second part focuses on nursing care during the labor and delivery process. Emphasis is placed on nursing assessment of labor progress. Nursing diagnoses are formulated, based on assessment data. Nursing interventions include some methods of facilitating maternal coping behaviors. Evaluation focuses primarily on assessment of maternal/fetal response and labor progress.

THE LABOR AND DELIVERY PROCESS

Theories of Labor

The causes of the onset of labor are still not completely understood. Although many theories have been postulated, it is not possible to explain the factor or factors that are responsible for the onset of labor in humans. Some of the theories that are currently most widely proposed are listed below.

Oxytocin Stimulation Theory. It has been hypothesized that oxytocin, which is secreted by the posterior pituitary gland, stimulates the uterine muscles to contract, thereby initiating and maintaining labor. Scientific data currently do not support this theory, although it is reinforced by the successful use of oxytocin to induce labor.[1]

Progesterone Deprivation Theory. Throughout pregnancy, there is a balance between estrogen and progesterone. Progesterone, which is produced by the placenta, is crucial to the maintenance of the pregnancy because it inhibits uterine muscular activity. If production of progesterone decreases near term, uterine contraction activity would increase, initiating labor. Since there is no documented evidence of decreased progesterone levels prior to labor, progesterone may have only an indirect effect on the onset of labor.

Organ Communication System. Theoretically, an organ communication system provides a mode through which a mature fetus possibly signals its mother to begin labor, thus controlling its own destiny with a timely birth. Scientific data supporting this theory are complex and incomplete. However, it is hypothesized that the fetal signal promotes an accelerated formation and release of prostaglandin from the maternal myometrium, causing labor contractions of the uterus. Most of the research has been done with animals, but many of the biochemical events appear to be similar in humans. Functional integrity of the fetal brain, pituitary and adrenal glands, kidneys, and membranes seems to be an important component of the organ communication theory as a cause of labor onset.[1] This explanation does recognize the fetus's production of cortisol, which is believed to stimulate the onset of labor.

• •

Review Question

List and briefly explain three theories of the cause of labor onset.

a. ______________________________

b. ______________________________

c. ______________________________

Answer

Currently accepted theories of the cause of labor are as follows:

a. *Oxytocin Stimulation Theory.* Oxytocin stimulates uterine contractions.
b. *Progesterone Deprivation Theory.* Progesterone inhibits uterine muscular activity. It is hypothesized that contraction activity increases as progesterone levels decrease toward term.
c. *Organ Communication System.* This system provides a communication mode from the fetus to its mother. A signal from the fetus possibly stimulates the mother's body to begin labor.

• •

Premonitory Signs of Labor

Although no one really knows the cause of labor, there are identifiable signs of approaching labor. They are called premonitory signs of labor. These signs are listed below.

Engagement. This is the passage of the largest diameter of the fetal presenting part (usually the biparietal diameter of the head) into the maternal pelvic inlet (brim). Engagement is assessed by pelvic and abdominal examination. In the primigravida (first pregnancy), engagement may occur as early as 2 weeks prior to the onset of labor (see the section on Descent Patterns in Chapter 4). In the multigravida (second or more pregnancy), engagement usually does not occur until labor is well established. Common discomforts following engagement are as follows: (1) leg pain owing to pressure on the sciatic nerve, and (2) urinary frequency owing to pressure on the bladder. Engagement should not be confused with the term *lightening,* which is the settling of the uterus and its contents into the pelvis. Lightening may occur prior to or concurrently with engagement and is a subjective sensation that is felt by the mother. Commonly, mothers "feel the baby drop."

Uterine Contractions. It is sometimes difficult to distinguish between Braxton Hicks contractions and the contractions of true labor. Contractions, which occur throughout pregnancy, may become increasingly uncomfortable just prior to labor. At this time, they are called Braxton Hicks contractions. They are irregular and do not increase in frequency, duration, or intensity. They do not cause significant cervical dilatation but may assist in ripening (i.e., softening and thinning/effacing of the internal cervical os) and moving the cervix forward/anterior in the pelvis. Such contractions are commonly termed "false labor." The discomfort of Braxton Hicks contractions can usually be lessened by walking or changing position. Walking usually intensifies the contractions of true labor (see the section on Ambulation as a Labor Stimulant in Chapter 5). True labor contractions are regular and tend to increase in frequency, duration, and intensity as labor progresses. These contractions bring about progressive cervical changes and cause discomfort in the lower back and abdomen.

Cervical Changes. True labor is diagnosed when regular, rhythmic contractions bring about progressive cervical effacement and dilatation. Cervical *effacement* is the gradual thinning of the internal cervical os. The thickness of the tissue is palpated and the degree is estimated in percentages. Effacement usually precedes dilatation in the primigravida and occurs concurrently with dilatation in the multigravida. Cervical *dilatation* is the gradual opening of the cervix to 10 cm. This is also termed *complete* or *full* dilatation.

Bloody Show. Prior to or during labor, the cervical mucous plug is expelled as a result of pressure from the presenting part of the fetus and some cervical effacement. Cervical capillaries may rupture, causing blood to be mixed with cervical mucus. Bloody show is thick, mucous, and pink or dark red in color. It may be scant in early labor and become copious as dilatation progresses. It must be differentiated from active vaginal bleeding, which is thin, watery, and bright red in color. Active bleeding may indicate abnormalities of the placenta such as placenta previa or abruptio placentae (see Chapter 8). Vaginal or rectal examination may be contraindicated when vaginal bleeding is present because examination may precipitate further bleeding.

Rupture of Membranes (ROM). Spontaneous rupture of membranes (SROM) may occur before true labor starts or anytime during labor. Approximately 12 percent of women experience SROM prior to the onset of labor.[2] Membranes may also be ruptured artificially (AROM). This procedure, called *amniotomy*, must be performed by a physician or midwife. Following ROM, nursing interventions include assessment of the fetal heart rate and of the color, consistency, and amount of fluid. In the absence of engagement, cord prolapse can occur with ROM. (See the section on Amniotomy as a Labor Stimulant in Chapter 5 for more detailed nursing interventions.)

Amniotic fluid may gush or slowly trickle from the vagina. Normal amniotic fluid is clear or cloudy and colorless or pale yellow. The odor should not be strong or foul (indicating infection). The fluid may be cloudy owing to the presence of vernix caseosa, which is a white, cheeselike substance that coats the fetal skin in utero. Meconium-stained (brown, black, or greenish color) amniotic fluid when the fetus presents head first indicates that at some point the fetus may have experienced distress causing anoxia. With anoxia, the anal sphincter relaxes, resulting in expulsion of feces into the amniotic fluid. This is likely to occur in the post-term pregnancy. (See Chapter 9 for the immediate care of the post-term infant.) Meconium-stained amniotic fluid may be normal only when the fetus presents buttocks first. In this case, expulsion of feces may be caused by cervical pressure on the fetal anus, not by anoxia.

The amount of amniotic fluid present in the term uterus is approximately 1000 ml. Some women fear that if the membranes rupture prior to the onset of labor, all the amniotic fluid will leave the uterine cavity and cause a "dry birth," that is, the baby will not have any lubrication during passage, thus making labor longer and more painful. This is a fallacy. Not all of the amniotic fluid leaves the uterine cavity at the time of ROM. Furthermore, throughout the remainder of labor, the placenta continues to produce amniotic fluid. Fluid is expelled, especially during contractions and when the woman moves or changes position. Amniotic fluid continues to provide moisture and lubrication throughout labor.

Amniotic fluid in excess of 2000 to 3000 ml is classified as *hydramnios* or *polyhydramnios.* It is often associated with fetal malformations in which the fetus is unable to swallow and/or urinate normally in utero. Hydramnios is also associated with multiple gestation and maternal disorders such as diabetes mellitus, Rh sensitization, and placental tumors.

Oligohydramnios is the term used to describe an extremely scant amount (less than 300 ml) of amniotic fluid that is very concentrated. The condition is rare and the cause is unknown, although it is associated with fetal renal disorders and postmaturity.

It is sometimes difficult to distinguish amniotic fluid from maternal urine. At term, pressure from the enlarged uterus on the bladder may cause involuntary leakage of urine, especially when the pregnant woman coughs or sneezes. Two tests are used most often to establish the presence of amniotic fluid:

NITRAZINE TEST TAPE. Amniotic fluid changes the color of nitrazine tape to blue-green, blue-gray, or dark blue—an alkaline reaction. Urine is acidic and does not change the color of the nitrazine tape. If a lubricant has been used for the vaginal exam prior to testing with nitrazine tape, false-negative results can be obtained, that is, the tape will remain yellow, olive, or olive-green in color. False results can also occur in the presence of bloody show or semen. If the tape does not change color and no lubricant has been used, this usually means probable intact membranes. Nitrazine tape is the most frequently used test to determine the presence of amniotic fluid.

FERNING OF CERVICAL MUCUS. During pregnancy, with the amniotic sac intact, cervical mucus is viscous and opaque. The mucus changes to a fernlike pattern of crystallization when mixed with amniotic fluid. Evidence of ferning of cervical mucus under a microscope indicates probable ROM.

Other Premonitory Signs of Labor. Additional subjective changes may occur just prior to the onset of labor. These changes may include a sudden burst of energy. Although the woman may want to use this energy for tasks she has neglected, she should refrain from doing so. This energy is needed for the work of labor. Other changes may include increased backache, increased vaginal secretions, a sudden 2- to 3-pound weight loss (from diuresis of retained fluid), and loose stools or diarrhea.

• •

Review Questions

1. The passage of the largest diameter of the fetal presenting part into the maternal pelvic inlet is called ______________________.
2. Differentiate between Braxton Hicks contractions and contractions that signal true labor by filling in the chart using the terms in column I.

COLUMN I	BRAXTON HICKS	TRUE LABOR
Discomfort		
Regularity		
Cervical dilatation		
Effect of walking		

3. During labor, cervical dilatation progresses to _____ cm.
4. Define effacement of the cervix. ______________________________
5. Describe the differences in color and consistency between bloody show (normal) and active vaginal bleeding (abnormal).
6. The procedure by which the membranes are artificially ruptured is called ______________________________.
7. In each of the following, what does the presence of meconium-stained amniotic fluid indicate?
   a. If the fetus presents head first, meconium may indicate:
   b. If the fetus presents buttocks first, meconium may indicate:
8. Approximately _____ ml of amniotic fluid is present in the term uterus.
9. An excessive amount of amniotic fluid associated with malformations in which the fetus is usually unable to swallow and/or urinate normally in utero is ______________________________.
10. Briefly describe two tests used to document ROM.
   a. ______________________________
   b. ______________________________

Answers

1. *Engagement* is the passage of the largest diameter of the fetal presenting part into the maternal pelvic inlet.
2. The differences between Braxton Hicks contractions and contractions that signal true labor are as follows:

COLUMN I	BRAXTON HICKS	TRUE LABOR
Discomfort	Occurs throughout pregnancy; may become uncomfortable just prior to labor	Increases in intensity and duration, causing discomfort in the lower back and abdomen

(continued)

COLUMN I	BRAXTON HICKS	TRUE LABOR
Regularity	Irregular	Regular
Cervical changes	Possibly some effacement—no progressive dilatation	Progressive dilatation and effacement
Effect of walking	May decrease discomfort	Intensifies contractions

3. Cervical dilatation progresses to 10 cm during labor.
4. Effacement is the gradual thinning of the internal cervical os.
5. Bloody show is thick, mucous, and pink or dark red in color. Active vaginal bleeding is thin, watery, and bright red in color.
6. *Amniotomy* is a procedure by which the membranes are artificially ruptured.
7. The significance of meconium-stained amniotic fluid is as follows:
   a. Meconium-stained amniotic fluid when the fetus presents head first may indicate that fetal anoxia (distress) may have occurred at some point.
   b. When the fetus presents buttocks first, meconium-stained amniotic fluid may be normal.
8. The term uterus contains approximately 1000 ml of amniotic fluid.
9. *Hydramnios* or *polyhydramnios* is an excessive amount of amniotic fluid associated with malformations in which the fetus is usually unable to swallow and/or urinate normally in utero.
10. Two tests used to document ROM are as follows:
    a. *Nitrazine test tape.* Amniotic fluid changes the pH, causing the tape color to become blue-green, blue-gray, or dark blue.
    b. *Ferning of cervical mucus.* Cervical mucus mixed with amniotic fluid changes to a fernlike pattern of crystallization.

• •

Stages of Labor

Stage I. This is the stage of dilatation that begins with the onset of regular contractions and ends with complete cervical effacement and dilatation (10 cm). Stage I is divided into two phases: (1) latent phase from 1 to 3 cm, and (2) active phase from 4 to 10 cm. Transition is the part of the active phase from 8 to 10 cm. The average length of the first stage of labor is 12½ to 14 hours for the primigravida and 6 to 7½ hours for the multigravida. (See Chapter 4 for more specific details.)

Stage II. This stage of expulsion begins with complete dilatation and effacement of the cervix and ends with delivery of the baby. The average length of time is 1½ to 2 hours for the primigravida and ½ hour for the multigravida. Although the woman has been in labor for many hours up to this point, during Stage II, she must actively push with contractions to assist the movement of the baby through the birth canal.

Stage III. The placental stage begins with delivery of the baby and ends with expulsion of the placenta. The average length of time is 20 minutes (⅓ hour).

Stage IV. The recovery stage is the first 1 to 4 hours after delivery of the placenta.

• •

Review Question

Using the following chart, indicate the beginning and end of each stage of labor. Include the approximate duration of labor for the primigravida (P) and the multigravida (M).

			HOURS DURATION	
STAGE	BEGINS WITH	ENDS WITH	P	M
I				
II				
III				
IV				

Answer

			HOURS DURATION	
STAGE	BEGINS WITH	ENDS WITH	P	M
I	Regular contractions	Complete dilatation and effacement	12½–14	6–7½
II	Complete dilatation and effacement	Delivery of the baby	1½–2	½

(continued)

STAGE	BEGINS WITH	ENDS WITH	HOURS DURATION P	HOURS DURATION M
III	Delivery of the baby	Delivery of the placenta	⅓	⅓
IV	Delivery of the placenta	1–4 hours after delivery of the placenta	1–4	1–4

Fetal Relationship to Maternal Pelvis

Fetal Lie. *Lie* refers to the relationship of the longitudinal axis (head to feet) of the fetus to the longitudinal axis of the mother. Ninety-nine percent of all lies are longitudinal; that is, the baby's longitudinal axis is parallel with the mother's. One percent are perpendicular, known as a *transverse lie* (shoulder presentation) or oblique (diagonal). Vaginal delivery of the fetus is not possible in the presence of transverse lie; cesarean delivery is necessary.

Fetal Attitude. *Attitude* refers to the relationship of the fetal parts to each other—the degree of flexion or extension. The normal fetal attitude is one of moderate flexion. The chin is flexed on the chest and the extremities are flexed on the abdomen, thereby taking up the smallest possible space in utero. (See Chapter 2, Adaptation of the Fetal Head.)

Presentation. *Presentation* refers to that part of the fetus that is lowermost in the pelvis. The part that first enters the pelvis is the presenting part. The most common (95 percent) presentation is cephalic (head). The degree of flexion or extension determines the type of cephalic presentation (Fig. 1–1). *Cephalic* presentations include the following variations: (1) *Occipital* or *vertex* presentation occurs when the head is fully flexed on the chest so that the occiput (O) is the presenting part in the lower segment of the uterus. This is the ideal presentation. (2) *Sinciput* presentation (military attitude)

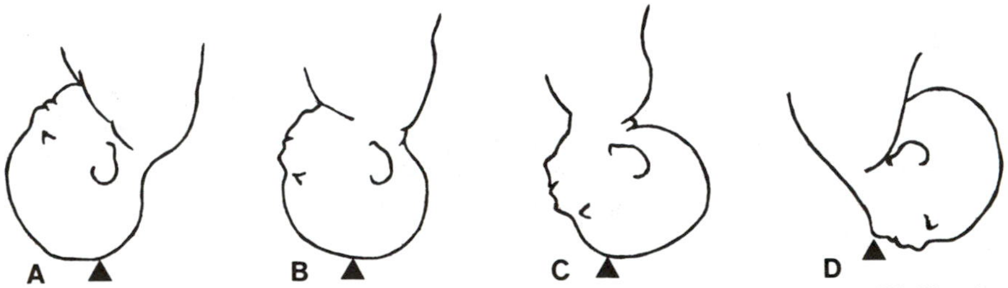

Figure 1–1. Cephalic (head) presentations. (*A*) Occipital or vertex. (*B*) Sinciput. (*C*) Brow. (*D*) Face or chin.

occurs when the head is neither flexed nor extended so that the anterior fontanel is the presenting part. This usually reverts to an occipital presentation for a normal vaginal delivery. (3) *Brow* presentation occurs when the head is extended so that the forehead (brow —B) is the presenting part. (4) A *face* or *chin* presentation occurs when the head is hyperextended so that the chin (mentum—M) is the presenting part. The latter two presentations—brow and face—require a larger pelvic diameter than the occipital for delivery.

Presentations in which the lower body parts present first are termed *breech* and occur in 3 percent of term deliveries. The sacrum (S) is the presenting part. There are three types of breech presentations. In a *frank* breech, the presenting part is the buttocks, with the thighs flexed on the abdomen and the legs extended onto the chest. A *complete* breech is characterized by flexion of the thighs on the abdomen and flexion of the calves on the thighs. In a single (or double) *footing* breech, one leg (or both) is extended at the knees and hips. (See Chapter 2 for more details.)

A *shoulder* presentation occurs when the fetus is in a transverse lie. The scapula (Sc) is the presenting part. This presentation is rare. If rotation (version) to longitudinal lie is not possible, cesarean delivery is necessary.

Position. *Position* is the relationship between the presenting part of the fetus and maternal pelvis. The maternal pelvis is divided into four quadrants: left anterior, left posterior, right anterior, and right posterior (Fig. 1–2). In a vertex presentation, if the occiput is directed toward the left anterior quadrant of the pelvis, then the fetal position is left occiput anterior (LOA). The most favorable position for delivery is occiput anterior (LOA or ROA). See Table 1–1 for

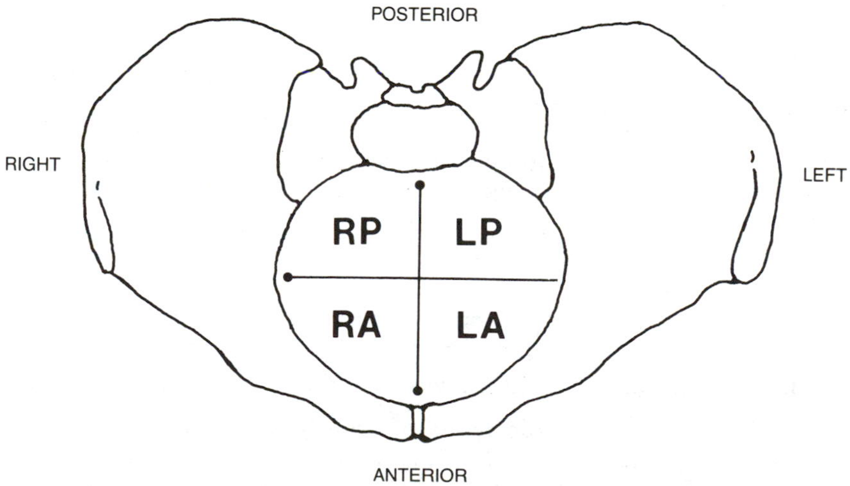

Figure 1–2. The four quadrants of the maternal pelvis: (RP) right posterior; (LP) left posterior; (RA) right anterior; (LA) left anterior.

Table 1–1. FETAL LIE, PRESENTATION, PRESENTING PART, AND POSITION

LIE/PRESENTATION	PRESENTING PART	SAMPLE POSITION
Longitudinal		
Cephalic		
Vertex	Occiput (O)*	Left Occiput Anterior (LOA)
Brow	Brow (B)*	Right Brow Posterior (RBP)
Face	Mentum (M)*	Left Mentum Anterior (LMA)
Breech	Sacrum (S)*	Right Sacrum Posterior (RSP)
Transverse		
Shoulder	Scapula (Sc)*	Left Scapula Anterior (LScA)

*Symbol for presenting part used in position.

examples of fetal positions as they relate to lie, presentation, and presenting part.

Station. The assessment of the level of descent of the presenting part in relation to the ischial spines of the maternal pelvis is termed *station* (see Chapter 2 for anatomy of the pelvis). When the presenting part, the bony prominence of the head, is at the level of the ischial spines, the station is zero (0), and engagement has occurred. The presenting part is said to be floating when it is entirely out of the pelvis and freely movable. The progression of descent is measured in centimeters, moving from a negative to a positive station. This is designated as −5 (at the level of the pelvic inlet), −4, . . . 0 . . . +4, +5 (pelvic outlet).

• •

Review Questions

1. The relationship of the longitudinal axis of the fetus to the longitudinal axis of the mother is termed ____________________.
2. The relationship of the fetal parts to each other is called ________.
3. Define presentation. ____________________
4. The most common cephalic presentation is ____________________.
5. Briefly describe the three types of breech presentations.
   a. ____________________

b. ____

____

____

c. ____

____

____

6. **Write in the correct name of the presenting part for each of the following presentations:**

PRESENTATION	PRESENTING PART
Cephalic: Vertex	
Brow	
Face	
Breech	
Shoulder	

7. **The relationship of the presenting part of the fetus to the maternal pelvis is called ______________.**

8. **Fetal descent is assessed in relation to the ischial spines of the maternal pelvis. This is called ______________.**

9. **Define the term *floating*.** ______________

____

____

Answers

1. *Lie* is the relationship of the longitudinal axis of the fetus to the longitudinal axis of the mother.
2. *Attitude* is the relationship of the fetal parts to each other.
3. Presentation refers to the part of the fetus that is lowermost in the pelvis.
4. The most common cephalic presentation is *occipital* (vertex).
5. Three types of breech presentations are as follows:
   a. *Frank breech*—thighs flexed on the abdomen with legs extended onto the chest.
   b. *Complete breech*—thighs flexed on the abdomen and calves flexed on the thighs.
   c. *Footling breech*—one or both legs extended at the knees and hips.
6. The presenting part for each of the following presentations:

PRESENTATION		PRESENTING PART
Cephalic:	Vertex	Occiput
	Brow	Brow
	Face	Mentum
Breech		Sacrum
Shoulder		Scapula

7. *Position* is the relationship of the presenting part of the fetus to the maternal pelvis.
8. *Station* is the assessment of the fetal descent in relation to the ischial spines of the maternal pelvis.
9. The presenting part is floating when it is freely movable above the pelvic inlet; above −5 station; not engaged.

• •

Mechanisms of Labor

The mechanisms of labor are maneuvers within the maternal pelvis that the fetus must accomplish so that vaginal delivery can occur (see Chapter 2 for a more in-depth description). These maneuvers are illustrated in Figure 1–3.

Descent. Initial descent occurs simultaneously with engagement. The head (in a vertex presentation) enters the pelvis with the occiput transverse (to the side) in the pelvic inlet. The fetus descends during each contraction and slightly retracts during relaxation so that the progression is slow.

Flexion. As the fetal head encounters resistance from the maternal pelvis and musculature, it flexes so that a smaller diameter of the head presents.

Internal Rotation. As the fetal head meets resistance from the maternal levator ani muscles, it usually rotates from occiput transverse to occiput anterior (90 degrees). This places the occiput beneath the symphysis pubis. This internal rotation usually occurs primarily during the second stage of labor.

Extension. The head is born during extension. The occiput emerges first, then the face, then the chin.

Restitution, External Rotation, and Expulsion. Once the head is delivered and is free from pressure and compression, it spontaneously rotates (restitution) 45 degrees, halfway back to the transverse position. The head is then rotated (external rotation) another 45 degrees, placing the shoulders in the anteroposterior diameter. Restitution and external rotation occur so close together that they are difficult to distinguish. The rest of the baby, which is smaller in diameter, is delivered spontaneously (expulsion).

• •

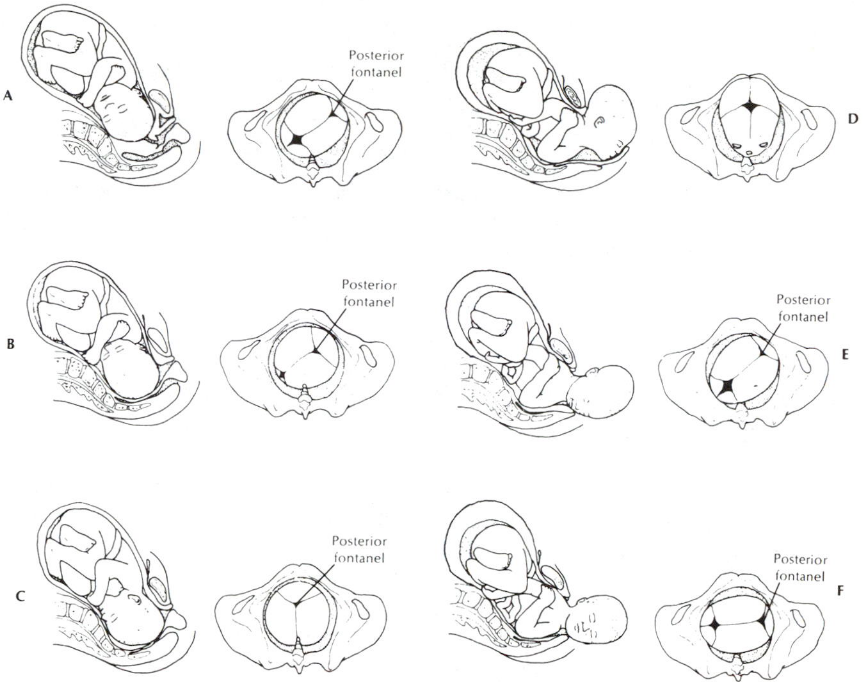

Figure 1–3. Mechanisms of labor for left occiput anterior (LOA) presentation. (*A*) Engagement and descent. (*B*) Flexion. (*C*) Internal rotation to occiput anterior (OA). (*D*) Extension. (*E*) Restitution. (*F*) External rotation. (From Bobak, IM and Jensen, MD: Essentials of Maternity Nursing: The Nurse and the Childbearing Family, ed 2. CV Mosby, St. Louis, 1987, p 362, with permission.)

Review Questions

Circle True or False and explain your answer.

1. T F The correct sequence of the mechanisms of labor is descent, flexion, extension, internal rotation, restitution, external rotation, expulsion.

____

____

2. T F Descent occurs simultaneously with engagement.

____

____

3. T F Restitution occurs as the head encounters resistance from the maternal pelvis.

____

____

Answers

1. False Internal rotation must occur before the baby's head can be born during extension.
2. True Initial descent occurs simultaneously with engagement.
3. False Flexion occurs as the head encounters resistance from the maternal pelvis. Restitution is the process of rotating 45 degrees mid-way to the transverse position after delivery of the head.

• •

NURSING CARE DURING THE LABOR AND DELIVERY PROCESS

This section emphasizes nursing care provided for the laboring woman. Actual and potential nursing diagnoses are provided throughout this section as a suggested focus for the reader. The nursing diagnoses should be kept in mind as they relate directly to the assessment data, nursing interventions, and rationale. Evaluation of labor progress is incorporated when appropriate. See Appendices A, B, and C for lists of all nursing diagnoses used throughout the book.

Recognition of the Onset of Labor

During the latter part of pregnancy, it is important that the nurse assess the woman's potential **knowledge deficit [of premonitory signs of labor] related to lack of exposure.** Based on assessment data, intervention would be to either provide a review or actually teach the woman to recognize the premonitory signs of labor. In review, they are engagement, uterine contractions, cervical changes, bloody show, rupture of membranes, sudden burst of energy, increased backache, increased vaginal secretions, sudden 2- to 3-pound weight loss, and loose stools or diarrhea. She should notify her physician or nurse-midwife when uterine contractions are regular and felt primarily in the lower back, are 5 to 10 minutes apart, last for at least 30 seconds, and continue despite walking. If membranes rupture spontaneously with or without contractions, the woman is usually advised to report this to her physician or midwife. She may be asked to come to the hospital as soon as possible for assessment of fetal well-being.

Nursing assessment of the laboring woman begins with the first verbal contact, usually a telephone notification that she is coming to the hospital. Adequate data collection followed by appropriate instructions are crucial at this time. By the time of labor onset, the following information should be available to the nurse:

1. Obstetric History
   a. Estimated date of delivery or confinement (EDD or EDC); Weeks gestation; Age; Gravida (the total number of times a woman has been pregnant, regardless of how long the pregnancy lasted); Para (the number of times the total contents of the uterus have been emptied after the age of viability); Abortions (the number of times pregnancy has ended prior to the age of viability); Stillbirths; Neonatal deaths; Living children (G_____, P_____, Ab_____, SB_____, ND_____, LC_____)
   b. Present pregnancy course: maternal vital signs, fetal heart rate, fundal growth pattern, maternal and/or obstetric complications such as pregnancy-induced hypertension, gestational diabetes, abnormal weight gain, infections (TORCH*) (Appendix D contains recommendations specific to the prevention of AIDS)
   c. Lab results: urine (protein, ketone, glucose) and blood (hemoglobin/hematocrit, type and Rh, VDRL, titers)
   d. Previous obstetric complications related to pregnancy, labor, and/or delivery
2. Medical history: conditions that would place the mother and/or fetus/newborn at risk (see Chapter 9)
3. Other Pertinent Information
   a. Method of preparation for labor/delivery
   b. Analgesia/anesthesia preference
   c. Birth preferences
   d. Cultural, religious, or ethnic influences
   e. Marital status
   f. Anxieties or fears
   g. Plans for breast- or bottle-feeding

If a woman has not received prenatal care, or if her records are unavailable, the above information will need to be obtained at the time of admission.

Admission Assessment

The initial admission assessment by the nurse or physician is performed to determine if the woman is in labor, how far she and the fetus have progressed, and her initial psychological response to labor. She may prefer to have her support person remain in the room during the assessment. Assistance may be needed to undress and put on a gown. This is a good time to obtain a urine specimen for urinalysis, protein, ketone, and glucose for comparison with pregnancy norms. An empty bladder further facilitates examination and causes the woman less discomfort. Vital signs are obtained for comparison with the prenatal baseline. Occasionally, the excitement of coming

---

*Toxoplasmosis, Other, Rubella, Cytomegalovirus, Herpes. "Other" is a broad category including syphilis, chlamydia, AIDS, and so forth.

to the hospital may cause the systolic blood pressure (BP) to be slightly elevated. If this occurs, the procedure should be repeated in 15 to 30 minutes for a more accurate reading.

Evaluation begins with assessment of the contractions. Ask the woman to describe her contractions. Where does she feel them? How do they feel? When did they begin? How frequently do they occur, and how long do they last? Palpate her contractions and compare what you feel with her perceptions (see Chapter 3).

Leopold's Maneuvers. Fetal position and presentation can be determined manually using Leopold's maneuvers (Fig. 1–4). With the woman in a supine position, drapes are applied exposing the abdomen. The following four maneuvers are performed.

FIRST MANEUVER. Facing the woman's head, place both hands on the fundus (the uppermost part of the uterus) and palpate to determine the contents. The fetal head is firm, round, and freely movable. In a cephalic presentation, the nodular buttocks should be identifiable in the fundus.

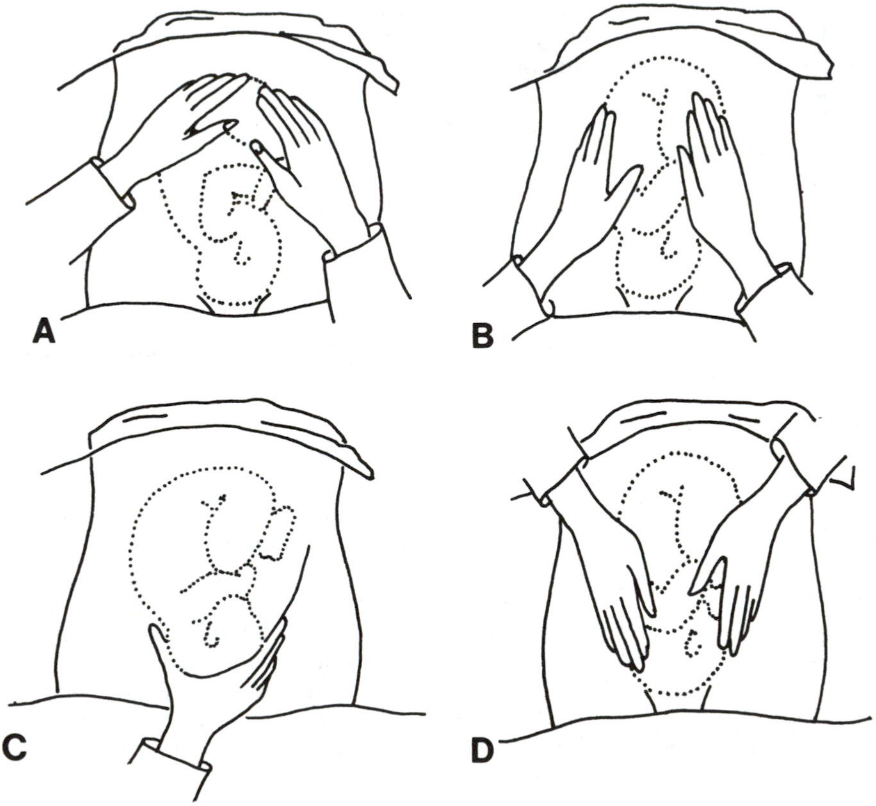

Figure 1–4. Leopold's maneuvers. (*A*) First. (*B*) Second. (*C*) Third. (*D*) Fourth.

SECOND MANEUVER. Move both hands at the same time down both sides of the abdomen to determine on which side of the uterus the fetal back lies. One hand remains stationary while the other palpates. The fetal back is identified as a smooth, curved, resistant plane. Opposite the back are the fetal front surface (concave and soft) and the small parts, that is, feet, hands, elbows, knees (irregular projections).

THIRD MANEUVER. Warn the woman that this maneuver may be uncomfortable. Gently grasp the bottom of the uterus, pressing slightly with thumb and fingers to determine which fetal part is presenting over the pelvic inlet. If the head is the presenting part, it will feel round and hard. If engagement has not occurred, the head can be gently rocked from side to side. The presence of the fetal head at the pelvic inlet provides the following information: longitudinal lie and cephalic presentation.

FOURTH MANEUVER. Stand near the woman's shoulders and face her feet. With the fingers of both hands, press in 2 inches on both sides of the abdomen just above the symphysis pubis. Exert gentle pressure downward (toward her feet). If one hand meets firm resistance, this is probably the fetal brow. If the fetal brow is felt on the same side as the small parts, then the head is well flexed. Only a small portion of the presenting part may be palpable if it has descended deeply into the pelvic inlet, that is, if engagement has occurred. This maneuver can be uncomfortable, particularly if the urinary bladder is not empty. Therefore, encourage the woman to empty her bladder prior to starting the maneuvers.

Auscultation of Fetal Heart Rate (FHR). The FHR is best heard through the fetal back in a vertex or breech presentation, and through the chest in a face presentation. In a vertex presentation, one would listen to the FHR below the maternal umbilicus on either the left or right side, depending on where the fetal back is located. (See Chapter 3 for further discussion of assessing FHR.)

Vaginal Examinations. Vaginal examinations are performed gently, using aseptic technique. Asepsis protects the woman from infection and protects the examiner from the possible contraction of infectious diseases. Palpation of the cervix provides dilatation and effacement data. Through a dilating cervix, the examiner will be able to determine fetal presentation (cephalic, breech, shoulder), station (degree of descent in relation to the ischial spines), and position. If the bag of waters (amniotic sac, membranes) is felt, this indicates that the membranes are intact. General assessment of the pelvis may also be performed at this time (see Chapter 2). The frequency of vaginal exams will be determined by labor progress. Vaginal exams should be kept to a minimum, particularly if the membranes are ruptured. Instruct the patient about the procedure in order to decrease anxiety and promote relaxation. It is important to share findings with the laboring couple so that they are aware of the progress being made. Vaginal exams may be contraindicated in the presence of any vaginal bleeding because of the possibility of placenta previa or abruptio placentae (see Chapter 8). Vaginal exams are also contraindicated in the presence of active herpes lesions.[3]

X-ray/Ultrasound. According to Muggah,[4] valid indications for pelvimetry include (1) previous difficult delivery; (2) abnormal or grossly contracted pelvis; (3) breech presentation; or (4) abnormal progress in second stage, undiagnosed fetal position, attitude, and station. A definite diagnosis of the above with pelvimetry would provide early indications for changing the management of labor and delivery.

If manual examination is inconclusive, x-ray pelvimetry may be performed to determine the presentation, position, lie, and attitude of the fetus. Since the effects of x-ray radiographic rays on the maternal ovaries and the fetus are not known, caution should be used in making this decision.

Fetal presentation and position are more commonly determined from pulsed-echo ultrasound. This procedure has replaced the use of x-ray pelvimetry in many institutions; however, valid indications for use are the same as those for pelvimetry. High-frequency sound waves are used to scan the mother's abdomen. The procedure is noninvasive and painless. There are no known contraindications to the use of ultrasound (see Chapter 9).

Admit or Send Home. Following assessment, if the woman is thought to be in labor, she should be admitted to the labor unit. If she is not in true labor, she may be sent home. If the distance is great, she may be asked to walk around for an hour and return for re-examination. If the woman is sent home, this can create feelings of great disappointment, which the nurse needs to take into consideration. If the woman is admitted too early, she may become discouraged with her lack of progress in the latent phase of labor. Allowing the couple to express their feelings and providing reassurance will help to decrease the disappointment

Vaginal Birth After Cesarean Section (VBAC). For many years, medical practice was governed by the old saying "once a C-section, always a C-section." Researchers[5–7] have found that many women experience a prolonged emotional pain following cesarean birth. These feelings include decreased self-esteem, failure to perform as a woman, regret, frustration, and shame. Maternal/fetal physical recovery is also more complex following cesarean delivery.

In 1980, the United States Department of Health and Human Services sponsored a conference on cesarean childbirth. The following statement was issued: "It is an acceptable practice to allow patients who have had a previous lower segment transverse cesarean to labor if there are no recurrent indications for cesarean birth."[8] No maternal or fetal morbidity cases following VBAC were noted in studies by Paul, Phelan, and Yeh[9] and Jarrell, Ashmead, and Mann.[10] Individual evaluation of each pregnant woman will determine whether or not she is eligible for VBAC.

• •

Review Questions

1. Mrs. Brown calls the labor unit and states that her membranes have ruptured but she is not in labor. The best response by the nurse would be:
   a. "You need to wait until your contractions start before coming to the hospital."
   b. "Come to the hospital as soon as possible so the doctor can check you and your baby."
   c. "Why don't you wait a few hours and call me back if anything happens."
   d. "You can come to the hospital if you want to, but it will be a while before your baby is born."
2. According to Mrs. Black's prenatal chart, she is G vii, P iv, Ab ii, SB i. Therefore, you might assume that Mrs. Black has carried _____ pregnancies past the age of viability.
3. During the admission assessment, urine is usually tested for which of the following?
   a. protein, hemoglobin, Rh factor
   b. VDRL, ketone, hemoglobin
   c. Rh, VDRL, glucose
   d. protein, ketone, glucose
4. Using Leopold's maneuvers, in a cephalic presentation the buttocks should be identifiable in the _____________________.
5. The FHR is best heard through the fetal back in a ___________ or ________ presentation.
6. Vaginal exams may be contraindicated in the presence of _________ _____________________________.
7. List three situations in which the use of pelvimetry is considered valid.
   a. _____________________
   b. _____________________
   c. _____________________

Answers

1. b. If membranes rupture spontaneously, with or without contractions, the woman is usually advised to report this to her physician or midwife as soon as possible for assessment of fetal well-being.
2. Mrs. Black has delivered four pregnancies past the age of viability (P iv). She has had six previous pregnancies; this is her seventh (G vii). Two pregnancies ended prior to the age of viability (Ab ii), and one resulted in a stillbirth (SB i). The stillbirth was counted as G i, P i.
3. d. Urine is tested for protein, ketone, and glucose.
4. Using Leopold's maneuvers, in a cephalic presentation the buttocks should be identifiable in the *fundus*.

5. The FHR is best heard through the fetal back in a *vertex* or *breech* presentation.
6. Vaginal exams may be contraindicated in the presence of *vaginal bleeding* or *active herpes lesions.*
7. Situations in which the use of pelvimetry is considered valid include: (a) previous difficult delivery; (b) abnormal or grossly contracted pelvis; (c) breech presentation; or (d) abnormal progress in second stage, undiagnosed fetal position, attitude, and station.

• •

Latent Phase of the First Stage of Labor

During the latent phase of the first stage of labor, progress is slow. The cervix dilates from 1 to approximately 3 cm. Effacement is often complete before dilatation begins in the primigravida and occurs simultaneously with dilatation in the multigravida. Contractions are usually mild and may be irregular, with a frequency of 5 to 20 minutes. The duration is 10 to 30 seconds.

During early labor, the woman may experience **anxiety [specify] related to uncertainty about the onset of labor.** She may be excited and talkative. She cannot believe labor has finally begun. She might be quiet and afraid. Although she wants the baby, she may not feel ready for labor and would like to make it go away; or, she may welcome labor. She and her partner may have some fear of the unknown and are usually open to instruction and directions. The pregnant adolescent may have little or no preparation for the labor/delivery experience. Fearfulness and shame may precipitate heightened anxiety leading to a greater perception of pain with contractions. The adolescent who has used denial extensively may present in the emergency room complaining of severe abdominal pain only to be confronted with the fact that she is pregnant and in labor. The older primigravida who has not had a genetic amniocentesis (amniotic fluid evaluation for detection of fetal abnormalities) may be very fearful of having a defective baby. (See Chapter 8 for nursing care of the pregnant adolescent and older primigravida.)

Emotional Fears Commonly Associated with Childbirth

Women who experience fear and anxiety during labor are more likely to have increased tension and prolonged labor. Fear related to childbirth falls into two categories: fears the woman has about herself and fears about the baby.

Fears the woman might have about herself include:

1. **Fear (of pain) related to labor; delivery; examinations; needles**
2. **Fear (of long labor) related to inability to tolerate the pain**
3. **Fear (of abandonment during labor) related to lack of understanding of usual routines**

4. **Fear (of internal injury or tears) related to intrusive procedures; body size**
5. **Fear (of losing self-esteem) related to doubtfulness of her ability to cope; loss of control during labor**
6. **Fear (of embarrassment: nudity; urinating and defecating in bed; messiness from amniotic fluid and vaginal discharge; the possibility of using foul language) related to uncertainty about acceptance of others**
7. **Fear (of helplessness) related to inability to control the onset or progress of labor; inability to control what others do to her during labor and delivery**

Fears the woman might have about the baby include:

1. **Fear (that the baby might not survive the labor/delivery process) related to lack of confidence in caretaker; predictive signs (fetal distress, early gestation)**
2. **Fear (that the baby might be injured during the delivery) related to use of forceps/vacuum extractor; relatively large size of baby**
3. **Fear (that the baby will have gross deformities) related to family history; advanced maternal age; maternal drug ingestion; unfounded myths**
4. **Fear (that the baby will not come out at all) related to the size of the baby in relation to the size of the pelvis**

Following assessment, these fears may be reduced by using the following nursing interventions:

1. Explain the process of labor to the unprepared mother and her support person in terms she understands. Review the process with educationally prepared couples. Frequent reinforcement of explanations or reviews is important in reducing fear and anxiety. Review emotions and sensations the mother is likely to experience as labor progresses.
2. Keep parents informed as labor progresses. Provide parents with opportunities for validation of health and progress; e.g., allow them to listen to the fetal heartbeat.
3. Praise and reinforce the mother's efforts to cope, and use this method of teaching to modify inappropriate behavior. Demonstrate desired breathing patterns for the laboring woman and, if necessary, perform breathing exercises with her during contractions.
4. Provide physically supportive care, thereby decreasing her discomfort and increasing her rapport with the nurse. Some physical comfort measures include: ambulation; bath/shower; comfortable positioning/position changes; back rubs; effleurage (a form of light abdominal massage); counterpressure to the back; appropriate coaching during and between contractions; wiping perspiration off with a cool, damp cloth; periodic mouth rinses; and the

application of lip emollients.[11] (See Chapter 7 for additional comfort measures.)

Orientation to Environment. Admission to the hospital labor unit usually occurs during early labor. Due to **anxiety [specify] related to unfamiliar surroundings,** orientation to the unit and the labor room will make the laboring woman and her support person feel more welcome and secure. The nurse should allow the woman in early labor to familiarize herself with the surroundings by encouraging her to walk around the room, sit in a chair, and locate necessary items for personal comfort. If the woman is tired and needs to rest or is in active labor, she should be encouraged to assume a side-lying position to facilitate placental oxygenation. The nurse should get to know the couple and explore their preparation and anticipations about their labor and delivery. The nurse should explain the purpose of the call light/intercom system and should place it within easy reach when leaving the room. The couple should know how to operate the television, radio, phone, and bed controls. Since most labor rooms include electronic fetal monitoring equipment, this is a good time to familiarize the couple with this equipment. (See Chapter 3 for an in-depth discussion of monitoring equipment.)

Perineal Preparation. A wide range of preps may be used from a full perineal shave to clipping of the pubic hair or just a thorough cleansing of the perineal area. If shaving is practiced, the nurse should avoid creating skin nicks with the razor since there is **infection, potential for related to inadequate primary defenses.** The nurse should wear gloves during the shaving procedure to protect both the woman and the nurse (see Appendix D). Many women complain of discomfort, burning, and itching following a perineal shave. Throughout labor, the perineum should be kept as clean and dry as possible. Use this time to assess the perineum for pre-existing problems such as purulent vaginal discharge, venereal warts, and so forth.

Vital Signs. Maternal vital signs provide data on the state of hydration and maternal/fetal status. Routinely, the BP and pulse are assessed at least every 1 to 2 hours considering the woman's antepartal baseline. There is potential **cardiac output, alteration in: decreased (maternal) related to dorsal recumbent position.** If the BP is low and the woman is lying on her back, she should be turned to her left side to increase circulation from the lower extremities. (See Chapter 3 for information about Vena Cava Syndrome.) Conversely, the BP may be elevated (e.g., greater than 140/90), or the pulse may be greater than 100 beats per minute. In these cases, more frequent assessment is necessary. Bleeding may cause an increased pulse and decreased BP. Assessment is done for bleeding (see Chapter 8) if these deviations occur. There is a potential for **hyperthermia related to infection; dehydration.** The temperature should be taken at least every 4 hours throughout labor. If it is greater than 37.2°C (99.0°F), it should be taken at least every 2 hours. This routine is altered following ROM (see Chapter 5). The implications of maternal vital signs on the fetal heart rate are discussed in detail in Chapter 3.

Fetal Heart Rate. FHR provides information for evaluating fetal response to labor and fetal well-being. Labor predisposes the fetus to **injury, potential for; (fetal) trauma related to decreased oxygenation.** FHR should be assessed at least every 30 minutes throughout the first stage of labor as long as the FHR remains between 120 to 160 beats per minute (see Chapter 3).

Contractions. Inherent in repeated labor contractions is potential **activity intolerance related to excessive expenditure of energy during contractions.** The nurse should palpate contractions and compare the assessment results (see Chapter 3) with the woman's perception of what she is feeling. Observation is made of her reactions. If she is expending too much energy, this is a good time to evaluate and possibly modify her coping behaviors. (See Chapter 7 for specific nursing interventions.)

Activity. Hospital policies will vary, but generally the woman may walk around or be in bed as she desires, provided all of the following are present: (1) uncomplicated pregnancy, (2) good fetal response to labor, (3) normal presentation, (4) engagement, and (5) intact membranes. If membranes are ruptured and engagement has occurred, ambulation may be permitted, even encouraged. The nurse should provide diversional activities as necessary and encourage the woman to relax. The couple usually functions well independently during the early (latent) phase; however, the nurse should use this time to create opportunities for answering questions and providing information.

Nutrition. Solid foods are usually not recommended during labor because of decreased gastrointestinal absorption. This is especially true if the woman has received narcotics. However, clear liquids and ice chips provide energy and maintain hydration. There is **fluid volume deficit, potential related to inadequate fluid intake.** If the woman becomes dehydrated and is experiencing nausea or vomiting during labor, fluids should be given intravenously. Many times, intravenous fluids are started when cervical dilatation is approximately 5 cm. If a cesarean delivery is anticipated, oral fluids should not be given because stomach contents may be aspirated during or after the procedure.

Elimination. A full bladder can cause **comfort, alteration in: pain, acute related to bladder distention,** and can interfere with the progress of labor and descent of the fetus. The nurse should assess the bladder status every 2 hours during labor. Hormones of pregnancy, pressure from the presenting part, and analgesia may cause decreased bladder tone so that the urge to void is not present. The woman needs to be encouraged to void as necessary. When she does, the amount should be recorded and the urine should be tested for protein, ketone, and glucose.

It is no longer routine to give every woman in labor an enema. However, if the woman has not had a bowel movement during the last 24 hours, or if fecal matter is felt in the rectum during examination, an enema may be indicated. Removing stool from the lower bowel makes the woman feel more comfortable, facilitates descent of the presenting part (see Chapter 4), and relieves inhibitions about pushing owing to embarrassment about expulsion of fecal matter.

Comfort Measures. **Comfort, alteration in: pain, acute related to the contraction frequency; contraction intensity; maternal position; tension** is common during labor. Ongoing assessment throughout labor will influence the type and amount of comfort measures needed. Prepared and/or experienced couples may only need reinforcement of what they were taught prior to labor. Inexperienced couples may need additional suggestions.

Position is probably the most important aspect of comfort. Whether the woman is standing, sitting, or lying down, she will need support to maintain her position during contractions. Pillows can be used to support the upper and lower back, head, and arms. Frequent position changes should be encouraged throughout labor; however, the woman should avoid the supine position, which may interfere with uteroplacental circulation and, consequently, compromise the fetus.

Conscious relaxation, breathing techniques, effleurage, pelvic rock, heat or cold to the lower back, back rubs, and counterpressure on the lower back may decrease the perception of pain with contractions (see Chapter 7). Couples should be taught to expend as little energy as possible in the process of promoting comfort during labor (e.g., use breathing techniques only during contractions).

Dry mouth and cracked lips can be very uncomfortable. Frequent fluids or ice chips help. Lip balm, lemon and glycerine swabs, or lollipops provide additional lubrication. Frequent mouth rinses help remove the bad taste that accompanies a dry mouth.

Comfort measures may not always be effective in decreasing the perception of pain. Intervention with analgesia/anesthesia may become necessary to facilitate coping and promote labor progression (see Chapter 6).

• •

Review Questions

1. Complete the following chart with the appropriate words to describe the latent phase of the first stage of labor.

LATENT PHASE

Dilatation ______________________

Contraction: frequency ______________________
duration ______________________
intensity ______________________

2. Identify fears a laboring woman might have:
   a. About herself:
      1. ____________________
      2. ____________________
      3. ____________________
   b. About the baby:
      1. ____________________
      2. ____________________
      3. ____________________

Answers

1.

		LATENT PHASE
Dilatation		1–3 cm
Contraction:	frequency	5–20 minutes
	duration	10–30 seconds
	intensity	mild

2. a. Fears the woman might have about herself:
      1. pain
      2. long labor
      3. abandonment
      4. internal injury
      5. losing self-esteem
      6. embarrassment
      7. helplessness
   b. Fears the woman might have about the baby:
      1. survival
      2. injury
      3. baby will not come out
      4. how baby will come out
      5. deformities

• •

Early Active Phase of the First Stage of Labor

During the early active (acceleration) phase of the first stage of labor, progress becomes more rapid. The cervix dilates from approximately 4 to 7 cm. Effacement is probably complete. Contractions are usually regular, are moderate in intensity, occur every 3 to 5 minutes, and last 30 to 45 seconds. Increased bloody show is present.

The woman may become apprehensive. She becomes doubtful of her ability to control the pain. She may be afraid to be alone. Her attention becomes more inner-directed. She may have difficulty following directions. Fatigue is evident. It becomes apparent that she is experiencing **coping, ineffective individual related to labor progression.**

Upon entering the room, the nurse should not interrupt the couple's concentration during contractions. Instead, the nurse evaluates the effectiveness of their coping mechanisms. The couple should be praised for their positive efforts. The coach needs to be relieved from time to time to decrease fatigue and provide a break. The nurse should promote an environment that is conducive to rest and relaxation. Complete relaxation between contractions should be encouraged. This will conserve energy and promote labor. Physical nursing care, including assessment of vital signs, FHR, contractions, nutrition, and elimination, and performing the comfort measures discussed above, must be provided, but with minimal disruption for the couple.

Transition Phase of the First Stage of Labor

During the transition (maximum slope) phase of labor, progress is most rapid. The cervix dilates from 8 to 10 cm. Contractions are usually regular and strong to expulsive, and they occur every 2 to 3 minutes and last for 45 to 60 seconds. Bloody show may be heavy, and intact membranes may rupture spontaneously.

A common complaint is **comfort, alteration in: pain, acute related to increased rectal pressure; strong contractions.** The woman will often lose control during transition. Irritability may take the form of anger or unwillingness to be touched. Communication is brief, with periods of amnesia between contractions. Response to contractions may include writhing, nausea and vomiting, and hyperventilation. Profuse perspiration (diaphoresis), as well as muscle cramps, leg tremors, chills, and generalized shaking, may occur. The urge to defecate is strong because of pressure of the presenting part on the rectum. This is experienced as an urge to push or bear down. Pain is described as severe, and many women express the feeling of not being able to make it. If ever they need support, it is now.

Preparations for birth can be made as the primigravida enters Stage II. During Stage II, the fetus descends so that the perineal area is bulging. Preparations for delivery for the multigravida may begin as early as at the beginning of transition (8 cm), since tissue and muscles of the birth canal are more relaxed from previous births. If transfer from a labor room to a delivery room is planned, it should be accomplished with as little disruption as possible. If transfer from bed to stretcher and/or delivery table is performed, attempts should be made to help the woman move between contractions.

Hospitals that offer a combination labor/delivery/recovery area are becoming popular today (see Chapter 7). The primary advantage is that there is no interruption for the laboring woman. She can continue to concentrate on coping with labor forces without a disruptive change in environment.

Regardless of where she is, maternal vital signs and FHR must continue to be assessed. Each contraction should be evaluated using very light touch. The nurse should encourage and assist with position changes, keeping the perineal area as clean and dry as possible. Perineal cleansing is routinely performed just before delivery. If severe back pain is present, firm pressure and/or heat may be applied. Nausea and vomiting may be alleviated by placing a cold, wet cloth on the neck. Frequent facial wipes and mouth care promote comfort. Regardless of how strong the urge, pushing is often not allowed until the cervix is completely dilated. Panting or blowing throughout each contraction may help to overcome the urge to push. Nursing interventions that promote descent are discussed in Chapter 2.

• •

Review Questions

1. Complete the following chart with the appropriate descriptive words for the early active and transition phases of the first stage of labor.

	EARLY ACTIVE PHASE	TRANSITION
Dilatation		
Contractions:		
frequency		
duration		
intensity		

2. Using a, b, or c, match the terms in column I with the appropriate phase of labor in column II.

COLUMN I	COLUMN II
a. Latent phase	_____ Irritable, unwilling to be touched
b. Early active phase	_____ Strong urge to push or bear down
c. Transition phase	_____ Becomes doubtful of ability to control pain
	_____ May not feel ready for labor
	_____ May be afraid to be alone
	_____ Open to instructions and directions
	_____ Periods of amnesia occur between contractions
	_____ Fatigue becomes evident
	_____ Period when the woman needs the most support

Answers

1.

	EARLY ACTIVE PHASE	TRANSITION
Dilatation	4–7 cm	8–10 cm
Contractions: frequency	3–5 min	2–3 min
duration	30–45 sec	45–60 sec
intensity	moderate	strong to expulsive

2. c, c, b, a, b, a, c, b, c
During the *latent* phase, the following may occur: may not feel ready for labor; open to instructions and directions. During the *early active* phase, the following may occur: becomes doubtful of ability to control pain; may be afraid to be alone; fatigue becomes evident. During the *transition* phase, the following may occur: irritable, unwilling to be touched; strong urge to push or bear down; periods of amnesia occur between contractions; period when the woman needs the most support.

• •

Second Stage of Labor

The following nursing diagnoses are appropriate for the second stage of labor:

1. **Comfort, alteration in: pain, acute related to stretching of the vagina; diaphoresis; heat production; bladder distention; strong uterine contractions**
2. **Cardiac output, alteration in: decreased related to dorsal recumbent position; analgesia; anesthesia**
3. Potential **Gas exchange, impaired (fetal) related to head compression; decreased placental perfusion; maternal anesthesia; malpresentation**
4. **Skin integrity, impairment of: potential related to uncontrolled expulsion of the fetus**
5. **Fluid volume deficit, potential related to decreased oral intake; diaphoresis; blood loss; vomiting; hyperventilation**

Labor is the expenditure of energy to accomplish delivery. The period of greatest energy flow is the second stage, the stage of expulsion. During the second stage, uterine contractions usually occur every 2 to 3 minutes, last 50 to 60 seconds, and are expulsive in strength. The urge to push or bear down is very strong. Coordinating involuntary uterine contractions and the voluntary contractions of pushing will promote progressive descent with *crowning* (the encircling of the largest diameter of the fetal head by the vulva) and delivery of the baby.

The couple is usually excited about the prospect of imminent delivery. At this time, any fatigue or discouragement will usually disappear and be replaced with a new surge of hope and feelings of accomplishment.

The nurse should be present throughout the second stage of labor in order to provide support and continuously monitor contractions. FHR should be taken at least after every other contraction or every 5 minutes. A drop in FHR may require specific nursing interventions, which are discussed in Chapter 3. Blood pressure and pulse are taken every 15 minutes and should be done between contractions. All of these vital signs should be recorded.

Cervical dilatation, effacement, and descent of the presenting part are determined by vaginal examination. The cervix usually must be completely dilated before pushing is allowed or encouraged since pushing prior to complete dilatation may result in cervical edema and may prolong labor. (See Chapter 4 for discussion of descent, Chapter 7 for coaching, and Chapter 2 for positions for pushing.) Pushing is encouraged until the presenting part (fetal head) is visible at the vaginal opening (introitus) with each contraction. If an *episiotomy* (surgical incision) is necessary to enlarge the vaginal opening, it will be performed at this time. (See Chapter 6 for anesthetics used at the time of delivery.) The woman may be encouraged to pant (stop pushing) so that the head is delivered gently with only the power of involuntary uterine contractions.

If a delivery-room birth is planned, transfer should be as nonintrusive as possible. Many hospitals are equipped with labor beds that can be used for transport, thus omitting the necessity of having the woman move to a stretcher. The practice of rushing to the delivery room while repeatedly telling the woman "don't push" causes a great deal of maternal anxiety. This can be omitted through careful planning and monitoring of labor progression.

If the father wishes to be present for the birth, the nurse should show him where to sit or stand in order to continue coaching and observe the birth. In addition to continual assessment of maternal/fetal status, the nurse must also prepare the mother physically. Her head and shoulders are supported with pillows, and if necessary, her legs are placed in stirrups, and the perineal area is cleansed. The woman is instructed to grasp her legs or the handles on the table. The nurse also needs to prepare the equipment for the delivery and assist the physician or midwife to don sterile gown and gloves.

Third Stage of Labor

Nursing diagnoses appropriate for the third stage include:

1. **Fluid volume deficit, potential related to bleeding from placental separation**

2. **Injury, potential for; (newborn) trauma related to improper positioning**
3. Potential **Family process, alteration in related to separation of parents and newborn**
4. **Comfort, alteration in: pain, acute related to fundal massage; perineal repair**

After delivery, the newborn should be placed at the level of the uterus or on the maternal abdomen prior to clamping the cord. If the baby is held below the level of the uterus, excess blood flow from the placenta to the baby may occur, causing an increased number of red blood cells which may affect the degree of physiologic jaundice of the newborn. Whether to clamp the cord immediately or wait for pulsations to cease is controversial because there may be benefits to the baby (e.g., decreased likelihood of anemia), as well as adverse effects (e.g., transfer of depressing drugs, or in diabetes, transfer of excessive red blood cells). The father may be allowed to cut the cord if he so desires.

Parents' reactions to this first sight of their baby are varied. They may stare in awe, scream, shout, laugh, or cry. The excitement is usually high. They involuntarily reach out to touch the baby. Occasionally, disappointment over the sex of the baby may be verbally expressed. The nurse should be accepting of all feelings that occur at this time. (Nursing care of the newborn immediately after delivery will be discussed later in this chapter.)

The third stage, the placental stage, is very short. It involves passively waiting for placental separation. The signs of placental separation are as follows: (1) the uterus becomes more global in shape and rises in the abdominal cavity; (2) the cord visibly lengthens outside the vagina; and (3) a trickle or gush of bright red blood exits the vaginal canal. Following signs of separation, the woman may be asked to push or bear down to facilitate placental expulsion.

The nurse may receive an order to administer an oxytocic drug (Pitocin, Methergine, Syntocinon) immediately following delivery of the placenta. Oxytocics stimulate uterine contractions and decrease blood loss from the placental implantation site. An oxytocic is administered earlier with the delivery of the anterior shoulder of the newborn for the same purpose. (See Chapter 5 for additional information about oxytocics.)

Delivery of the placenta followed by the contraction or clamping down of the uterus may be painful and unexpected by the mother. Encourage her to use her breathing techniques. Support and reassurance are important during this time.

Fourth Stage of Labor

The following nursing diagnoses are appropriate for the fourth stage:

1. **Fluid volume deficit, potential related to excess blood loss; distended bladder causing fundal relaxation**
2. **Comfort, alteration in: pain, acute related to perineal trauma; uterine contractions; exhaustion**
3. Potential **Family process, alteration in related to separation of parents and newborn**

Following examination of the vagina and cervix, and episiotomy repair, the mother may need to be transferred to a separate recovery area. Positive identification (footprinting, fingerprinting and/or identification bands with matching numbers) of mother and baby must be done before the transfer.

Nursing assessment of the mother is performed every 15 minutes during the first hour and every 30 minutes for at least the second and third hours. Nursing assessment includes:

Vital Signs. BP and pulse provide significant data regarding the new mother's circulatory status. They are initially assessed every 15 minutes. The temperature should be taken at least once during the recovery period, unless predisposing factors for infection have occurred. In that case, the temperature should be taken every 2 hours. Temperature elevation during the first 24 hours postpartum is usually related to dehydration.

Fundus. The fundus should be firm, midline, and at the level of or below the umbilicus. If it is not firm, massage is indicated to prevent hemorrhage from the placental implantation site. If clots are present, they must be expressed if the fundus is to remain firm. Manual expression is accomplished by placing one hand above the symphysis pubis to anchor the bottom of the uterus. With the other hand, massage the fundus until it is firm, then exert downward pressure on the fundus while continuing to anchor the bottom of the uterus. If the fundus does not remain firm, or if it is above the umbilicus and/or deviated from midline, bladder distention should be suspected.

Lochia. Check for color, amount, and presence of clots. Lochia should be red and moderate in amount. Saturating one pad during the period of an hour constitutes normal lochia flow during Stage IV. Saturating more than one pad per hour is considered excessive. Jacobson[12] developed the following standard for nurses to facilitate accuracy in observing and reporting lochia amount: (1) *scant*—pad stain of less than 1 inch or blood present only when the perineum is wiped with tissue; (2) *moderate*—pad stain of less than 6 inches; (3) *heavy*—pad saturated within 1 hour. The presence of solid particles may indicate either retained placental fragments or relaxation of the fundus. A cervical or vaginal wall laceration may be suspected if the lochia flows in spurts or continuously trickles in the presence of a firm fundus.

Perineum. Whether or not an episiotomy has been performed, the perineum should be inspected for signs of excessive trauma, swelling, bruising, or tears. Some edema may occur following episiotomy repair or delivery over an intact perineum. Intermittent ice packs/cold compresses to the perineum during the first 24 hours postpartum will help prevent undue bruising, swelling, and pain.

Urinary Bladder. Immediately following delivery, the bladder has increased capacity, decreased tone, and decreased sensitivity. The bladder should be palpated for urinary retention and the woman encouraged to void as necessary. Catheterization may be necessary.

• •

Review Questions

1. The period of greatest energy flow for the woman in labor is the ________ stage of labor.
2. Pushing is allowed/encouraged when the cervix is dilated:
   a. 5 cm c. 9 cm
   b. 7 cm d. 10 cm
3. A surgical incision sometimes used to enlarge the vaginal opening is an ________.
4. List three components of nursing assessment of maternal/fetal status during the second stage of labor:
   a. ________
   b. ________
   c. ________
5. List three signs of placental separation:
   a. ________
   b. ________
   c. ________
6. All but one of the following drugs are oxytocics used to stimulate uterine contractions and may be administered following delivery of the placenta:
   a. Pitocin c. AquaMEPHYTON
   b. Methergine d. Syntocinon
7. Following delivery, the fundus is assessed every 15 minutes during the first hour. It should be firm and:
   a. midline and above the umbilicus
   b. midline and at the level of the umbilicus
   c. deviated to the right and above the umbilicus
   d. deviated to the right and at the level of the umbilicus
8. Following episiotomy repair, perineal bruising, swelling, and pain can be decreased with the application of ________.
9. Which of the following has increased capacity, decreased tone, and decreased sensitivity following delivery?
   a. pituitary gland c. urinary bladder
   b. liver d. heart

Answers

1. The *second* stage of labor is the period of greatest energy flow for the woman in labor.
2. d. Pushing is allowed/encouraged when the cervix is dilated 10 cm.
3. *Episiotomy* is a surgical incision sometimes used to enlarge the vaginal opening.
4. Nursing assessment of maternal/fetal status during the second stage of labor includes: (a) continuous monitoring of contractions; (b) FHR after every contraction or every 5 minutes; and (c) BP and pulse every 15 minutes.
5. Three signs of placental separation are: (a) the uterus becomes more global in shape and rises in the abdomen; (b) the cord visibly lengthens outside the vagina; and (c) a trickle or gush of bright red blood exits the vagina.
6. c. AquaMEPHYTON is not an oxytocic drug. Pitocin, Methergine, and Syntocinon are all oxytocics.
7. b. Following delivery, the fundus should be firm, midline, and at or below the level of the umbilicus.
8. *Cold compresses* or *ice packs* applied to the perineum after episiotomy repair will decrease bruising, swelling, and pain.
9. c. The urinary bladder has increased capacity, decreased tone, and decreased sensitivity following delivery.

• •

Immediate Care of the Newborn

The following are nursing diagnoses that are appropriate for the newborn immediately after delivery:

1. Potential **Gas exchange, impaired (newborn) related to cold stress; excess mucus; ineffective respiratory effort; intrauterine hypoxia**
2. Potential **Hypothermia related to change in environment; body size; inadequate subcutaneous fat; absence of shiver response**
3. **Injury, potential for; trauma (to newborn) related to eye prophylaxis; hemorrhage; cold stress; resuscitation**

Following delivery, Apgar scores are noted at 1 minute and 5 minutes. The Apgar score chart (Table 1–2) was developed by Dr. Virginia Apgar as a method of evaluating the newborn's adaptation from intrauterine to extrauterine environment at 1 minute after birth. The 5-minute score evaluates the newborn's responsiveness to resuscitation measures and correlates with later neurologic development. A score of 7 to 10 means good condition; 4 to 6 means moderately depressed; and 1 to 3 means severely depressed. Resuscitative measures are indicated if the score is less than 7. There is a direct correlation between the 5-minute Apgar score and newborn morbidity/mortality.

Table 1–2. APGAR SCORE CHART*

	SCORE		
OBSERVATION	***0***	***1***	***2***
Heart rate	Absent	Slow (below 100)	Over 100
Respiratory effort	Absent (apneic)	Slow, irregular shallow	Good, sustained cry; regular respirations
Reflex irritability	No response	Grimace, frown	Sneeze, cough, cry
Muscle tone	Limp, completely flaccid	Some flexion of extremities; some resistance to extension of extremities	Active motion, good muscle tone, spontaneous flexion
Color	Cyanotic, pale	Body pink, extremities blue	Completely pink

*From: Apgar, V: A proposal for a new method of evaluation of the newborn infant. Curr Res Anesth Analg 260–267, 1953, with permission.

The newborn should be dried immediately and placed either under a radiant warmer or skin to skin with the mother and covered with warm blankets to prevent heat loss. Since the newborn's head is the most difficult area to dry thoroughly, a knit or stockinette cap will help to reduce heat loss. Following Apgar scoring and a cursory physical assessment, the newborn may be weighed and measured (head and chest circumferences, length). AquaMEPHYTON (vitamin K) may be administered intramuscularly at this time or later to facilitate normal blood clotting. Positive identification of mother and baby should be established with matching bands and newborn footprints and mother's fingerprint/thumbprint. If the condition of the newborn is stable, he or she may be bundled and held by the father until physical care of the mother is complete.

A woman who plans to breast-feed should be encouraged to nurse her baby soon after delivery. Newborns are usually alert for about 30 minutes after birth. This is labeled as the first period of reactivity. Their vision is thought to be within an 8-inch field. Encouraging mother-father-baby face-to-face interaction at this time is important.

Prophylaxis against eye infection of the newborn is a legal requirement in the United States and is governed by state law. Prophylaxis is used to prevent gonococcal infection of the conjunctiva (ophthalmia neonatorum), which is a potentially blinding disease.

Although silver nitrate (1 percent) is still used, it has been largely replaced because it is not effective against chlamydia, which is an infectious agent that may also cause ophthalmia neonatorum. Tetracycline (1 percent) or erythromycin (0.5 percent) may be used for eye prophylaxis, but erythromycin ointment is more effective against chlamydia.[13]

The Committee on Ophthalmia Neonatorum of the National Society to Prevent Blindness recommends that eye prophylaxis for all newborns should be performed within 1 hour after birth.[14] The nurse should try to delay the newborn's eye treatment within the safe time period to prevent clouding of vision during the first hour of life and perhaps facilitate parent-infant attachment. In contrast, Butterfield, and colleagues[15] indicated that maternal response to the newborn's decreased vision following eye prophylaxis was of no consequence; that is, the mother's pleasure and excitement during the first hour after birth were not altered. He concluded that newborn eye openness may encourage more attention from the father than from the mother.

Emergency Delivery— A Nursing Responsibility

In an emergency delivery, the following nursing diagnoses may be appropriate:

1. **Anxiety [specify] related to delivery in an unplanned environment**
2. **Injury, potential for; trauma (to mother) related to lacerations; hemorrhage; infection**
3. **Comfort, alteration in: pain, acute related to fear; anxiety; hysteria; lack of medical support; rapid labor progression**
4. **Injury, potential for; trauma (to fetus/newborn) related to rapid uncontrolled delivery of the head; cord compression; inappropriate care; contamination; prematurity**

Occasionally, a woman's labor may progress more rapidly than expected. The nurse may find herself in the position of having to assist with the delivery of the baby. This can occur either outside of the hospital setting or within the hospital before the doctor or midwife arrives. Regardless of the setting, the laboring woman will usually experience a sense of panic about the imminent delivery. When a woman shouts "The baby's coming!" speed and calmness on the part of the nurse are essential. The nurse should first observe the perineum to determine how much preparation time exists. While helping the woman to assume a comfortable position, it is essential to decrease her panic. Short, positive verbal commands are best. Using a calm voice, the nurse must convey an understanding of the woman's fears and the intention to help make this as safe and positive an experience as possible. The woman should be encouraged to pant during each contraction to decrease the urge to push. It may be necessary to pant with her in this anxious situation.

If time permits, the nurse's hands should be washed thoroughly. Sterile gloves and drapes are available in the hospital setting. With the increased incidence of infectious diseases, gloves serve as a protection for the nurse as well as for the delivering woman. Outside of the hospital, clean sheets, blankets, towels, clothing, or unread newspapers may be used to provide a clean surface.

As the woman pants through her contractions, the nurse may facilitate stretching of the perineum by applying warm compresses and/or gently massaging the perineal tissue with the forefinger (inside the posterior vaginal wall) and thumb (directly on the perineum). As the head begins to emerge, the woman will need constant support and reassurance. The nurse should apply gentle pressure to the fetal head to keep the fetal head flexed and facilitate slow delivery. The nurse should *never* attempt to delay delivery by applying forceful pressure on the fetal head or by having the woman hold her legs tightly together. Delivery of the head should be slow and controlled and is best achieved in between contractions, while supporting the perineum. Rapid delivery of the head may cause maternal perineal tears and fetal subdural or dural tears.

The fetal cord may be wrapped around the neck (*nuchal cord*). To check for this before the shoulders are delivered, the nurse slides one or two fingers between the back of the baby's head and the vaginal wall. If one or two loops exist, the cord may be pulled out and slipped over the baby's head. If the loop is too tight, the cord should be clamped in two places, cut between the clamps, and then unwrapped from the baby's neck.

Following delivery of the head, the mouth and nose should either be suctioned with a bulb syringe (or DeLee mucus trap, if available) to remove the fluid, mucus, and blood or wiped out with a clean cloth or finger. To deliver the shoulders, the nurse's hands are placed on both sides of the baby's head, and gentle downward pressure is exerted to deliver the anterior shoulder from under the symphysis pubis. Using upward pressure, the posterior shoulder will deliver next. The nurse then encourages the mother to bear down for delivery of the rest of the baby.

The baby is held at the level of the uterus or placed on the maternal abdomen for clamping and cutting the cord. The clamps are placed approximately 4 to 6 inches from the abdomen, and the cord is cut between the two clamps. Outside of the hospital setting, clean shoelaces or strong cord may be used for clamping (do not use wire). It is not necessary to cut the cord if transport to a hospital is possible. If the cord must be cut, a sterilized razor, knife, or scissors is recommended. Placing the baby on the mother's abdomen or allowing the newborn to nurse at the mother's breast will facilitate contraction of the uterus, enhancing separation of the placenta. Following spontaneous expulsion of the placenta, if the cord has not been cut, the placenta may be wrapped in clean newspaper and then wrapped with the baby. The placenta will provide warmth if the shiny (fetal) side is placed against the baby and they are wrapped together. Care should be taken to avoid any tension on the cord if it is still attached to the baby.

If the newborn does not breathe spontaneously following suctioning, the baby should be placed in a head-down position. Gently rubbing the baby's back or flicking the soles of the feet may be sufficient to initiate respirations. If respirations still do not occur, ventilation with bag and mask or mouth-to-mouth resuscitation should be started.

Prevention of heat loss is important. The baby must be thoroughly dried as soon as possible, doing the head and trunk first since these will be the areas of greatest heat loss. Placing the infant directly against the mother's skin and covering both mother and baby may be sufficient to maintain the infant's temperature.

The nurse must record important information such as time of delivery, Apgar scores at 1 and 5 minutes, time of placental expulsion and its condition, presence of a nuchal cord (cord wrapped around the neck), color of the amniotic fluid, and mother's blood type and Rh factor, if known. Mother and baby should be positively identified before transporting to the hospital. Identification bands (tape or strips of cloth) should include mother's name, date and time of delivery, and sex of the infant.

Maternal safety is maintained by promoting uterine contractions to decrease blood loss following delivery of the placenta. Allowing the baby to nurse will stimulate the release of oxytocin, which causes the uterus to contract. If nursing at the breast is not possible, gentle fundal massage should be continued until the uterus becomes firm. Mother and baby should be transported to the nearest hospital as soon as possible for further evaluation and care. Words of praise to the mother, recognizing her courage in a trying situation, will help to decrease her anxiety and possible guilt feelings.

Conclusion

Labor and delivery can be an exciting and meaningful experience. The nurse is the key person in providing permission, direction, and support for the expectant couple. Sensitivity to the couple's needs and provision for expression of individual desires can decrease feelings of helplessness and enhance feelings of control. Encouraging mother and father to explore their new baby can foster the bonds of attachment and positively influence life-long relationships.

• •

Review Questions

1. Referring to Table 1–2 as necessary, provide the appropriate Apgar score for each of the following:
   a. _____ heart rate: absent
   b. _____ muscle tone: active motion
   c. _____ reflex irritability: grimace

d. _____ respiratory effort: slow—irregular
e. _____ color: completely pink

2. There is a direct correlation between the 5-minute Apgar score and newborn:
   a. mortality c. development
   b. growth d. mental ability

3. The most frequently used prophylactic for gonococcal and chlamydia infections of the conjunctiva is _______________.

4. When a woman in labor shouts "The baby's coming!" the first action by the nurse should be to:
   a. control the woman's panic c. call the doctor
   b. observe the perineum d. wash his or her hands

5. Warm compresses and/or gently massaging the perineal tissue just prior to delivery will facilitate perineal _______________.

6. Which of the following is the most appropriate method of safely promoting slow delivery of the fetal head?
   a. applying gentle pressure to the fetal head
   b. tightly crossing the woman's legs
   c. applying forceful pressure to the fetal head
   d. encouraging the woman to push with her contractions

7. The umbilical cord wrapped around the fetal neck is called a _____ cord.

8. Prior to clamping the umbilical cord, the newborn should be placed:
   a. on the mother's abdomen
   b. at the level of the mother's heart
   c. below the level of the uterus
   d. in a head-elevated position on the mother's abdomen

Answers

1. The appropriate Apgar score for each of the following is:
   a. 0 heart rate: absent
   b. 2 muscle tone: active motion
   c. 1 reflex irritability: grimace
   d. 1 respiratory effort: slow—irregular
   e. 2 color: completely pink

2. a. There is a direct correlation between the 5-minute Apgar score and newborn *mortality*.

3. *Erythromycin ointment* is most frequently used prophylactically for gonococcal and chlamydia infections of the conjunctiva.

4. b. When a woman in labor shouts "The baby's coming!" the first action by the nurse should be to observe the perineum.

5. Warm compresses and/or gently massaging the perineal tissue just prior to delivery will facilitate perineal *stretching*.

6. a. The most appropriate method for safely promoting slow delivery of the fetal head is by applying gentle pressure to the fetal head.

7. The umbilical cord wrapped around the fetal neck is called *nuchal* cord.

8. a. Prior to clamping the umbilical cord, the newborn should be placed on the mother's abdomen.

• •

REFERENCES

1. Pritchard, JA, McDonald, PC, and Gant, NF: Williams Obstetrics, ed 17. Appleton-Century-Crofts, Norwalk, Connecticut, 1985, p 295.
2. Olds, SB, London, ML, and Ladewig, PA: Maternal Newborn Nursing: A Family-Centered Approach, ed 2. Addison-Wesley, Menlo Park, California, 1984, p 415.
3. Haun, N: Nursing care during labor. Canadian Nurs 80(9):26, 1984.
4. Muggah, HF: Ultrasonography and radiography. In Oxorn, H: Oxorn-Foote: Human Labor and Birth, ed 5. Appleton-Century-Crofts, Norwalk, Connecticut, 1986, p 650.
5. Cox, BE and Smith, EC: The mother's self esteem after a cesarean delivery. Matern Child Nurs J 7:309, 1982.
6. Hawkins, J and Gorvine, B: Postpartum Nursing: Health Care of Women. Springer, New York, 1985, p 56.
7. Mercer, RT: The nurse and maternal tasks of early postpartum. Matern Child Nurs J 6:341, 1981.
8. United States Department of Health and Human Services: Cesarean childbirth. National Institutes of Health, Bethesda, MD, 1981.
9. Paul, RH, Phelan, JP, and Yeh, S: Trial of labor in the patient with a prior cesarean birth. Am J Obstet Gynecol 151:297, 1985.
10. Jarrell, MA, Ashmead, GG, and Mann, LI: Vaginal delivery after cesarean section: A five year study. Obstet Gynecol 65(5):628, 1985.
11. Lederman, RP: Evaluating uterine contractions. In Malinowski, JS, et al: Nursing Care of the Labor Patient. FA Davis, Philadelphia, 1978, p 13.
12. Jacobson, H: A standard for assessing lochia volume. Matern Child Nurs J 10(3):174, 1985.
13. Bryant, BG: Unit dose erythromycin ophthalmic ointment for neonatal ocular prophylaxis. J Obstet Gynecol Neonatal Nurs 13(2):83, 1984.
14. National Society to Prevent Blindness: Prevention and treatment of ophthalmia neonatorum. Revised 4/81.
15. Butterfield, PM, et al: Does the early application of silver nitrate impair maternal attachment? Pediatrics 67(5):738, 1981.

BIBLIOGRAPHY

Avery, MD and Burket, BA: Effect of perineal massage on the incidence of episiotomy and perineal laceration in a nurse-midwifery service. J Nurse-Midwife 31(3):128, 1986.

Collins, BA: The role of the nurse in labor and delivery as perceived by nurses and patients. J Obstet Gynecol Neonatal Nurs 15(5):412, 1986.

Doenges, ME, Kenty, JR, and Moorhouse, MF: Maternal/Newborn Care Plans: Guidelines for Client Care. FA Davis, Philadelphia, 1988.

Haun, N: Nursing care during labor. Canadian Nurs 80(9):26, 1984.

Holmes, J and Magiera, L: Maternity Nursing. Macmillan, New York, 1987.

Howe, C: Physiologic and psychosocial assessment in labor. Nurs Clin N Amer 17(1):49, 1982.

Kintz, DL: Nursing support in labor. J Obstet Gynecol Neonatal Nurs 16(2):126, 1987.

Klaus, MD and Kennel, JH: Maternal-Infant Bonding. CV Mosby, St. Louis, 1982.

Kogut, EA: The nurse's role in antepartum fetal assessment. J Perinat 6(2):108, 1986.

Laufer, A, et al: Vaginal birth after cesarean section. J Nurse-Midwife 32(1):41, 1987.

McKay, S and Roberts, J: Second stage labor: What is normal? J Obstet Gynecol Neonatal Nurs 14(2):101, 1985.

Miller, CF and Sutter, CS: Vaginal birth after cesarean. J Obstet Gynecol Neonatal Nurs 14(5):383, 1985.

Neeson, JD and May, KA: Comprehensive Maternity Nursing: Nursing Process and the Childbearing Family. JB Lippincott, Philadelphia, 1986.

Oxorn, H: Oxorn-Foote Human Labor and Birth, ed 5. Appleton-Century-Crofts, Norwalk, Connecticut, 1986.

Phillips, CR and Anzalone, JT: Fathering: Participation in Labor and Birth. CV Mosby, St. Louis, 1978.

Pritchard, JA, McDonald, PC, and Gant, NF: William's Obstetrics, ed 17. Appleton-Century-Crofts, Norwalk, Connecticut, 1985.

Reeder, SJ and Martin LL: Maternity Nursing: Family, Newborn, and Women's Health Care, ed 16. JB Lippincott, Philadelphia, 1987.

Standards for Obstetrics, Gynecologic, and Neonatal Nursing, ed 3. The Nurse's Association of the American College of Obstetricians and Gynecologists, 1986.

Taylor, K and Copstick, S: Psychological care in labour. Nurs Mirror 161(4):42, 1985.

Williams C: Emergency childbirth. Nursing 16(3):33, 1986.

POST-TEST 1

1. Match column I with column II.

COLUMN I		COLUMN II
a. Oxytocin Stimulation Theory	(1) _____	A signal from the fetus stimulates the mother's body to begin labor.
b. Progesterone Deprivation Theory	(2) _____	Uterine contraction activity increases as progesterone production decreases near term, initiating labor.
c. Organ Communication System	(3) _____	Uterine contractions are caused by oxytocin from the posterior pituitary gland.

2. Identify the premonitory signs of labor using a check (✓).

_____ a. engagement in the primigravida
_____ b. flexion
_____ c. transverse lie
_____ d. internal rotation
_____ e. extension
_____ f. bloody show
_____ g. SROM
_____ h. increased backache
_____ i. −3 station
_____ j. increased vaginal secretions
_____ k. occiput posterior
_____ l. loose stools
_____ m. 2–3 pound weight loss
_____ n. hydramnios
_____ o. AROM

3. The settling of the uterus and its contents into the pelvis is called ____.

4. The passage of the largest diameter of the fetal presenting part into the maternal pelvic inlet is called _______________________.

5. Match column I with column II.

COLUMN I		COLUMN II
a. True labor	(1) _____	Walking decreases the discomfort of contractions.
b. False labor	(2) _____	Contractions do not increase in frequency, intensity, or duration.
	(3) _____	Contractions progressively increase in frequency and duration.
	(4) _____	Contractions do not cause cervical dilatation.
	(5) _____	Walking usually intensifies contractions.
	(6) _____	Progressive cervical changes occur.

6. Gradual thinning of the internal cervical os is called __________.

7. Gradual opening of the cervix to 10 cm is called __________.

8. Vaginal discharge that occurs prior to or during labor and is thick, mucous, and pink or dark red is called __________.

9. Use a check (✓) to identify the following normal characteristics of amniotic fluid when the fetus is in a vertex presentation.
   _____ a. clear or cloudy
   _____ b. meconium stained
   _____ c. pale yellow
   _____ d. greenish color
   _____ e. strong odor
   _____ f. 1000 ml
   _____ g. greater than 2000 ml

10. The presence of meconium may be considered normal in which of the following presentations?
    a. vertex
    b. breech
    c. occipital
    d. cephalic

11. Excessive amniotic fluid is often associated with fetal malformations in which the fetus is unable to swallow and/or urinate normally in utero. This is called __________ or __________.

12. Use a check (✓) to identify which of the following tests are used to establish the presence of amniotic fluid obtained from the vagina.
    _____ a. nitrazine test tape
    _____ b. amniotomy
    _____ c. vaginal examination
    _____ d. cervical mucus ferning
    _____ e. ultrasound

13. Identify the appropriate stage of labor (I, II, III, IV) for each of the following:
    _____ a. the placental stage
    _____ b. ends with complete dilatation
    _____ c. 1 to 4 hours after delivery of the placenta
    _____ d. begins with regular contractions
    _____ e. fundal and lochia assessments are performed every 15 minutes
    _____ f. average length of time for the primigravida is 12½ to 14 hours
    _____ g. the stage of expulsion
    _____ h. ends with delivery of the baby

_____ i. pushing is encouraged with contractions
_____ j. the period of greatest energy flow for the woman in labor
_____ k. signs of placental separation normally occur
_____ l. contractions bring about progressive dilatation and effacement of the cervix and descent of the fetus

14. Match column I with column II.

COLUMN I		COLUMN II
a. Attitude	(1) _____	Relationship between the presenting part of the fetus and the maternal pelvis.
b. Lie		
c. Presentation	(2) _____	Relationship of the longitudinal axis of the fetus to the longitudinal axis of the mother.
d. Position		
e. Station	(3) _____	Relationship of the fetal parts to each other — the degree of flexion or extension.
	(4) _____	Refers to the fetal part that is lowermost in the pelvis.
	(5) _____	The level of descent of the presenting part in relation to the ischial spines of the maternal pelvis.

15. Identify the appropriate landmark on the fetus that is used to determine position with each of the following:

PRESENTING PART	PRESENTATION
a. occiput	(1) _____ face
b. forehead	(2) _____ frank breech
c. mentum	(3) _____ vertex
d. sacrum	(4) _____ complete breech
e. scapula	(5) _____ shoulder
	(6) _____ footling breech
	(7) _____ brow

16. Using the terms *descent, flexion, internal rotation, extension, restitution, external rotation,* and *expulsion,* identify the mechanism of labor that each of the following statements describes:
    a. _____ The fetal head rotates from OT to OA, which places the occiput beneath the symphysis pubis.
    b. _____ The fetal head enters the pelvis OT.
    c. _____ Following delivery, the head rotates, placing the shoulders in the A-P diameter.
    d. _____ Resistance from the maternal pelvis forces the fetal head to present its smallest diameter.
    e. _____ Spontaneous delivery of the baby's body.
    f. _____ Delivery of the head occurs with this mechanism.
    g. _____ Spontaneous rotation of the fetal head (after delivery) back to the transverse position.

17. Mrs. Smith, a 20-year-old G i, P 0 with a term pregnancy, is complaining of intermittent low back pain that has increased in frequency, duration, and intensity during the past 4 hours. Prior to admission to the labor area, which of the following might the nurse perform in assessing Mrs. Smith. Place a check (✓) in front of the appropriate actions.
    _____ a. Palpate contractions for frequency, duration, and intensity.
    _____ b. Obtain vital signs, including FHR.
    _____ c. Obtain an x-ray pelvimetry.
    _____ d. Perform Leopold's maneuvers.
    _____ e. Administer an enema and perineal prep.
    _____ f. Obtain a catheterized urine specimen.
    _____ g. Assess cervical dilatation and effacement via vaginal examination.

18. Leopold's maneuvers are used to manually determine fetal position and presentation. Identify the appropriate maneuver (first, second, third, fourth) for each of the following:
    a. _____ The head is the presenting part over the pelvic inlet.
    b. _____ The buttocks are identifiable in the fundus.
    c. _____ The flexed fetal brow may be identified if engagement has not yet occurred.
    d. _____ The fetal back is outlined and small parts are identified.

19. Solid foods are not recommended during labor because of decreased:
    a. renal retention
    b. gastrointestinal absorption
    c. use of routine enemas
    d. liver function

20. A full bladder during labor may:
    a. cause urinary incontinence
    b. interfere with labor progress
    c. be ignored, since it is not significant
    d. cause nausea and vomiting

21. Use a check (✓) to identify appropriate nursing measures that may be employed during labor to promote comfort.
    _____ a. reinforcement of learned coping patterns
    _____ b. support to maintain position during contractions
    _____ c. encouraging the supine position during contractions
    _____ d. forcing oral fluids to combat dry mouth
    _____ e. teaching conscious relaxation and pelvic rock
    _____ f. providing back rubs and counterpressure
    _____ g. encouraging continual ambulation

22. List three fears for each of the following:
    a. Fears the woman might have about herself:
        (1) ______________________________
        (2) ______________________________
        (3) ______________________________

b. Fears the woman might have about her baby:
(1) ______
(2) ______
(3) ______

23. Using the chart below, fill in the appropriate response for each phase of the first stage of labor.

	DILATATION	FREQUENCY	DURATION
Latent			
Early Active			
Transition			

24. During which phase of the first stage of labor (latent, early active, transition) is each of the following most likely to occur?
a. ______ Irritable, unwilling to be touched.
b. ______ Strong urge to push or bear down.
c. ______ Becomes doubtful of ability to control pain.
d. ______ May not feel ready for labor.
e. ______ May be afraid to be alone.
f. ______ Open to instructions and directions.
g. ______ Periods of amnesia occur between contractions.
h. ______ Fatigue becomes evident.
i. ______ Period when the woman needs the most support.

25. List three signs of placental separation following delivery.
a. ______
b. ______
c. ______

26. Baby Smith has been evaluated by the nurse at 1 minute after birth. The following observations were noted: Heart rate—over 100; Respiratory effort—slow, irregular, shallow; Reflex irritability—grimace, frown; Muscle tone—some flexion of extremities, some resistance to extension of extremities; Color—body pink, extremities blue. Using the Apgar scoring method, provide the appropriate score for each of the five areas plus the sum of scores to determine Baby Smith's Apgar score at 1 minute after birth.
a. ______ Heart rate
b. ______ Respiratory effort
c. ______ Reflex irritability
d. ______ Muscle tone
e. ______ Color
f. ______ Total Apgar score at 1 minute after birth

27. Baby Smith's total Apgar score at 1 minute provides an index for nursing care. Which of the following is the most appropriate immediate nursing intervention?
    a. initiate resuscitative measures
    b. prevent heat loss by bundling the baby securely
    c. facilitate attachment with parents
    d. weigh, measure, and apply eye prophylaxis

28. Circle True or False and explain your answer:
    a. T F The most frequently used prophylactic for gonococcal infection of the conjunctiva in the newborn is erythromycin ointment.

    ____
    ____
    ____

    b. T F The laboring woman who thinks the baby is coming is usually feeling pressure, which causes her to panic; therefore, the most appropriate nursing action is to help her decrease her panic.

    ____
    ____
    ____

    c. T F Warm compresses and/or gently massaging the perineal tissue just prior to the delivery will facilitate perineal stretching.

    ____
    ____
    ____

    d. T F The most appropriate method of safely promoting slow delivery of the head is to apply forceful pressure to the fetal head.

    ____
    ____
    ____

    e. T F Immediately following delivery, but prior to clamping the cord, the newborn should be placed at the level of the uterus.

    ____
    ____
    ____

    f. T F Following emergency delivery outside the hospital setting, the placenta should always be separated from the baby to prevent contamination.

    ____
    ____
    ____

Answers to Post-Test

1. (1) c, (2) b, (3) a
   (1). Organ Communication System — the fetus transmits a signal to its mother to initiate the onset of labor.
   (2). Progesterone Deprivation Theory — a decrease in progesterone production near term causes an increase in uterine contraction activity, initiating labor.
   (3). Oxytocin Stimulation Theory — oxytocin causes uterine contractions.

2. a, f, g, h, j, l, m
   The following are premonitory signs of labor: engagement, uterine contractions, bloody show, SROM, increased backache, increased vaginal secretions, loose stools, 2- to 3-pound weight loss.

3. *Lightening* is the settling of the uterus and its contents into the pelvis.

4. *Engagement* is the passage of the largest diameter of the fetal presenting part into the maternal pelvic inlet.

5. (1) b, (2) b, (3) a, (4) b, (5) a, (6) a
   True labor is characterized by the following: contractions progressively increase in frequency and duration; walking usually intensifies contractions; progressive cervical changes occur. False labor is characterized by the following: walking decreases the discomfort of contractions; contractions do not increase in frequency, intensity, or duration; contractions do not cause cervical dilatation.

6. *Effacement* is the gradual thinning of the internal cervical os.

7. *Dilatation* is the gradual opening of the cervix to 10 cm.

8. *Bloody show* is the vaginal discharge that occurs prior to or during labor. It is thick, mucous, and pink or dark red in color.

9. a, c, f
   Amniotic fluid should be clear or cloudy, pale yellow, and approximately 1000 ml.

10. b. Meconium may be considered normal in a breech presentation.

11. *Hydramnios* or *polyhydramnios* is the presence of excessive amniotic fluid. It is often associated with fetal malformations in which the fetus is unable to swallow and/or urinate normally in utero.

12. a, d
    The following tests are used to establish the presence of amniotic fluid in the vagina: nitrazine test tape and cervical mucus ferning.

13. a. III, b. I, c. IV, d. I, e. IV, f. I, g. II, h. II, i. II, j. II, k. III, l. I
    Stage I includes the following: ends with complete dilatation; begins with regular contractions; average length of time for the primigravida is 12½ to 14 hours; contractions bring about progressive dilatation and effacement of the cervix and descent of the fetus. Stage II includes the following: the stage of expulsion; ends with delivery of the baby; pushing is encouraged; the period of greatest energy flow for the woman in labor. Stage III includes the following: the

placental stage; signs of placental separation normally occur. Stage IV includes the following: 1 to 4 hours after delivery of the placenta; fundal and lochia assessments are performed every 15 minutes.

14. (1) d, (2) b, (3) a, (4) c, (5) e
    (1) Position—relationship between the presenting part of the fetus and the maternal pelvis.
    (2) Lie—relationship of the longitudinal axis of the fetus to the longitudinal axis of the mother.
    (3) Attitude—relationship of the fetal parts to each other—the degree of flexion or extension.
    (4) Presentation—refers to the fetal part that is lowermost in the pelvis.
    (5) Station—the level of descent of the presenting part in relation to the ischial spines of the maternal pelvis.

15. (1) c, (2) d, (3) a, (4) d, (5) e, (6) d, (7) b
    The occiput is the presenting part in a vertex presentation. The forehead is the presenting part in a brow presentation. The mentum is the presenting part in a face presentation. The sacrum is the presenting part in frank breech, complete breech, and footling breech presentations. The scapula is the presenting part in a shoulder presentation.

16. The mechanisms of labor are as follows:
    a. Internal rotation—the fetal head rotates from OT to OA, which places the occiput beneath the symphysis pubis.
    b. Descent—the fetal head enters the pelvis OT.
    c. External Rotation—following delivery, the head rotates placing the shoulders in the A-P diameter.
    d. Flexion—resistance from the maternal pelvis forces the fetal head to present its smallest diameter.
    e. Expulsion—spontaneous delivery of the baby's body.
    f. Extension—delivery of the head occurs with this mechanism.
    g. Restitution—immediate rotation of the fetal head (after delivery) back to the transverse position.

17. a, b, d, g
    Nursing assessment prior to admission to the labor area might include: palpate contractions for frequency, duration, and intensity; obtain vital signs, including FHR; perform Leopold's maneuvers; assess cervical dilatation and effacement via vaginal examination.

18. Leopold's maneuvers include:
    a. Third—the head is the presenting part felt over the pelvic inlet.
    b. First—the buttocks are identifiable in the fundus.
    c. Fourth—the flexed fetal brow may be identified if engagement has not yet occurred.
    d. Second—the fetal back is outlined and small parts are identified.

19. b. Solid foods are not recommended during labor because of decreased gastrointestinal absorption.

20. b. A full bladder during labor may interfere with labor progress.

21. a, b, e, f
Nursing measures that may promote comfort during labor are: reinforcement of learned coping patterns, support to maintain position during contractions, teaching conscious relaxation and pelvic rock, providing back rubs and counterpressure.

22. a. Fears the woman might have about herself are: fear of pain, long labor, abandonment, internal injury, losing self-esteem, embarrassment, and helplessness.
 b. Fears the woman might have about the baby are: fear of survival, injury, deformity, how the baby will get out, or that the baby will not come out.

23.

PHASE OF STAGE I	DILATATION	FREQUENCY	DURATION
Latent	1–3 cm	5–20 min	10–30 sec
Early Active	4–7 cm	3–5 min	30–45 sec
Transition	8–10 cm	2–3 min	45–60 sec

24. Latent—d, f; Early Active—c, e, h; Transition—a, b, g, i
During the latent phase, the following may occur: may not feel ready for labor; open to instructions and directions. During the early active phase, the following may occur: becomes doubtful of ability to control pain; may be afraid to be alone; fatigue becomes evident. During transition, the following may occur; irritable, unwilling to be touched; strong urge to push or bear down; periods of amnesia occur between contractions; period when the woman needs the most support.

25. The three signs of placental separation are: (a) the uterus becomes more global in shape and rises in the abdomen; (b) the cord visibly lengthens outside the vagina; and (c) a trickle or gush of bright red blood exits the vagina.

26. Using the Apgar scoring method, the nurse would evaluate Baby Smith as follows:
 a. 2 Heart rate—over 100
 b. 1 Respiratory effort—slow, irregular, shallow
 c. 1 Reflex irritability—grimace
 d. 1 Muscle tone—some flexion of extremities; some resistance to extension of extremities
 e. 1 Color—body pink, extremities blue
 f. 6 Total Apgar score at 1 minute after birth

27. a. Since Baby Smith's 1-minute Apgar score is 6, the most appropriate intervention is initiation of resuscitative measures. A score of 3 to 6 means the baby is moderately depressed.

28. a. T The most frequently used prophylactic for gonococcal and chlamydia infections of the conjunctiva in the newborn is erythromycin ointment.
 b. F The woman in labor who thinks the baby is coming is usually feeling pressure, which causes her to panic; however, the most appropriate

nursing intervention is to first observe the perineum for signs of imminent delivery.

c. T Warm compresses and/or gentle massage of the perineal tissue just prior to delivery will facilitate perineal stretching.

d. F The most appropriate method of safely promoting slow delivery of the head is not by applying forceful pressure to the fetal head, which may cause damage. Slow delivery of the fetal head is best accomplished by applying gentle pressure to the fetal head.

e. T Immediately following delivery, but prior to clamping the cord, the newborn should be placed at the level of the uterus or on the maternal abdomen. This prevents an increased amount of blood from the placenta to the newborn, which may occur when the baby is held below the level of the uterus.

f. F Following emergency delivery outside the hospital setting, it is not necessary to cut the cord if transport to a hospital is possible. Clamp the cord with clean shoelaces or strong cord and wrap the placenta in newspaper and then bundle with the baby.

2 MECHANISMS OF LABOR

Janet S. Malinowski

OBJECTIVES

Upon completing this chapter, you will be able to:

- ▶ Briefly describe three adaptive processes that the fetal head must undergo as it moves through the maternal pelvis.
- ▶ List the eight mechanisms of labor in proper sequence and identify the pelvic planes in which they occur.
- ▶ Describe the passage of the fetus through the normal female pelvis by:
  - a. identifying the pelvic bones, the significant landmarks, and the normal female pelvic type
  - b. identifying the significant characteristics of each plane, the pelvic diameters that are manually measurable, and the mechanisms of labor as they occur in each plane
- ▶ Complete a pelvic measurements chart, listing the ideal findings that would allow the normal mechanisms of labor to occur.
- ▶ Compare the normal mechanisms of labor with those of a fetus in occipital posterior position and breech presentation.
- ▶ Identify two ways to convert fetal presentation from breech to cephalic.
- ▶ Use given data to predict the presence or absence of normal mechanisms of labor.
- ▶ Apply four physical principles that influence fetal descent.
- ▶ Explain three ways to promote changes in fetal position.

This chapter presents the anatomy of the bony pelvis and its relationship to the movement of the fetus during the birth process. The chapter is divided into four parts: (1) the normal mechanisms of labor through a normal female pelvis, (2) mecha-

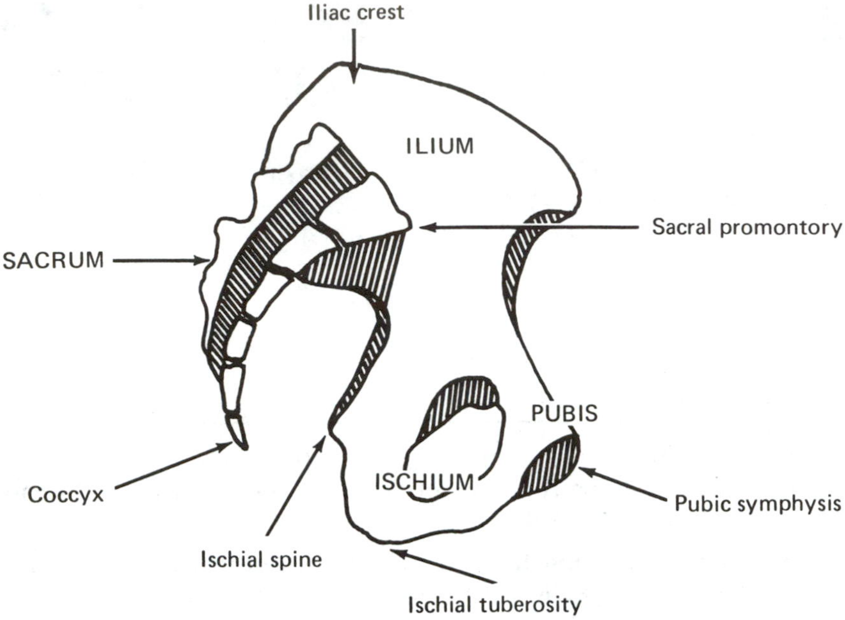

Figure 2–1. Anatomy of the bony pelvis.

nisms for occipital posterior position and breech presentation, (3) conversion to cephalic presentation, and (4) nursing implications related to the mechanisms of labor.

Before beginning the first part, it is beneficial to review the anatomic terms of the pelvis in Figure 2–1. The reader needs to be well acquainted with these terms to understand the chapter's contents.

THE NORMAL MECHANISMS OF LABOR THROUGH A GYNECOID PELVIS

Adaptation by the Fetal Head

The fetus passively adapts to the relatively unyielding maternal pelvic architecture by molding, flexing, and rotating to fit through the passageway in a vaginal birth. The head, the largest fetal diameter, normally enters the pelvis first. Occiput (vertex) presentations occur in about 95 percent of all labors.[1]

The five bones that form the head are loosely joined by membranes covering the sutures (Fig. 2–2). These bones *mold* or override, thereby readjusting the head's diameter so that it fits into and through the bony pelvis despite some resistance. This is not to say that all fetal heads will fit through the pelvis. Some are too large. In that case cephalopelvic disproportion (CPD) exists. But in the pres-

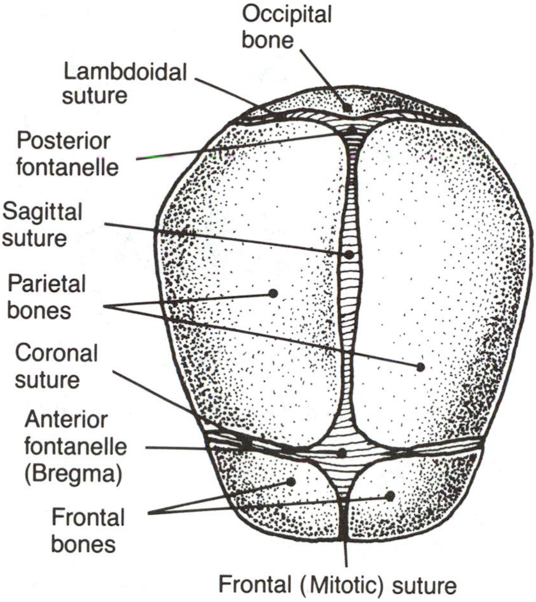

Figure 2–2. Superior view of the fetal skull.

ence of slight disproportion, given time, the head usually molds into a small enough diameter to permit passage through the pelvis.

As the head enters the pelvis it is usually in a nonflexed military attitude. There is usually room for the occipitofrontal diameter, which is 11.0 cm, to fit into the inlet of the pelvis (Fig. 2–3). As the head moves through the pelvis a smaller diameter is necessary. This is accomplished by *flexion* of the neck, placing the chin on the chest. The result is a reduced diameter of 9.5 cm and is called the suboccipitobregmatic diameter—the area below the occipital bone moving around the head to the bregma (anterior fontanel) (Fig. 2–4). Normally, the fetal head enters the pelvis with the occipital bone aimed toward the left or right side of the pelvis—in an occiput transverse (OT) or oblique (tilted diagonally) position. Upon meeting resistance, internal *rotation* occurs. The head rotates approximately 90 degrees aiming the occipital bone occiput anterior (OA)—toward the front of the pelvis—where the pelvic space is more accommodating.

• •

Review Questions

Briefly describe the following adaptive processes that the fetal head goes through:

1. Molding: ______________________________

____

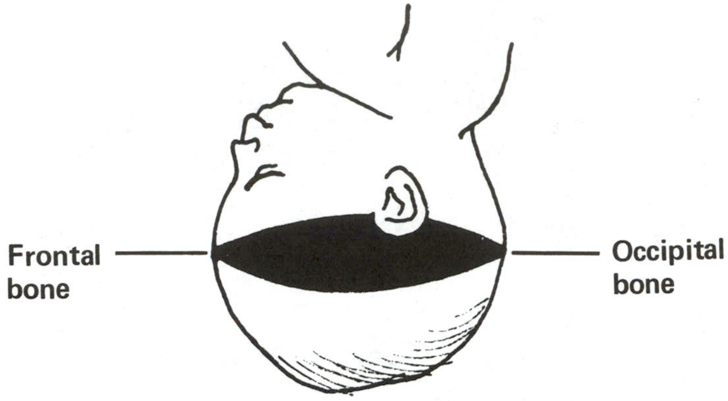

Figure 2–3. Occipitofrontal diameter.

2. Flexion: ______________________________
____

3. Rotation: ______________________________
____

Answers

1. Molding: The bones in the fetal head overlap (mold), forming a smaller diameter.
2. Flexion: The fetal head normally enters the pelvis nonflexed with an 11 cm occipitofrontal diameter. By flexing the head it presents a 9.5 cm suboccipitobregmatic diameter.
3. Rotation: The fetal head rotates from OT to OA because that way it finds less resistance.

• •

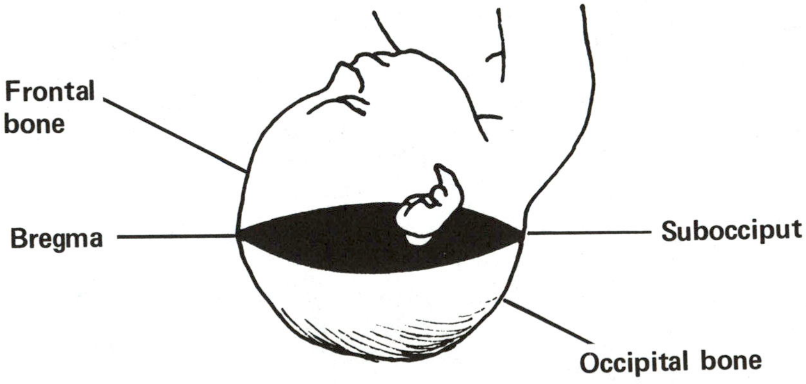

Figure 2–4. Suboccipitobregmatic diameter.

Pelvic Characteristics

The characteristics of the pelvis are usually assessed by the physician or nurse during the initial prenatal visit, and often reassessed near term or in labor to determine the effect of ligament softening that normally occurs. The woman's obstetric record is likely to have a chart such as this:

PELVIC MEASUREMENTS: D.C.________		Spines ________
Sacrum ________	Arch ________	Bitubs ________
Coccyx ________________	Type ________________	

It is recommended that the reader fill in the blanks on this chart, using the norms that are identified in italics in the succeeding sections of the text.

There are four basic pelvic types essentially referring to the shape of the pelvic inlet: gynecoid (normal female), android (normal male), anthropoid (long anterior-posterior diameter), and platypelloid (wide transverse diameter) (Fig. 2–5). In each one of the three pelvic planes (inlet, midpelvis, and outlet), each pelvic type has

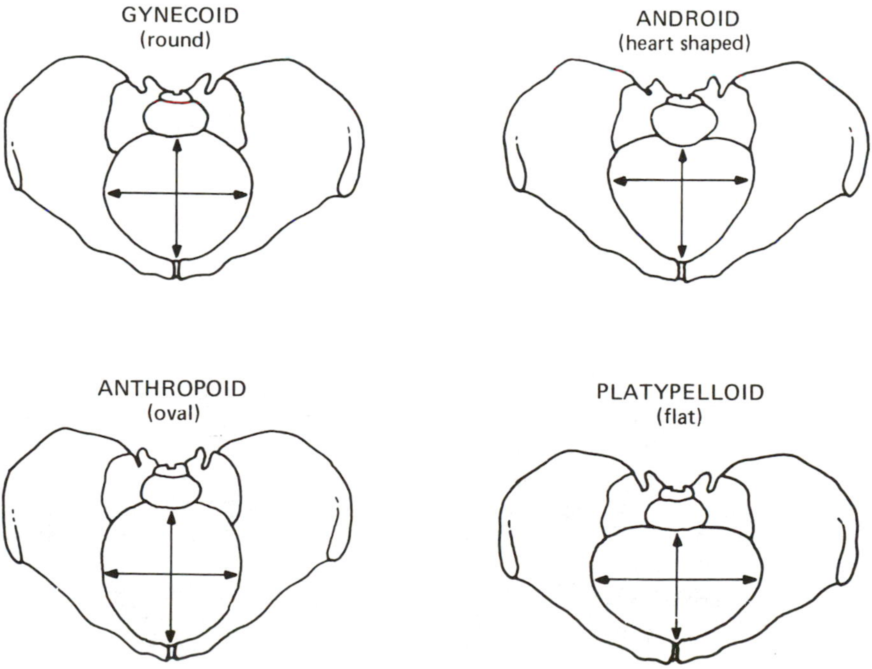

Figure 2–5. Pelvic types; shapes of pelvic inlets.

certain features that are characteristic of that type. Many women have a mixture of these features and therefore have a "mixed" type of pelvis.

The true (consistently) *gynecoid* pelvis is the most desirable pelvic type for childbirth. As the fetus passes through the pelvis, it undergoes the eight mechanisms of labor, that is, engagement, descent, flexion, internal rotation, extension, restitution, external rotation, and expulsion (see Fig. 1–3). In the following sections, which deal with fetal movement through the various pelvic planes, each mechanism has been capitalized to attract the attention of the reader.

• •

Review Questions

1. The normal female type pelvis is called ______________.
2. The three planes of the pelvis are: (a) ______________, (b) ______________, and (c) ______________.
3. Referring to Chapter 1 as necessary, the eight mechanisms of labor are: (a) ______________, (b) ______________, (c) ______________, (d) ______________ ______________, (e) ______________, (f) ______________, (g) ______________ ______________, (h) ______________.

Answers

1. The normal female type pelvis is called *gynecoid.*
2. The three planes of the pelvis are: (a) *inlet,* (b) *midpelvis,* and (c) *outlet.*
3. The mechanisms of labor in proper sequence are: (a) *engagement,* (b) *descent,* (c) *flexion,* (d) *internal rotation,* (e) *extension,* (f) *restitution,* (g) *external rotation,* and (h) *expulsion.*

• •

The Pelvic Inlet

The mechanisms of labor begin in the pelvic inlet. Depending on which source is used, the first mechanism of labor is engagement or descent. Pritchard[1] says engagement is first. Oxorn[2] says descent, which includes engagement, is the first mechanism. For simplicity, the mechanisms are explained as if they occur separately and independently. Actually all mechanisms require that descent occurs simultaneously.

The pelvic inlet, or brim, is bordered by the symphysis pubis in front, the iliopectineal lines on the innominate bones on the sides, and the sacral promontory in the back (Fig. 2–6). As the greatest transverse diameter (occipitofrontal) of the head passes through the pelvic inlet, engagement occurs followed by descent.

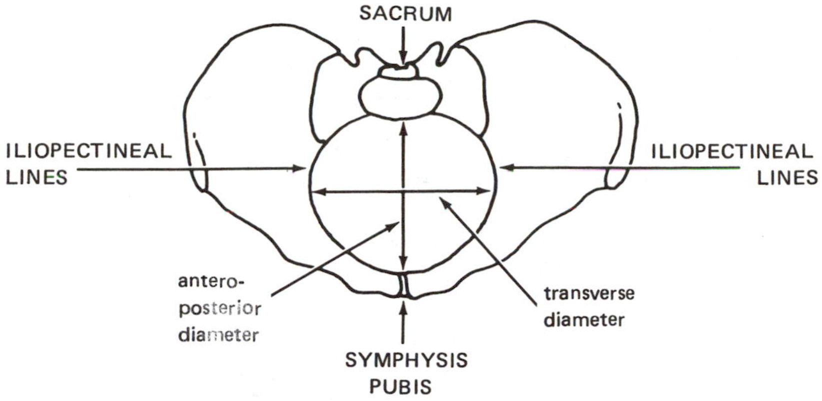

Figure 2–6. Inlet of gynecoid pelvis.

The pelvic diameter from front to back (anterior-posterior [AP]) can be measured by the examiner. One or two gloved fingers are inserted into the vagina and extended from below the symphysis pubis to the middle of the sacral promontory, which is a distinct projection on the upper portion of the sacrum. Upon palpating the sacral promontory, the examiner's free hand can indicate where the symphysis pubis rests on the gloved hand. The length from this point to the fingertip that touched the promontory is measured. This distance from the prominence to the outside lower margin of the pubis is the *diagonal conjugate* (DC) and is normally 12.5 cm. In instances when the sacral promontory cannot be reached, the conclusion may be greater than (>) 11 cm if the examiner knows the fingers can reach 11 cm or NR for "not reached."

The actual AP diameter that the fetus moves through is the inside measurement, the *obstetric conjugate* (OC), which is the distance from the posterior superior aspect of the symphysis pubis to the sacral promontory (Fig. 2–7). This diameter cannot be measured manually but is estimated by subtracting 1.5 cm from the DC. Therefore, if the DC is 12.5 cm, the OC is 11.0 cm ($12.5 - 1.5 = 11.0$). The actual space available to the fetus in the AP diameter of the inlet (the OC) normally is 10 cm or greater. Less than 10 cm is classified as a contracted pelvic inlet.[3]

It is not possible to measure the transverse diameter of the inlet of the pelvis without using x-ray pelvimetry. Since a gynecoid pelvis has a round or slightly transverse oval inlet, and a circle (round) has consistently equal diameters, it can be assumed that if the AP diameter is 11 cm, the transverse diameter is also 11 cm; if the inlet is slightly oval, the transverse diameter is slightly longer.

The fetal head normally descends into the pelvic inlet in a transverse position (OT) or, less frequently, an oblique position—halfway between transverse and anterior or posterior. When the position of the head is OT, the sagittal suture, which connects the anterior and posterior fontanels, is in the transverse diameter of the pelvis. The nonflexed head presents its occipitofrontal diameter,

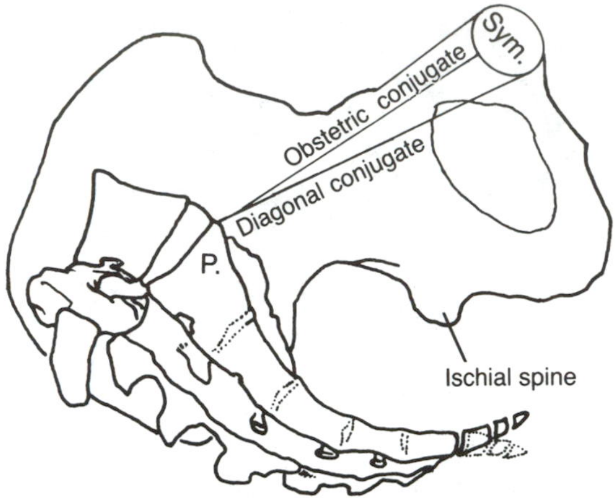

Figure 2–7. Anteroposterior diameters of the pelvic inlet: the obstetrically important obstetric conjugate, and the clinically measurable diagonal conjugate. (P. = sacral promontory; Sym. = symphysis pubis.

which is 11 cm. If the pelvic OC is also 11 cm, some molding of the fetal head will undoubtedly occur.

• •

Review Questions

Fill in the blanks or circle the correct response:

1. The boundaries of the pelvic inlet are: ______________, ______________, and ______________.
2. The (anteroposterior or transverse) diameter of the pelvic inlet is measurable manually. This diameter is called ______________. Its length normally is ______________ cm and is measured from ______________ ______________ to ______________.
3. The mechanisms of labor that occur/begin in the inlet are ______________ and ______________.
4. The position of the head as it enters the inlet is (anteroposterior or transverse).
5. The diameter of the head that presents in the inlet is ______________, which measures ______________ cm.
6. What assumption can you make about the diameter of the head if it is to descend through the inlet of a gynecoid pelvis?
____
____
____

Answers

1. The boundaries of the pelvic inlet are the *symphysis pubis*, the *iliopectineal lines*, and the *sacral promontory*.
2. The manually measurable *anteroposterior* diameter of the inlet is called the *diagonal conjugate* and normally measures 12.5 cm from the *subpubic arch* to the *middle of the sacral promontory*.
3. *Engagement* occurs in the inlet and *descent* begins.
4. The head normally enters the inlet in a *transverse* or *oblique* position.
5. The *occipitofrontal* diameter presents in the inlet and measures *11* cm.
6. The occipitofrontal diameter must be slightly smaller than the pelvic inlet (usually transverse) diameter if the head is to move through this plane.

The Midpelvis

The midpelvis (or midplane) boundaries include the lower margin of the symphysis pubis in front, the ischial spines on the sides, and the sacrum (S3–S4) in back (Fig. 2–8). The head must bypass these boundaries to successfully negotiate the midpelvis. There should be as few protrusions into the pelvis as possible to provide sufficient room for fetal descent. Therefore, upon palpation, the *sacrum* should be *curved* (outward—concave, hollow, deep) instead

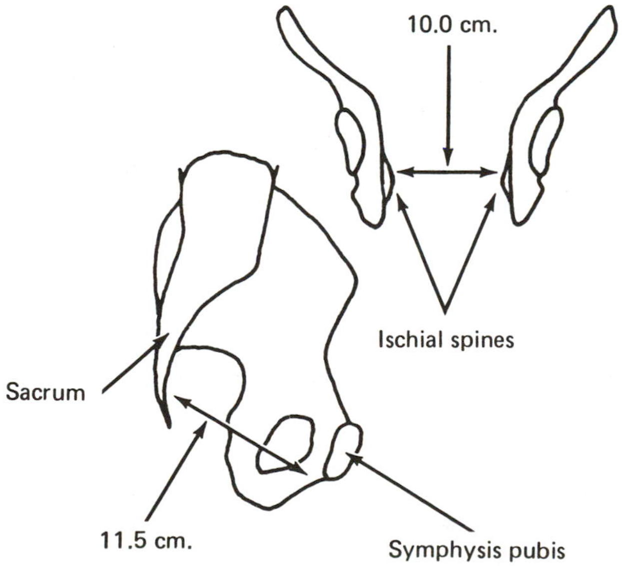

Figure 2–8. Midpelvis of gynecoid pelvis.

of flat, convex, or inwardly inclined. The *ischial spines* should be *nonprominent* or *blunt,* and the side walls parallel or nonconvergent.

Actual measurements of the midpelvis are not taken except by x-ray pelvimetry, although an experienced clinician can make an educated estimate about the diameters. A normal AP diameter is 11.5 to 12.0 cm, and a normal transverse (between the ischial spines) diameter is 10.0 to 10.5 cm. Since the transverse diameter of the midplane in its lower portion is somewhat smaller than the transverse diameter of the inlet, the fetal neck experiences FLEXION, causing the smaller (9.5 cm) suboccipitobregmatic diameter to present. Further flexion may occur when the presenting head reaches the muscles of the pelvic floor.

INTERNAL ROTATION of the head (from transverse to anterior position—OT to OA) occurs near or when the head reaches the muscles and fascia of the pelvic floor in the midpelvis. This usually takes place during Stage II.

• •

Review Questions

1. The three bones that border the midpelvic plane are: (a) ________, (b) ________________, and (c) ________________.
2. Indicate the ideal characteristics about the following bony parts that can be determined by palpation:
   sacrum: ________________
   ischial spines: ________________
   side walls: ________________
3. Circle the correct responses: The transverse diameter of the midpelvis is (smaller than, the same as, larger than) the transverse diameter of the inlet. Therefore, the (occipitofrontal, suboccipitobregmatic) diameter of the fetal head presents in this plane. In order for this to occur (descent, flexion, internal rotation) must take place. Since the AP diameter is larger than the transverse, the head internally rotates from ________________ to ________________.

Answers

1. The bones that border the midpelvis are: (a) the *lower margin of the symphysis pubis*; (b) the *ischial spines*; and (c) the *sacrum.*
2. The sacrum should be *curved*; the spines, *nonprominent*; the side walls, *nonconvergent.*
3. The transverse diameter of the midpelvis is *smaller than* that of the inlet. Therefore, the *suboccipitobregmatic* diameter presents as a result of *flexion.* Since the AP diameter is larger, the head rotates from *OT* to *OA.*

• •

The reader should remember to go back to the Pelvic Measurements Chart. Using the ideal normal findings, the *spines are nonprominent* and the *sacrum is curved.* Did you remember to fill in the normal pelvic type (gynecoid) and the normal DC (11.5 cm or greater)?

The Pelvic Outlet

The outlet is the last pelvic plane the fetal head must pass through. It is bordered in front by the pubic arch, on the sides by the bi-ischial tuberosities, and in the back by the tip of the sacrum (coccyx or tailbone). The transverse diameter is manually measurable between the *bi-ischial tuberosities* (bitubs). It usually measures about 11 cm. The anteroposterior diameter is determined by the *subpubic arch* (the angle under the symphysis pubis) and the coccyx. The diameter is adequate if a *90-degree angle* (Fig. 2–9) and a *movable coccyx* exist.

By the time the head passes through the outlet, it normally is flexed (a diameter of 9.5 cm) and rotated so the occiput (OA) lies beneath the symphysis pubis, and the sagittal suture (the suture line between the anterior and posterior fontanels) is in the anteroposterior diameter of the outlet. As the base of the occiput comes into direct contact with the inferior margin of the symphysis pubis, the occiput moves away from the sacrum. The resultant mechanism is EXTENSION, and the head (caput) appears at and moves through the vaginal opening. The brow and face advance rapidly and appear in succession over the anterior margin of the perineum (posterior wall of the vagina extending to the rectum).

The head then falls back toward the anus. Once the head is out of the vagina, the neck spontaneously untwists, turning the head in the direction it came from. This is called RESTITUTION. If the head originally was turned to the left, it now rotates toward the left ischial tuberosity. (Restitution is sometimes omitted as a separate mechanism of labor and is considered to be a part of external rotation.) Next the head is assisted to EXTERNALLY ROTATE completely to a transverse position as the shoulders rotate (anteroposterior) internally by essentially the same process that rotated the head internally. This orients the remainder of the body for the birth process. The anterior shoulder emerges under the pubic arch, followed by the

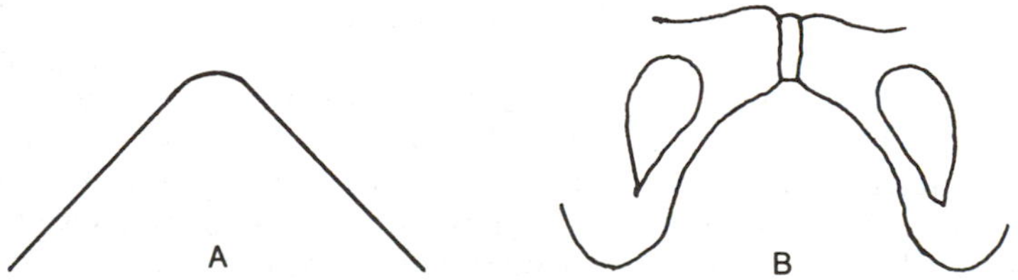

Figure 2–9. A 90-degree angle. (*A*) Geometric shape. (*B*) Anterior angle of pelvic outlet.

posterior shoulder. The remainder of the body, which is smaller in diameter, then delivers spontaneously. This EXPULSION is the last mechanism of labor.

• •

Review Questions

1. Engagement, descent, flexion, and internal rotation have already occurred. What remaining mechanisms occur in or near the outlet?

   (a) ______________ (c) ______________
   (b) ______________ (d) ______________

2. The pelvic measurements of concern in the outlet are associated with the following; give their ideal characteristics:
   a. bi-ischial tuberosities = _____ cm
   b. subpubic arch = _____ degrees
   c. coccyx = ______________.

Answers

1. The mechanisms that occur in or near the outlet are: (a) *extension*, (b) *restitution*, (c) *external rotation*, and (d) *expulsion*.
2. Ideally, a. the bi-ischial tuberosities are *11* cm, b. the subpubic arch is *90* degrees, and c. the coccyx is *movable*.

• •

Now you are ready to fill in the remaining blanks of the Pelvic Measurements Chart. Your last answer (2, above) provides you with the correct information.

MODIFIED MECHANISMS

Occipital Posterior Position

The mechanisms of labor are modified somewhat for the fetus who is occiput posterior (OP); that is, the occiput is directed toward the posterior segment of the pelvis. Rather than *engaging* in the inlet and beginning *descent* in the normal OT position, the fetus is OP. The usual explanation of why a fetus assumes an OP position is the existence of an abnormal configuration in the pelvis, as in the android and anthropoid pelvises. These pelvises have a narrow anterior segment so the occiput tends to move to the posterior segment.

As the fetus descends further in the pelvis, only partial *flexion* of the OP head usually occurs in the midplane. More flexion occurs when the head meets resistance from the pelvic floor in the outlet. Assuming that few fetuses are directly OP but more likely left or right OP (LOP or ROP), the fetal head can *internally rotate* one of two ways: the long arc of approximately 135 degrees to directly OA or the short arc of approximately 45 degrees to directly OP. For the fetus who rotates to OA, the mechanisms thereafter are the same as previously presented for the normal mechanisms (extension, external rotation, and expulsion).

The fetus who rotates directly OP is said to be *persistent occipitoposterior* (POP). In this case, the anterior fontanel (bregma) descends behind the pubic bone. In order to maneuver the subpubic arch, the head needs to flex further. The degree of flexion determines whether the presenting suboccipitofrontal diameter is 10.5 or 11.5 cm. This is 1 to 2 cm larger than that in the OA position. Upon delivery of the top and back of the head, the occiput *extends* or falls back toward the anus. Then the nose, mouth, and chin are born. *Restitution, external rotation* and *expulsion* then occur in their usual ways. In the presence of abnormal progress in labor, forceps assisted or cesarean delivery may be warranted.

Several problems for the mother and fetus are inherent in the OP position. Among them are the following:

1. **Anxiety [specify] related to more painful and longer than usual labor.**
2. **Comfort, alteration in: pain, acute related to descent of OP fetal head down maternal back bones and extended period of uterine contractions.**
3. **Injury, potential for; trauma (to the maternal birth canal [perineum, urethra and anus]) related to abnormal OP fetal position, larger than usual fetal diameters presenting, and possible use of forceps to assist in the delivery.**
4. **Injury, potential for; trauma (to the fetus) related to longer than usual labor, precipitating fetal distress and difficult delivery.**

Additional nursing concerns and interventions dealing with fetal descent and prolonged labor are discussed later in this chapter and in Chapter 4.

• •

Review Questions

Fill in the blanks for questions 1, 2, and 3:
When the fetal position is persistent occiput posterior:

1. The fetus enters the pelvis in ______________ position due to ______________.

2. Flexion is only ______________ in the midpelvis but more extensive in the ______________________________.

3. Internal rotation involves approximately ______________ degrees to ______________ occiput posterior.

Put words in the parentheses in the proper sequence for question 4:

4. **During extension (the mouth, the chin, and the nose) become visible.**
5. **Explain why a woman experiencing POP is likely to experience a longer and more painful labor:** ______________________________
____
____
____

Answers

1. The fetus enters the pelvis in *occiput posterior (OP)* position because of *the narrow anterior pelvic segment.*
2. Flexion is only *slight or partial* in the midpelvis but more extensive in the *outlet.*
3. The internal rotation involves approximately *45* degrees to *directly* occiput posterior.
4. During extension the *nose, mouth and chin (in that sequence)* are born and become visible.
5. A longer than usual labor is likely when POP is due to a larger than 9.5 cm suboccipitofrontal diameter descending the posterior segment of the pelvis. This usually prolongs the labor, increases the mother's anxiety, and causes pain as the fetal head moves down her "back" bones.

• •

Breech Presentation

With a breech presentation, the fetus goes through somewhat modified mechanisms of labor three times. Each time the succeeding presenting parts are progressively larger. The buttocks and lower limbs come first. The buttocks (or breech) is a poor cervical dilator. Thus, labor progress is often slow. (Labor progression curves are discussed in Chapter 4.) Often descent does not occur until complete cervical dilatation and rupture of membranes.[4] After descent of the buttocks and lower limbs, the shoulders and arms descend, followed by the head.

During the first series of mechanisms of labor, *engagement* occurs when the trochanters of the femurs have passed through the pelvic inlet. Lateral (sideways) *flexion* then occurs at the waist. The anterior hip leads the way. Upon reaching the pelvic floor, the anterior hip meets resistance and *internally rotates* toward the anterior pelvic segment, directing the sacrum transversely in the pelvis. The posterior buttocks are then in position to be born and as they fall (*extends*) toward the anus, the anterior hip slips out under the symphysis, completing the *expulsion* of the buttocks and legs.

The shoulders and arms are then ready to *engage* in the pelvic inlet and *internally rotate* 45 degrees from transverse to anterio-posterior. The sacrum, now outside of the mother's body, *externally rotates* from anterior to transverse. Then lateral *flexion* occurs in the shoulders. When the anterior shoulder is under the symphysis, the posterior shoulder is born as the baby's body is flexed upward. Then the body is lowered and the anterior shoulder and arms are born (*expelled*).

Finally, the head undergoes the mechanisms of labor. When the shoulders are at the outlet, the head *engages* in the pelvic inlet usually with the occiput in the normally large anterior pelvic segment. *Flexion* occurs. At the pelvic floor, the head *internally rotates* placing the occiput under the symphysis, and the sacrum (outside of the mother) anterior. The nape of the neck moves under the symphysis and then the head *flexes,* presenting the face—chin first, forehead last—as the birth (*expulsion*) is completed.

Some variations of the above occur if the presentation is a footling or kneeling breech. It should be apparent that inherent in the breech presentation is the risk of **injury, potential for; trauma (to the fetus [intracranial hemorrhage, central nervous system damage, fractures, anoxia from compression of umbilical cord]) related to the numerous manipulations and the progressive size of the fetal diameters.** Likewise, there is **injury, potential for; trauma (to the mother [genital tract lacerations, hemorrhage]) related to the vaginal delivery of a breech presentation.**

• •

Review Questions

1. Identify the correct order of the anatomic fetal parts that undergo the mechanisms of labor in a breech presentation:
   (a) ______________________, (b) ______________________
   ______________________, and (c) ______________________.

2. Explain why there is concern about the pelvic size even though the first set of mechanisms can be successfully completed:______________
   ____

3. For both the mother and the fetus, list two types of trauma likely during vaginal delivery of a breech presentation:
   Mother: (a) ______________________, (b) ______________________.
   Fetus: (a) ______________________, (b) ______________________.

Answers

1. The fetal parts progress through the birth canal in the following order: (a) *the buttocks and lower limbs,* (b) *the shoulders and arms,* and (c) *the head.*

2. Each succeeding presenting part/s is/are larger, and, therefore, the last part, the head, may be too large to be vaginally delivered.

3. Maternal trauma during vaginal delivery of a breech presentation can involve *genital tract lacerations* and *hemorrhage.* Fetal trauma can involve *intracranial*

hemorrhage, central nervous system damage, fractures, and anoxia from umbilical cord compression.

• •

CONVERSION TO CEPHALIC PRESENTATION

The normal mechanisms of labor as described involve a head first, or cephalic, presentation. Vaginal delivery is feasible, although the mechanisms are more complex, as already mentioned, when the breech is presenting. Because mortality and morbidity are greater with vaginal breech deliveries, cesareans are often preferred. Although still controversial, numerous studies[5–13] document the successful use of external cephalic version (ECV) to rotate breech or shoulder to cephalic presentation, thereby avoiding cesarean delivery. Although ECV is often done during the prenatal period, it may be done during early labor. In order to consider ECV, certain conditions are desirable, such as a low-risk pregnancy, near-term gestation, and intact membranes. Before, during, and after the ECV procedure performed by the physician, real time ultrasound scanning and electronic fetal monitoring are done. Usually uterine stimulation is inhibited by a tocolytic agent.[14] Intravenous terbutaline is used most frequently, although subcutaneous administration is also reported. Nurses are responsible for knowing the institution's protocol and assuring that it is carried out.

Except for some certified nurse-midwives, nurses do not do ECV but may recommend an antepartal exercise that can convert the breech presentation to vertex. Beginning around 32 weeks' gestation, women with a breech presentation can be taught to lie down with one hip tilted up and the buttocks slightly elevated for 10 to 15 minutes twice a day. This position may encourage the fetus to spontaneously rotate its buttocks into the fundus, placing the head in the pelvis. Figure 2–10 illustrates a slightly different position that DeSa Souza, the originator, recommended. Through either EVC or this exercise, the fetal head may assume a position that is then compatible with the normal mechanisms of labor.

• •

Review Question

Attempts to alter fetal presentation from breech to cephalic can include:

a.____________________

b.____________________

Answer

Alteration of fetal presentation from breech to cephalic can be done by:

a. external cephalic version usually performed by a physician

b. an antepartal positional exercise done at home by the pregnant woman

• •

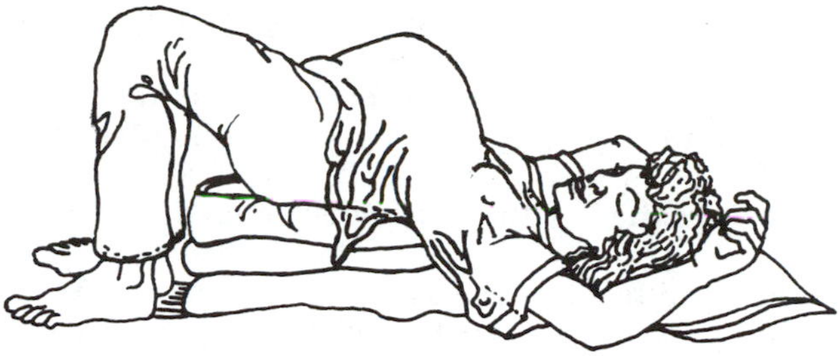

Figure 2–10. Postural exercise to convert breech presentation to vertex.

NURSING IMPLICATIONS RELATED TO THE MECHANISMS OF LABOR

Using Predictive Assessment Data

Despite the lack of recognition in medical literature, nurses can influence the normal progression of the mechanisms of labor. Through the process of assessment, the nurse has access to data that are predictive of whether the normal mechanisms of labor are likely to occur or already are occurring. The following areas of assessment provide the needed data:

Obstetric History. The woman's obstetric history is one source of data. The chart may not contain the desired information, and unless the nurse asks the right questions, she might not get the necessary information. Consideration should be given to the size of her previous babies, the duration of those labors, and the occurrence of injury to the woman or babies during previous births. Since fetal weight and size usually have a direct relationship, a woman who has safely delivered an 8½ pound baby is not expected to have a difficult delivery in the future, unless the estimated fetal weight (EFW) is much larger. Conversely, the woman whose largest baby had a birth weight of 5 pounds, even though the labor was a short five hours, may have difficulty with an EFW of 7 pounds.

Pelvic Measurements. The pelvic measurements recorded on the woman's chart are a source of information about possible pelvic contractures. Likewise, radiologic and ultrasonic techniques are used with varying degrees of success. Once the fetus passes a plane where difficulty was expected, the characteristics of the next plane need to be considered.

If the DC of the pelvic inlet is less than 12.5 cm, the fetus may continue to "float" above the pelvic inlet. A contracted pelvic inlet often results in abnormal presentation. Face and shoulder presentations occur three times more frequently, while prolapse of the cord and of the extremities occurs four to six times more frequently.[15] If the fetal head cannot enter the inlet, labor is likely to be prolonged and ineffective. The alert nurse recognizes that if engagement does not occur at the usual time (see Chapter 4), the DC on the chart should be noted, and this legitimate concern about lack of progress reported to the responsible physician.

In the midpelvis, if the spines are prominent or the sacrum flat or inwardly inclined, the fetus may have difficulty moving beyond zero station, that is, below the ischial spines. Contraction of the midpelvis is a frequent cause of transverse (OT) arrest of the fetal head.

If the pubic arch is less than 90 degrees, the coccyx nonmovable, or the bituberosities less than 11 cm, the outlet may be difficult for the normal size fetus to maneuver. In such a case, at the time of delivery, perineal tears are likely. An extensive episiotomy is usually indicated even if the laboring woman requests otherwise. A midline episiotomy may be adequate, although because of the potential for third- or fourth-degree lacerations, a mediolateral episiotomy may be done. Nurses need to explain the medical necessity of episiotomy when it is done and to realize that forceps are inappropriate "aids" in this case because they require even more space in an already tight outlet.

Vaginal Examination. Vaginal examinations provide further data about the fetal movement within the pelvis. In the presence of good uterine contractions, there should be progressive cervical dilatation and fetal descent consistent with the norms established in the Friedman curves (see Chapter 4). Cervical effacement should occur without cervical edema, which is often due to pushing prior to complete dilatation. Molding of the fetal head is a normal finding. Caput succedaneum, the development of edema on the scalp, is a frequently seen deviation from normal. The fetal position is also noted. Ideally, it moves from OT to OA. The presence of asynclitism may indicate a small pelvis or a large head. *Asynclitism* occurs when the biparietal diameter is tilted rather than parallel to the pelvic planes. The tilt should be spontaneously corrected if the normal internal rotation to OA position is to occur. Any discrepancies from the norms should be communicated in the chart and reported to the physician.

Client Symptoms. Another source of data is the woman's expression of pain and tension. Both the nurse and the woman's designated support person should respond to these. Severe pain in the back is consistent with a fetal position of persistent occiput posterior (POP), which was discussed earlier in this chapter. Some back relief may be obtained by assuming a position other than supine—lateral, sitting, or knee-chest. Applying constant or intermittent sacral pressure may provide comfort. Heat (a moist towel) or cold (an ice pack) may also be beneficial when applied to the site of discomfort. A woman who is tense tightens her muscles, including those that line and support the pelvis. This causes resistance to fetal movement in a downward direction. Signs of emotional tension are uneven voice patterns, appearance of tears, inability to concentrate, or timid, fearful behavior. The nurse should try to coach the woman in relaxation techniques such as those used in Lamaze (see Chapter 7) before resorting to medications.

• •

Review Questions

1. Why is it significant for the nurse to note the size and outcome of a woman's previous deliveries? ____

2. Circle the abnormal findings determined during a vaginal exam.
   a. cervix dilating
   b. cervix effacing
   c. cervical edema
   d. fetal head molding
   e. fetal scalp edema
   f. fetal position of POP

3. What measures can be taken to relieve back discomfort?
   a. ________________________________
   b. ________________________________
   c. ________________________________

Answers

1. A woman who has delivered a baby of the same or smaller birth weight without adverse effects is expected to do the same this time.
2. During a vaginal exam it is abnormal to find: (c) cervical edema, (e) fetal scalp edema, and (f) fetal position of POP.
3. To relieve back discomfort: (a) change to positions other than supine; (b) apply sacral pressure; and (c) apply heat and/or cold to the site of discomfort.

• •

Nursing Interventions That Promote Descent

Nurses should consider several physical principles when attempting to promote fetal descent: (1) proper body alignment facilitates normal functioning; (2) empty space will be filled; (3) gravity moves things downward; and (4) decreased resistance promotes progress. An illustration of each principle in regard to labor follows.

(1) The fetus must be in a longitudinal attitude (up and down, or vertical axis) in order to be expelled through the pelvic outlet. This has implications for maternal, as well as fetal, alignment. Pushing is more effective if the woman's shoulders are in line with her pelvis, rather than if she is tilted to one side. Therefore, the nurse needs to ensure good maternal alignment, especially when the mother is supine and attempting to push. For the woman who has experienced many childbirths and/or excessive weight gain, the abdomen may be pendulous. If the abdominal muscles fail to align the fetus in the birth canal, the fetal head cannot press against the cervix. As a result the head is useless as a dilating wedge and the effectiveness of the uterine contractions is lost. Alignment of the long axis of the fetus with the long axis of the mother will alter this phenomenon, as well as promote descent. An old, but useful method from the past is to apply a many-tailed Scultetus binder (Fig. 2–11) and leave it in

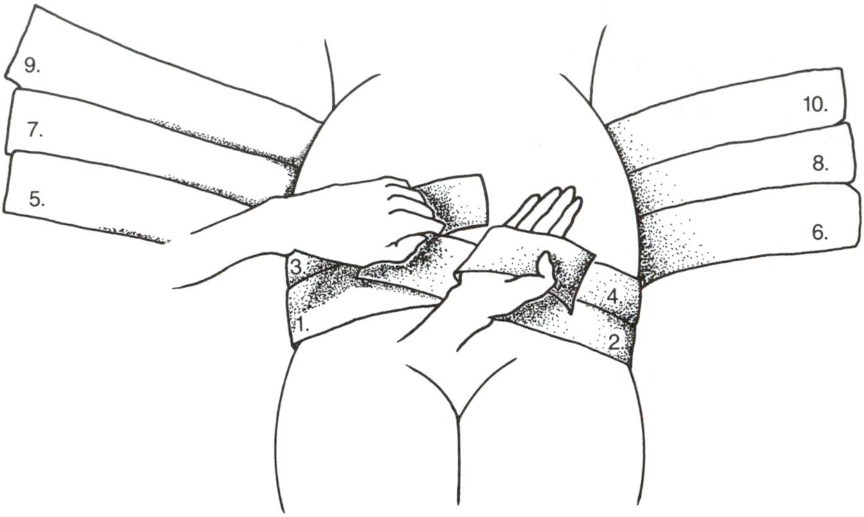

Figure 2–11. Application of the scultetus binder. (Courtesy of Gay P. Hall, LtC, USAF NC, CNM.)

place until delivery. The binder serves to realign the fetus from oblique to longitudinal lie and acts as a mechanism for repositioning the uterus into the pelvic girdle.[16]

(2) The nurse can promote empty space by encouraging emptying of the bowel and bladder. When filled, these organs take up considerable space in the pelvis. The bowel can be emptied with an enema if necessary. This might also stimulate labor (see Chapter 5). During labor, the bladder should be emptied every 2 to 3 hours. If the bladder is palpable and the woman is unable to empty it on her own, catheterization is necessary.

(3) In the past few years, there has been increased acceptance of the effect of gravity on fetal descent—namely, the use of standing and sitting postures in labor. These upright positions also bring the fetus forward so that the presenting fetal part is better aligned with the pelvic inlet and, therefore, able to move more easily into the pelvis. Standing can be done in a number of ways: leaning against a wall, holding onto a side rail, or walking. One can stand or sit in a shower. Sitting can be done (a) in bed with pillows and the head of the bed supporting the back, or leaning forward supported by a padded bedside stand; (b) in a comfortable chair, preferably a rocking chair; or (c) on a bed pan, toilet, shower stool, or in a jacuzzi. Sitting in water (a tub or jacuzzi) may be contraindicated when membranes are ruptured. None of these positions should be assumed for a long period of time because they become tiring.

Squatting, an infrequently used position in some geographic areas, utilizes the principle of gravity. An upright position is assumed with thighs flexed and abducted, and as flat footed as possible. Figure 2–12 depicts this position using a "labor" or "squat bar" on a delivery table. The squatting position facilitates descent and birth of the fetus because it enlarges the pelvic outlet an average of 28 percent over its dimensions in the supine position.[17] Furthermore, while squatting the urge to push is usually efficient because the abdominal wall relaxes and the pelvis tilts forward. The longitudinal axis of the birth canal is thereby straightened and fetal descent facilitated. Squatting is also effective in promoting spontaneous rotation of the fetal head.[18,19]

In a study done by nurse-midwives Rossi and Lindell[20] in which women could assume the position of their choice during Stage II, women favored reclining, side-lying, and lateral reclining. The choice of position was thought to be due to cultural conditioning and the physical presence of a bed in the birthing room. In non-Western cultures women preferred upright positions, for example, standing or squatting for birth. The implication for nurses is that women in Western cultures are unlikely to spontaneously assume the squatting position unless they are encouraged to use this alternative position.

(4) The final physical principle—decreased resistance promotes progress—suggests another alternative to the traditional delivery position. Instead of lithotomy with the legs up in stirrups, Lehrman[21]

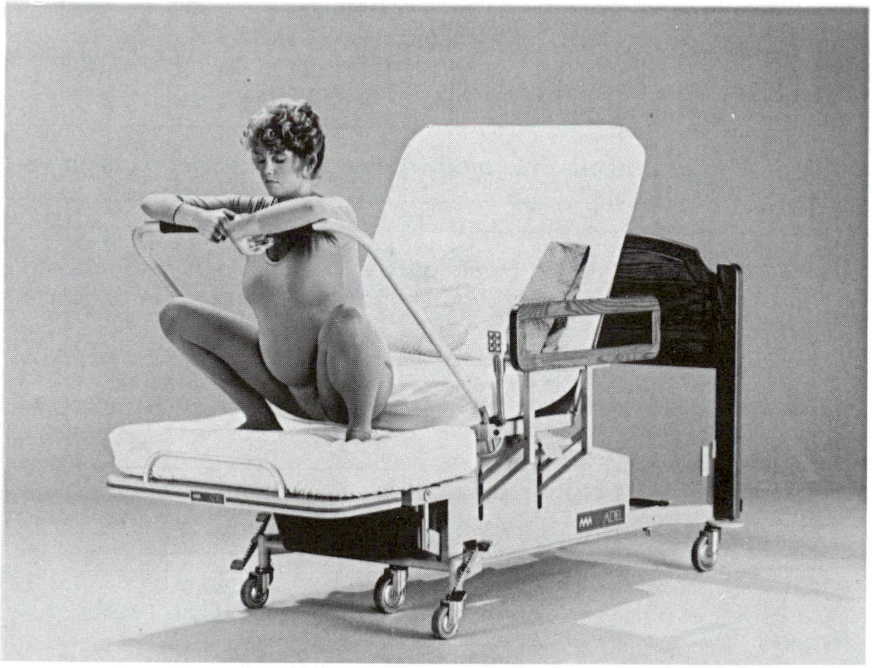

Figure 2–12. Labor Bar. (Photo courtesy of Adel Medical Ltd., Clackamas, Oregon.)

recommends the left lateral position. Due to the decreased resistance of the perineal muscles in that position, descent of the fetus may be facilitated. Furthermore, the lateral position requires no special equipment on the delivery table or bed.

In conclusion, there is one other consideration that nurses should make when promoting fetal descent. Until the fetal head reaches a certain point spontaneously, pushing is unlikely to be effective. Roberts [22,23] suggests that laboring women who do not have the urge to push, even when completely dilated, *not* be encouraged to bear down until the fetal head is 0 to +1 station. The reason is that the fetal head may not be in a position compatible with assisted descent (bearing down) until it spontaneously descends further in the pelvis. Roberts further says that when a woman has an irresistible urge to push—although *only* 8 to 9 cm dilated with a soft cervix, 0 to +1 station and OT to OA position—the woman should be permitted to bear down. Roberts found that cervical lacerations are not likely to result from pushing with the urge to do so. She does caution that, regardless of station, bearing down should not occur if the cervix is dilated only 6 to 7 cm. Although Roberts' viewpoints are not widely accepted, they do logically imply that a station at or below 0 is likely to be consistent with effective bearing down attempts.

• •

Review Questions

1. What is the rationale for aligning the fetus longitudinally with the laboring woman's body? ______________________________

____

2. How is fetal descent promoted by having a laboring woman void every 2 to 3 hours? ______________________________

____

3. If a woman is tired of being on her feet, identify two alternate positions that nurses could suggest that might promote fetal descent.
   a. ______________________________
   b. ______________________________

4. Besides taking advantage of the force of gravity, squatting promotes descent by:
   a. ______________________________
   b. ______________________________

5. Delivery in the left lateral position exemplifies the principle of ______________________________

Answers

1. The fetus needs to be aligned in an up and down position so that descent will be promoted.

2. Frequent voiding provides space that is otherwise occupied by a filling bladder.
3. In addition to standing, a nurse could suggest sitting (a) in a shower or jacuzzi, (b) in a bed leaning backward supported with pillows, (c) in bed leaning forward, (d) in a chair, or (e) on a bedpan or toilet, to promote fetal descent.
4. Squatting promotes descent by: (a) enlarging the pelvic outlet, (b) relaxing the abdominal wall, and (c) tilting the pelvis forward.
5. Delivery in the left lateral position is an example of the principle of decreased resistance promotes progress.

• •

Nursing Interventions That Provide Changes in Fetal Position

For many years nurses have recognized the benefits of altering a woman's position during labor. The patient is more comfortable, and position changes often spontaneously rotate the fetus to a more desirable position.

There are sound reasons why a fetus rotates when the mother assumes certain postures. Except for the head, the back is the heaviest, densest part of the fetal body. Given time, the fetal back will rotate to the lower side of the maternal abdomen placing the lighter more buoyant small parts of the fetus on the upper side. A woman who lies on her back is likely to cause the fetus to assume a posterior (OP) position. By assuming a Sims' or knee-chest position, the mother facilitates fetal rotation to OA. (Sims' position is semiprone on one side [e.g., left] with the [left] arm behind the back, and the chest inclined forward, the legs flexed with the upper [right] knee closest to the chest.) This position also promotes less pain associated with uterine contractions and greater efficiency from the contractions.

Andrews,[24] a nurse-midwife, recommends additional nursing measures to rotate a fetus to OA. The mother can be placed in a hands-and-knees posture with hands fisted to prevent wrist fatigue and perform a pelvic rock 10 times slowly and rhythmically. With lower back arched towards the ceiling, the mother or coach can gently but deeply stroke 10 times from back to front on the side of the fetal back (which is the same as the occiput), continuing as far as possible to the other side. This combination of pelvic rocking and stroking is continued for 10 minutes at a time. Rest periods are taken with the mother lying in Sims' position and then the above exercises are repeated. For the fetus who is ROT, the mother rests in Sims' position on her left side to encourage the fetus to rotate 90 degrees forward to OA. For the fetus who is ROP, she rests in Sims' position on her right side to encourage the fetus to rotate less than 180 degrees to OA.

- If ROP or ROT, stroke from right to left.

- If OP, stroke right to left.
- If LOP or LOT, stroke from left to right.

The directions in which the strokes are made are dependent on the fetus's original position.

If rotation is necessary, Andrews recommends that it should be attempted early in labor to promote comfort. In some instances, for example, if the inlet has a contracted anterior segment, rotation from OP should be attempted until the head has passed the inlet. In other pelvises, a position other than OA may be advantageous for fetal movement through the pelvis, for example, OP in anthropoid and OT in platypelloid.

• •

Review Question

Explain three ways to promote changes in fetal position:

a. ______________________________

____

b. ______________________________

____

c. ______________________________

____

Answer

To promote changes in fetal position, do the following:

a. Have the mother lie on the side to which the heavy back (occiput) ideally would turn; for example, for OA have her be as near prone as possible (via Sims' or knee-chest position).

b. Have her pelvic rock while on hands and knees.

c. Have mother (or someone else) stroke the fetal back in the direction in which the fetus should turn.

• •

CONCLUSION

Most readers benefit from seeing a fetus go through the mechanisms of labor. If the reader has access to models of a fetal head and pelvis, it is recommended that they be used to demonstrate the motions that have been described in this chapter. The real test of understanding of the mechanisms of labor will come in application of this knowledge—whether it be during the care of a woman in labor or in explaining the mechanisms to another person.

REFERENCES

1. Pritchard, JA, MacDonald, PC, and Gant, NF: Williams Obstetrics, ed. 17. Appleton-Century-Crofts, Norwalk, Connecticut, 1985, p 323.

2. Oxorn, H: Oxorn-Foote: Human Labor and Birth, ed 5. Appleton-Century-Crofts, Norwalk, Connecticut, 1986, p 94.
3. Pritchard, JA, MacDonald, PC, and Gant, NF: Williams Obstetrics, ed 17. Appleton-Century-Crofts, Norwalk, Connecticut, 1985, p 677.
4. Oxorn, H: Oxorn-Foote: Human Labor and Birth, ed 5. Appleton-Century-Crofts, Norwalk, Connecticut, 1986, p 228.
5. Dyson, DC, Ferguson, JE 2II, and Hensleigh, P: Anterpartum external cephalic version under tocolysis. Obstet Gynecol 67:63, 1986.
6. Ferguson, JE 2d and Dyson, DC: Intrapartum external cephalic version. Am J Obstet Gynecol 152:297, 1985.
7. Hofmeyr, GJ, et al: External cephalic version and spontaneous version rates: ethnic and other determinants. Br J Obstet Gynaecol 93:13, 1986.
8. Kasule, J, Chimbira, TH, and Brown, IM: Controlled trial of external cephalic version. Br J Obstet Gynaecol 92:14, 1985.
9. Morrison, JC, et al: External cephalic version of the breech presentation under tocolysis. Am J Obstet Gynecol 154:900, 903, 1986.
10. O'Grady, JP, et al: External cephalic version: A clinical experience. J Perinat Med 14:189, 1986.
11. Rabinovici, J, et al: Impact of a protocol for external cephalic version under tocolysis at term. Isr J Med Sci 22:34, 1986.
12. Savona-Ventura, C: The role of external cephalic version in modern obstetrics. Obstet Gynecol Surv 41:393, 1986.
13. Stine, LE, et al: Update on external cephalic version performed at term. Obstet Gynecol 65:642, 1985.
14. Bhat, N, Seifer, D, and Hensleigh, P: Paradoxical response to intravenous terbutaline. Am J Obstet Gynecol 153:310, 1985.
15. Pritchard, JA, MacDonald, PC, and Gant, NF: Williams Obstetrics, ed 17. Appleton-Century-Crofts, Norwalk, Connecticut, 1985, p 678.
16. Hall, GP: The scultetus binder. J Nurse-Midwife 30(5):290, 1985.
17. Russell, JGB: Molding of the pelvic outlet. J Obstet Gynaecol Br Commonw 76:817, 1969.
18. Kurokawa, J and Zilkoski, MW: Adapting hospital obstetrics to birth in the squatting position. Birth 12:88, 1985.
19. McKay, S: Squatting: An alternate position for the second stage of labor. Matern Child Nurs J 9:181, 1984.
20. Rossi, MA, and Lindell, SG: Maternal positions and pushing techniques in a nonprescriptive environment. J Obstet Gynecol Neonatal Nurs 15(3):207, 1986.
21. Lehrman, E: Birth in the left lateral position: An alternative to the traditional delivery position. J Nurs-Midw 30(4):193, 1985.
22. Roberts, J, et al: A descriptive analysis of involuntary bearing-down efforts during the expulsive phase of labor. J Obstet Gynecol Neonatal Nurs 16(1):53, 1987.
23. McKay, S and Roberts, J: Second stage labor: What is normal? J Obstet Gynecol Neonatal Nurs 14(2):103, 1985.
24. Andrews, CM: Changing fetal position. J Nurse-Midwife 25(1):7, 1980.

BIBLIOGRAPHY

Bobak, IM and Jensen, MD: Essentials of Maternity Nursing: The Nurse and the Childbearing Family, ed 2. CV Mosby, St. Louis, 1987.

Kurokawa, J and Zilkoski, MW: Adapting hospital obstetrics to birth in the squatting position. Birth 12(2):87, 1985.

McKay, S and Roberts, J: Second stage labor: What is normal? J Obstet Gynecol Neonatal Nurs 14(2):101, 1985.

McKay, S: Squatting: An alternate position for the second stage of labor. Matern Child Nurs J 9(3):181, 1984.

Oxorn, H: Oxorn-Foote: Human Labor and Birth, ed 5. Appleton-Century-Crofts, Norwalk, Connecticut, 1986.

Pritchard, JA, MacDonald, PC, and Gant, NF: Williams Obstetrics, ed 17. Appleton-Century-Crofts, Norwalk, Connecticut, 1985.

Roberts, JE, et al: A descriptive analysis of involuntary bearing-down efforts during the expulsive phase of labor. J Obstet Gynecol Neonatal Nurs 16(1):48, 1987.

Romund, JL and Baker, IT: Squatting in childbirth: A new look at an old tradition. J Obstet Gynecol Neonatal Nurs 14:406, 1985.

Rossi, MA and Lindell, SG: Maternal positions and pushing techniques in a nonprescriptive environment. J Obstet Gynecol Neonatal Nurs 15:203, 1986.

POST-TEST 2

1. The following landmarks are significant in the various planes of the pelvis. Identify the plane in which each landmark is located and which diameter (anteroposterior or transverse) it influences.

	PLANE	DIAMETER
Bi-ischial tuberosities		
Posterior superior margin of symphysis pubis		
Coccyx		
Ischial spines		
Subpubic arch		

2. Describe the ideal passage of the fetus through the pelvis. Include the eight mechanisms of labor and three diameters of the pelvis.

____
____
____
____
____
____
____
____
____
____

3. When only six mechanisms of labor are listed, engagement and restitution are omitted. In which mechanisms are they included? Engagement is within ______________. Restitution is within ______________.

4. Put a check mark (✓) in front of those items that indicate ideal characteristics of the pelvis:

_____ DC of 10.5 cm
_____ hollow sacrum
_____ blunt (ischial) spines
_____ movable coccyx
_____ convergent side walls
_____ bituberosities of 7.5 cm
_____ arch of 80 degrees
_____ android type

5. Mrs. Beebe appears comfortable, although vaginal examination indicates she is 5 cm, 0 station, ROP. Her previous labor had an uncomplicated delivery of a 4-pound baby; the current EFW is 6 pounds. Her pelvic measurements are: DC 11 cm, spines nonprominent, sacrum hollow, arch 85 degrees, bitubs 11 cm, coccyx movable, type gynecoid.

   a. Give at least three reasons why you anticipate she will undergo the normal mechanisms of labor despite a few problematic data:
      (1) _______________
      (2) _______________
      (3) _______________
   b. Indicate four ways you might encourage fetal descent:
      (1) _______________
      (2) _______________
      (3) _______________
      (4) _______________
   c. What three measures might a nurse take to promote ideal fetal position?
      (1) _______________
      (2) _______________
      (3) _______________

6. In the chart below, briefly compare the mechanisms of labor as they occur for the fetus in the normal occiput anterior (OA), occiput posterior (OP), and breech presentation.

	OA	OP	BREECH
ENGAGEMENT			
DESCENT			
FLEXION			
INTERNAL ROTATION			
EXTENSION			
RESTITUTION			
EXTERNAL ROTATION			
EXPULSION			

Answers to Post-Test

1. The given landmarks are in the following plane and diameter:
   Bi-ischial tuberosities: outlet, transverse
   Posterior superior margin of symphysis pubis: inlet, anteroposterior
   Coccyx: outlet, anteroposterior
   Ischial spines: midpelvis, transverse
   Subpubic arch: outlet, anteroposterior.

2. Engagement occurs as the greatest diameter of the fetal head passes through the pelvic inlet. The occipitofrontal diameter of the head descends into the transverse diameter (occasionally oblique) of the inlet of the gynecoid pelvis. It descends further into the midplane, flexing to the smaller suboccipitobregmatic diameter. The head usually internally rotates from transverse to anteroposterior diameter near the floor of the midpelvis. In the outlet, the occiput moves under the symphysis pubis and extends, bringing the head out through the vaginal opening. Then restitution of the head occurs and the head externally rotates to a transverse position, orienting the remainder of the body for expulsion.

3. If descent, flexion, internal rotation, extension, external rotation, and expulsion are listed as the mechanisms of labor, engagement is within *descent* and restitution is within *external rotation*.

4. Ideal characteristics of the pelvis that are listed are hollow sacrum, blunt spines, and movable coccyx. Ideal characteristics that are not given are DC of 12.5 cm, nonconvergent side walls, bituberosities of 11 cm, arch of 90 degrees, and gynecoid type.

5. a. Although the baby is approximately 2 lb larger than her previous one, the baby has (1) already moved through the inlet (past the small DC) and is in the (2) midpelvis (zero station), which appears adequate (considering the spines and sacrum). The other slightly small area is the 85-degree arch; (3) a relatively small baby (6 lb) should be accommodated by this (4) pelvic outlet, since all the other measurements (bitubs and coccyx) are ideal. The OP fetal position is not ideal but is (5) not creating any apparent discomfort. (The Friedman curve should be assessed for abnormal cervical dilatation and descent patterns.)
   b. Fetal descent could be encouraged by (1) promoting maternal and fetal alignment, (2) providing more pelvic space by keeping the bowel and bladder empty, (3) allowing the force of gravity to work (have the mother stand, sit or squat), and (4) using a nontraditional left lateral position for delivery.
   c. The fetus should be rotated from ROP to OA. The nurse should encourage the mother to (1) lie frequently on her right side in a Sims' position. Periodically, the mother can (2) get up on her hands and knees and pelvic rock. She can also (3) stroke her abdomen (fetus) from right to left encouraging rotation.

6. A chart comparing the mechanisms of labor in OA and OP positions and breech presentation should look like this:

	OA	OP	BREECH
ENGAGEMENT	In inlet, OT position	In inlet, OP position	In inlet, three separate times, buttocks, shoulders, head
DESCENT	Begins in inlet, continues throughout pelvis		
FLEXION	In midpelvis, of head—chin on chest	In midpelvis, of head, partial	In outlet, lateral, at waist, shoulders; chin on chest
INTERNAL ROTATION	OT to OA	OP 45 degrees to directly OP	Hips, shoulders, occiput turn anteriorly
EXTENSION	In outlet Forehead first	In outlet Forehead first	In outlet Chin before forehead
RESTITUTION	← Outside of outlet →		
EXTERNAL ROTATION	← Outside of outlet →		
EXPULSION	← Outside of outlet →		

3 MATERNAL-FETAL MONITORING

Janet S. Malinowski

OBJECTIVES

Upon completing this chapter, you will be able to:

- Identify the anatomic parts of the pregnant uterus at term.
- Use the following terms correctly:
  UC—fundal dominance, pathologic retraction ring, increment, acme, decrement, tonus, frequency, duration, intensity, rest interval, primary and secondary uterine dysfunction, hypotonic and hypertonic, tetanic, incoordinate, coupling.
  FHR—funic and uterine souffles, baseline, tachycardia and bradycardia, decelerations (early, late, variable), shoulders, accelerations, overshoots, long- and short-term variability, sinusoidal, saltatory.
- Assess UC and FHR using acceptable techniques and differentiate normal from abnormal.
- Demonstrate awareness of the need for alternative methods of assessment, for example, intermittent versus continuous, external versus internal monitoring.
- Explain the rationale for nursing interventions during fetal monitoring.
- Demonstrate sound nursing judgment and promote patient comfort when monitoring UC and FHR.
- Document nursing care related to UC and FHR.

The two components of *fetal monitoring* are assessment of uterine contractions (UC) and assessment of fetal heart rate (FHR). Their interrelationship is important. An overall objective of nursing care during labor is to promote a healthy environment for both mother and fetus. Normal UC and FHR patterns provide reassurance that a healthy environment most likely exists. It is the responsibility of the nurse to assess and document both UC and FHR at least every 30 minutes during Stage I and at least every 15 minutes during Stage II. Intervention is necessary when abnormalities exist. This chapter addresses the current practices in fetal monitoring including the prudent interventions in the presence of abnormalities. (See Chapter 9 for other methods of determining fetal well-being.)

UTERINE ACTIVITY

Anatomy and Physiology of the Uterus During Labor

Rhythmic contractions in the uterus occur at the onset of Stage I of labor. The contractions are involuntary—independent of the laboring woman's will and of extrauterine control. The uterus is a muscular sac made up of three layers: (1) the *perimetrium*—the outer covering; (2) the *myometrium*—the thick muscular layer; and (3) the *endometrium*—the inner glandular, supportive tissue layer (Fig. 3–1).

The myometrium is composed of three types of muscle fibers illustrated in Figure 3–2: (1) a longitudinal layer on the outside, (2) an interlacing pattern of muscle fibers and blood vessels in the middle, and (3) an inner layer of circular fibers. As the pregnant uterus contracts the longitudinal muscle fibers straighten the fetus so that one fetal pole (usually the buttocks) is at the top of the uterus, and the other (the head) presses on the bottom of the uterus. The fetus is then in a longitudinal lie (see Chapter 1) as opposed to a transverse lie, which is incompatible with vaginal birth.

Involuntary uterine contractions begin, last longest, and are strongest in the uppermost portion of the uterus, the *fundus.* Con-

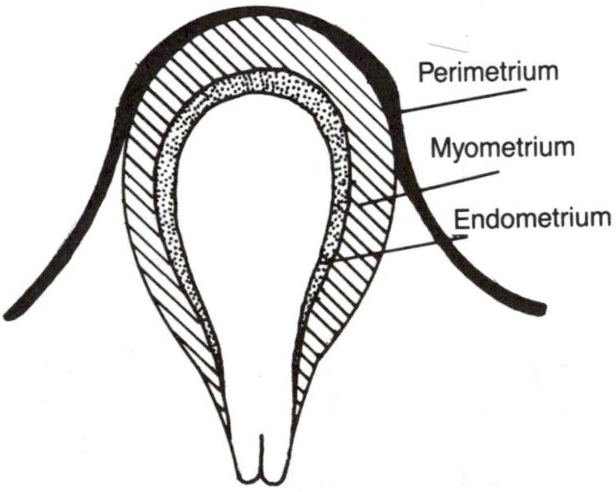

Figure 3–1. Tissue layers of the uterus.

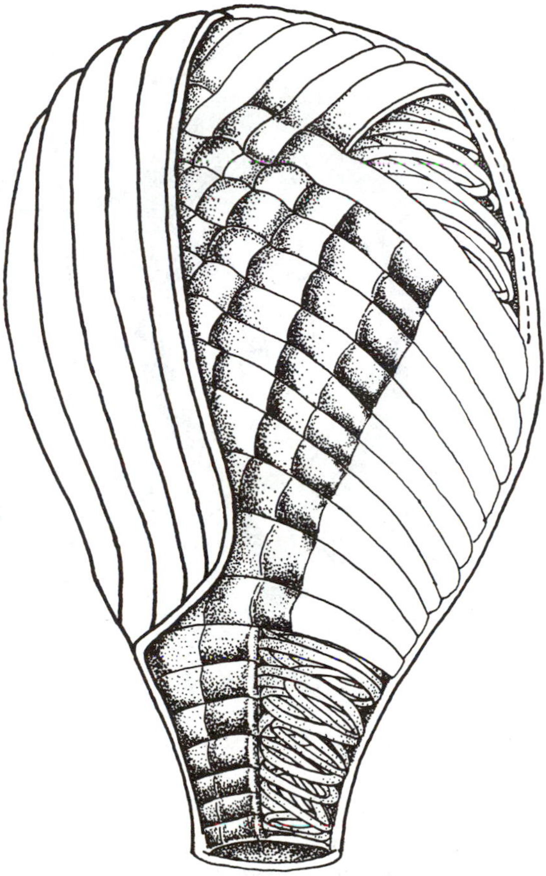

Figure 3–2. Uterine muscle fibers. (Adapted from Childbirth Graphics Ltd.)

tractions are therefore *fundal dominant.* They radiate downward over the body of the uterus. With each UC the actively contracting muscles in the fundus shorten and retract, gradually pushing the fetus downward, and thinning and expanding the more passive lower portion, the *cervix* (Fig. 3–3). As a result, the fetus descends, and the cervix effaces and dilates (terms defined in Chapter 1). Upon complete effacement (100 percent) of the *internal os* (Fig. 3–4) and complete dilatation (10 cm) of the *external os,* the cervix is no longer palpable and Stage II begins. It is then that the involuntary UC are supplemented by the voluntary forces of the abdominal and diaphragmatic muscles to expel the fetus through the birth canal.

Normally a nonpalpable *physiologic retraction ring* (Fig. 3–5) separates the upper thickening portion of the uterus from the lower thinning portion. In labor obstructed by conditions such as fetopelvic disproportion and malpresentation, the physiologic ring becomes

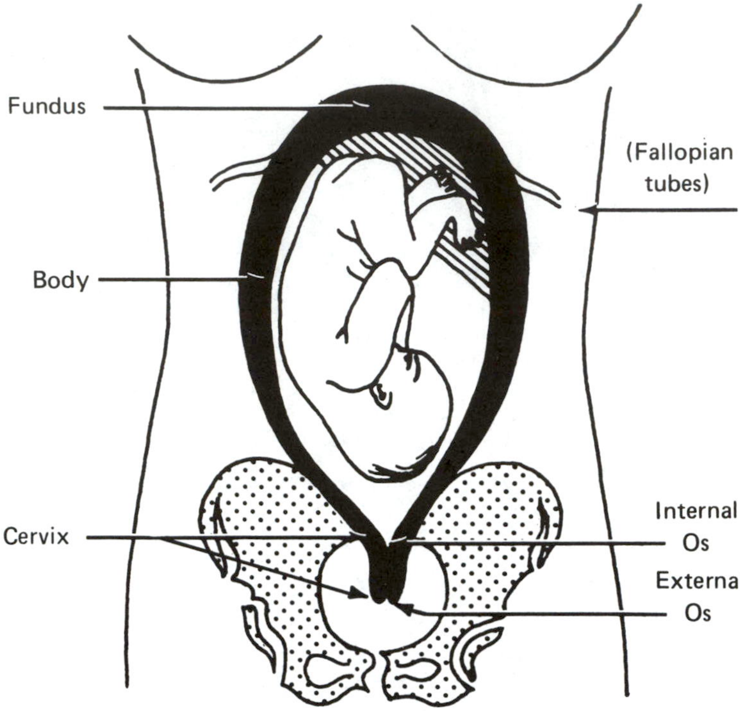

Figure 3–3. Anatomy of pregnant uterus at term.

exaggerated and on rare occasions palpable through the abdominal wall. It is then termed a *pathologic retraction (Bandl) ring.* In this abnormal situation, nurses need to seek medical intervention, recognizing that unless the obstruction is relieved, the myometrium is likely to become exhausted and/or rupture. Nurses may suspect the

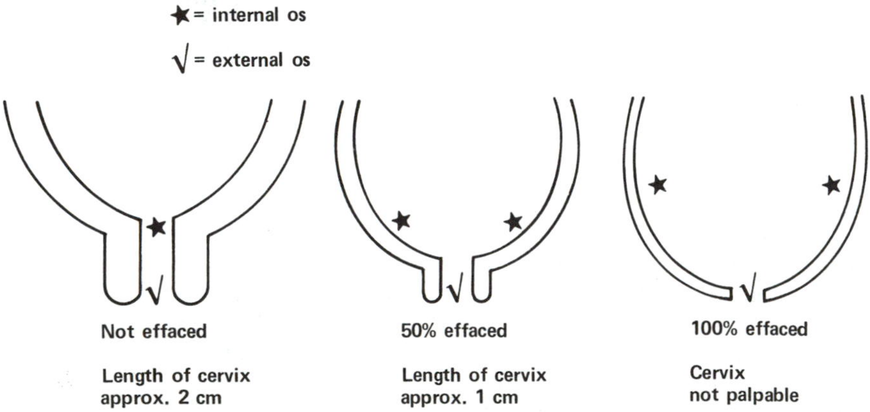

Figure 3–4. Cervical effacement.

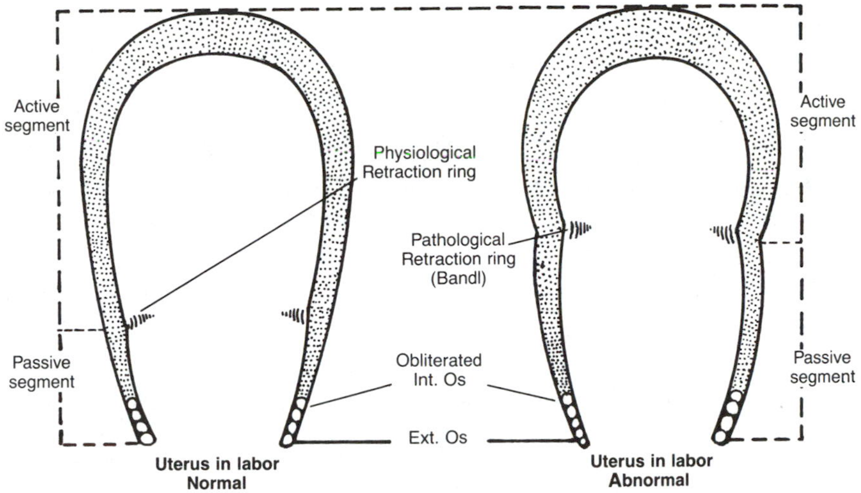

Figure 3–5. Retraction ring: physiologic and pathologic. (Adapted from Oxorn-Foote.)

presence of Bandl ring when labor arrests or is prolonged (see Chapter 4).

• •

Review Questions

1. Between the perimetrium and endometrium is the middle layer of the uterus called the ______________. It is composed of the following types of muscle fibers: (a) ______________, (b) ______________, and (c) ______________.

2. A primary function of the longitudinal uterine muscles is to ______________.

3. The upper portion of the uterus is called the ______________, the middle uterine portion is called the ______________, and the lower uterine portion is called the ______________, which is made up of the (a) ______________ and (b) ______________.

4. Fundal dominance refers to ______________

5. Circle the correct term in the parentheses: The muscles in the fundus (actively, passively) contract and retract; the muscles in the cervix (actively, passively) expand/dilate; a normal, physiologic retraction ring (can, cannot) be felt between the upper and lower portions of the uterus.

Answers

1. The middle layer of the uterus is called the *myometrium*, which is composed of (a) *longitudinal*, (b) *interlacing*, and (c) *circular* muscle fibers.
2. The longitudinal uterine muscles straighten the fetus so it is longitudinal in the uterus.
3. The upper portion of the uterus is the *fundus*, the middle is the *body*, and the lower is the *cervix*. The cervix is made up of the (a) *internal* os and (b) *external* os.
4. Fundal dominance refers to UC beginning and being longest and strongest in the fundal portion of the uterus.
5. The muscles in the fundus *actively* contract and retract; the muscles in the cervix *passively* expand/dilate; a physiologic retraction ring *cannot* be felt through the abdominal wall. On rare occasions a pathologic ring may be palpable.

• •

Terms Used to Describe Uterine Contractions

During early labor the actual onset of UC may be difficult to determine. The *increment,* a steep crescent-like slope, is from the beginning of the UC until its peak strength. The *acme,* or peak, is the period of greatest uterine contractility—an increase of 30 to >100 millimeters of mercury (mm Hg) of intrauterine pressure. The *decrement* is the diminishing intensity or termination of the contraction. The decrement is initially steep but becomes more horizontal, reflecting a gradual transition to the *tonus* (resting tone). Between contractions the uterus normally assumes a tonus ranging from as much as 5 to 15 mm Hg or, according to Oxorn,[1] 8 to 12 mm Hg. The characteristic pattern of UC is diagramed in Figure 3–6. Uteroplacental circulation usually is decreased or compromised during the peak of the contraction and returns to normal during the rest interval. Most fetuses tolerate this transient period of stress without an adverse response.

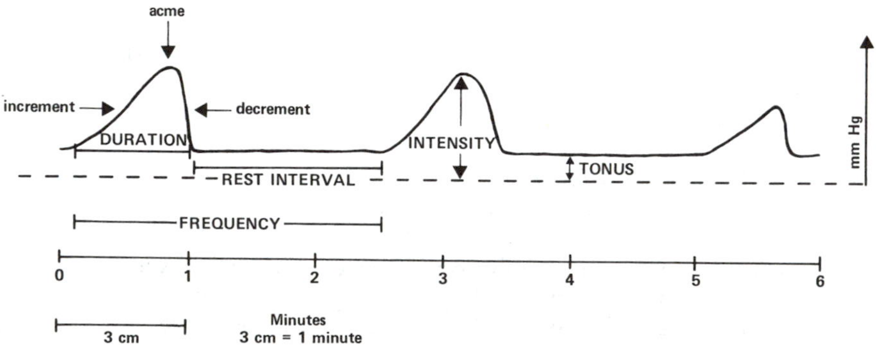

Figure 3–6. Pattern of uterine contractions.

When describing the UC, the *frequency* is the time in minutes from the onset of one UC (beginning of the increment) until the onset of the next UC. Rarely do UC occur at exactly the same frequency (e.g., every 3 minutes), so several UC need to be timed and compared. At the onset of labor, UC may be every 10 to 20 minutes, but typically the frequency becomes every 2 to 3 minutes during the active phase of labor. Another definition of UC frequency is the number of UC in 10 minutes. This method of describing UC frequency lacks specificity. Therefore, it is not recommended that nurses describe UC in this manner on labor charts.

The *duration* is the time in seconds between the onset of the increment until the completion of the decrement—that is, from the beginning until the end of one contraction. In early labor the duration may be 15 to 20 seconds, but it eventually becomes approximately 60 seconds. When the duration is longer than 90 seconds, the physician must be informed, because the contraction may be harmful to both mother and fetus. Exceedingly long contractions are not only very painful for the mother but may cause uterine rupture. For the fetus, long contractions may interfere with uteroplacental blood flow, causing fetal hypoxia. Figure 3–7 provides a schematic comparison of internal monitor, manual palpation, and patient's perception of the apparent contraction. The most objective, internal monitor, is considered to be the most accurate.

The *intensity* is the strength of the contraction at the acme. The intensity can be compared with the degree of indentation possible when pressing against the uterus through the abdominal wall. For example, it can be mild like a soft nose, moderate like the somewhat resisting chin, or strong like the nonindentable forehead. A more precise measurement can be obtained with mm Hg via an internal uterine catheter.

The normal *rest interval* (relaxation period) between the end of

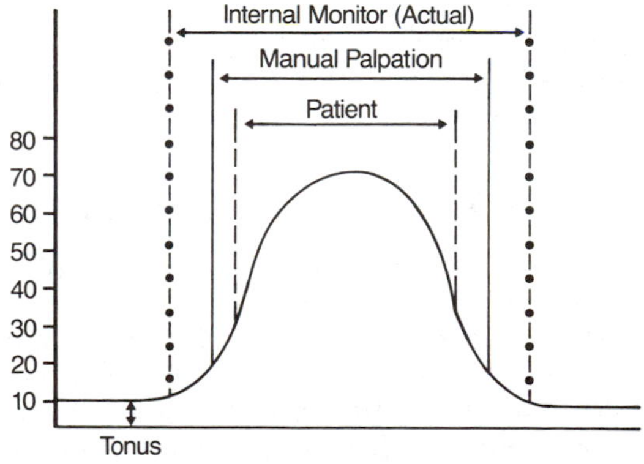

Figure 3–7. Comparison of internal monitor, manual palpation, and the patient for determining apparent duration of contraction. (Courtesy of Lois Vice.)

one UC and beginning of the next UC is ideally at least 60 seconds. The minimum acceptable rest interval is 20 seconds. During the rest interval the fetus receives the maximum oxygen supply from the placenta.

• •

Review Questions

Fill in the blanks with the correct terms:

1. The interval from the beginning of the UC until its peak is the ________________________________.
2. The peak of the UC is the ____________________.
3. The interval from the peak to the end of the UC is the ________________________________.
4. The resting tone of the uterus is its ____________________.
5. The period of time from the beginning of one contraction to the beginning of the next is the UC ____________________. What unit of time is this measured in? ____________________
6. The period of time from the beginning of one contraction to its end is its ____________. What unit of time is this measured in? ____________.
7. By indenting the fundus during the peak of a contraction or noting the pressure displayed in mm Hg via an internal monitor, the UC ______________________________ is determined.
8. The interval between the end of one UC and the beginning of the next is the ________________. It normally lasts at least ______ seconds.

Answers

The correct terms are (1) *increment*; (2) *acme*; (3) *decrement*; (4) *tonus*; (5) *frequency, minutes*, (6) *duration, seconds*, (7) *intensity*, (8) *rest interval, 20*.

• •

Uterine Contraction Assessment Methods

Although there are several ways to assess UC, objective data is considered to be much more reliable than subjective. The laboring woman usually provides a *subjective* description. It may be vague or detailed. It usually includes where the pressure is felt—in the back, in the suprapubic area, or beginning in the lower back and circling around to the abdomen. An intermittent *objective* assessment is done by the nurse or physician using light fingertip *palpation of the fundus*. Care must be taken to differentiate between the uterine wall and adipose tissue. Palpation between contractions provides a basis for normal uterine tonus. With a UC, gradual tensing of the fundus can be felt and the frequency, duration, and intensity determined. As the woman nears Stage II, she may be irritated by palpation and complain that it is painful. *Electronic monitoring* eliminates the need for frequent palpation and provides a continuous objective assessment of UC. Despite these advantages, electronic monitoring is not necessary in the presence of normal labor patterns. Electronic monitoring can be done externally or internally.

For *external* monitoring of UC a transducer (also called tocotransducer or tocodynamometer) is positioned on the abdominal wall over the uterine fundus. Efforts should be made to place the transducer's pressure sensing button as close as possible to the fundal surface. The transducer is held in place by an elastic belt (or band) that fits snugly around the abdomen. No conductive paste or gel is necessary because this is a sensor not a conductor. When the transducer is cleaned, soapy water is used, not alcohol, which would damage the transducer by removing the adhesive glue. A rubber coated lead wire is attached from the transducer to the electronic monitor, which graphically records the UC frequency and duration, as well as other movements such as maternal coughing or vomiting and fetal activity. The external monitor does not record the intensity of the contractions but merely frequency and duration. In the presence of normal uterine activity the monitoring device can be removed intermittently. This is advisable, so that the laboring woman can ambulate to the bathroom rather than use the bedpan. Periodically, the belt needs to be readjusted and the skin underneath massaged. When the monitor is in place, the mother is usually in a (preferably left) lateral, sitting or semisitting position. Portable machines are available that permit ambulation without discontinuing the tracing. Although the external electronic method of monitoring UC is reliable, it has disadvantages. (1) Upon movement by the mother, the transducer frequently requires repositioning. Therefore, there is a tendency to discourage movement, including ambulation. (2) Accurate recording in an obese mother or very active fetus is difficult because good contact with the uterine wall cannot be maintained.

For *internal* monitoring of UC the cervix ordinarily must be at least 2 to 3 cm dilated and the membranes ruptured. Using sterile technique, an intrauterine pressure catheter (abbreviated IUC or IUPC) is placed through the vagina into the uterus between the presenting fetal part and the lower uterine segment. According to the 1981 NAACOG standards, it was inappropriate for nurses to insert intrauterine catheters. The 1986 standards state that the qualified nurse can apply electronic fetal monitor components. A qualified nurse is one who is deemed competent in the pertinent knowledge base and clinical skills by the employing hospital.

The IUC, which is fluid filled, is secured to the mother's thigh by tape and connected to the monitor. Periodically, the catheter, or closed system, may need to be flushed with sterile water to remove substances (e.g., vernix, mucus, air bubbles) that might clog the catheter. For accurate readings, the distal end of the catheter and the proximal end (attached to the monitor) should be level with the transducer, and the catheter should be connected to a strain gauge apparatus via a 3-way stopcock. Calibration should be performed according to the manufacturer's instructions.

Use of the IUC is not routine. The benefits should outweigh the risks. It is desirable in the presence of questionable UC—those thought to be potentially harmful to the maternal/fetal unit (see next section). The internal monitoring device provides more accuracy than the external method, because the internal monitor is not affected by extraneous movements and adipose tissue. It is often applied in an obese woman receiving oxytocin stimulation. The internal monitor accurately records frequency, duration, intensity, and tonus. By comparing the recorded tonus (resting tone) with the pressure during the UC acme, the internal monitor can be used to determine the UC intensity. An increase of approximately 25 mm is mild, 50 mm is moderate, and 70 mm or greater is strong intensity. The absence of abdominal belts provides less restrictions in movement for the mother, although she is usually confined to bed as a result of the physical constraints of the monitoring device. The IUC should not be used unnecessarily. Since insertion of a catheter into the uterus is an invasive procedure, there is a slight risk of uterine infection and perforation.

• •

Review Questions

1. When palpating UC where and how is it done?

2. What nursing interventions are necessary when an external monitor is used to assess UC?

3. What advantages exist when an internal monitor replaces an external monitor?

Answers

1. When palpating UC:
   - use fingertips gently on the uterine fundus
   - determine the tonus and rest interval between contractions
   - determine the frequency between onset of contractions, duration of each contraction, and intensity (by indenting at the acme)

2. When using an external UC monitor:
   - position the transducer over the greatest fundal surface and reposition as necessary
   - secure the transducer with an elastic band
   - interpret the UC frequency and duration using the graphic recording
   - palpate the UC acme to assess the intensity
   - (usually) position the mother on her side
   - discourage excessive movement by the mother
   - provide skin care under the transducer and band as necessary
   - in the presence of normal uterine activity and no other complications, periodically remove the monitor device to permit ambulation to the bathroom and elsewhere

3. Advantages that exist when an internal monitor replaces an external monitor include:
   - more accuracy exists despite movement or adipose tissue
   - UC intensity and tonus, as well as frequency and duration, can be determined by the graphic recording rather than by palpation
   - more movement is permitted

• •

Abnormal Uterine Contraction Patterns

Dystocia is abnormal or difficult labor. One of the causes of dystocia is uterine dysfunction (sometimes called uterine dystocia). Uterine dysfunction can involve very weak contractions or very intense contractions. The nurse's role is to differentiate normal from abnormal UC patterns (Fig. 3–8) and to respond accordingly. Normally, contractions become more frequent, longer in duration, and stronger in intensity as labor progresses.

Primary uterine dysfunction involves a slow moving labor from the onset. It may be due to weak, short duration, irregular, or infrequent UC (Fig. 3–8,*B* and *C*). Well-established, efficient (i.e., causing cervical changes) contractions should not become weak or cease. If they do, *secondary uterine dysfunction* exists. (See Chapter 4 for abnormal labor curves.)

Whether caused by primary or secondary uterine dysfunction, weak ineffective contractions are called *hypotonic contractions.* The nurse's role is to assess and support. The nurse must assess for infection, dehydration, exhaustion, and discouragement in the

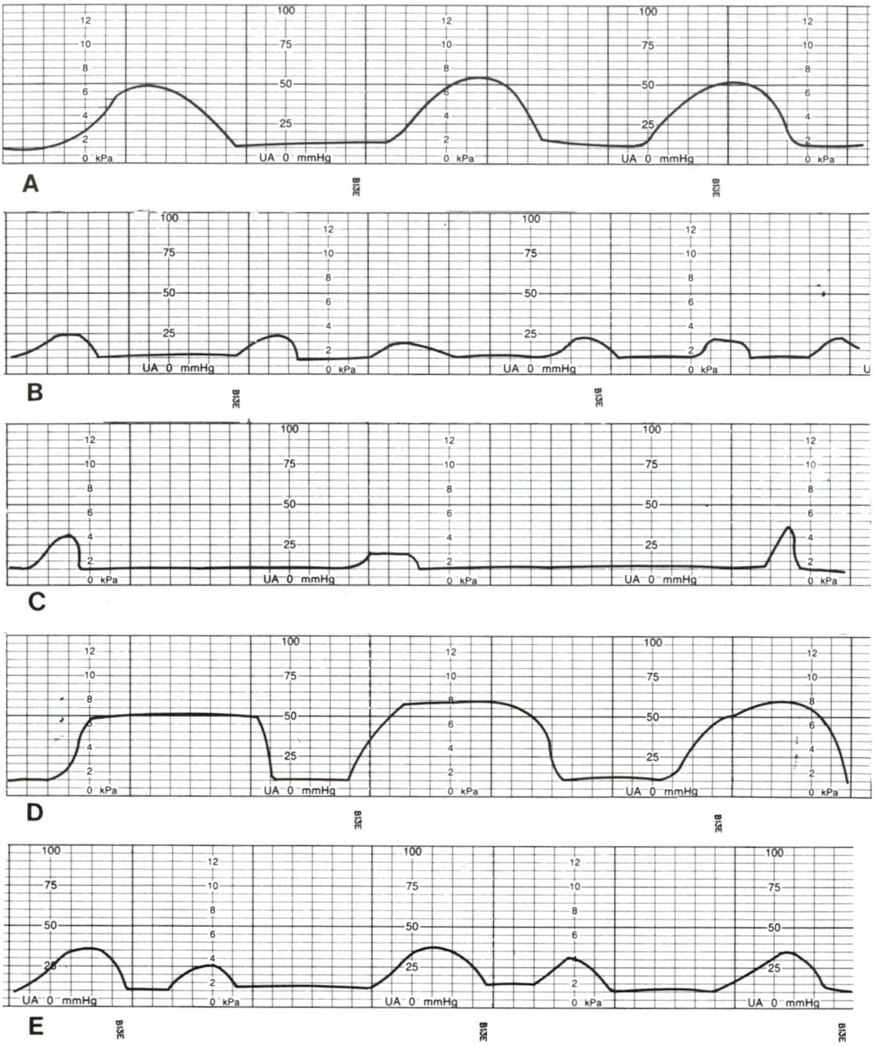

Figure 3–8. Normal UC (*A*) compared with abnormal UC seen in hypotonic UC (*B, C*) and hypertonic UC (*D, E*). (*A*) Normal. (*B*) Weak intensity, short duration. (*C*) Irregular, infrequent. (*D*) Tetanic. (*E*) Coupling.

woman, and infection and distress in the fetus. In the presence of some labor progress without maternal or fetal complications, nursing interventions such as position change, comfort measures, and ambulation can be tried (see Chapter 1). Medical intervention is not required although oxytocin, prostaglandin, or nipple stimulation of labor is often begun.

Conversely, contractions can be *hypertonic,* that is, excessive in frequency, duration, or intensity. Three hypertonic states are tetanic, incoordinate, and coupling.

Contractions of 90 seconds or more duration are called *tetanic* (Fig. 3–8*D*). These contractions can cause insufficient placental exchange and, therefore, fetal distress. Hypertonic contractions are very painful and could cause uterine rupture if allowed to continue. Hospital protocol should identify what interventions can be taken. The following interventions may be effective for tetanic UC:

1. Turn off IV oxytocin if infusing. By stopping oxytocin, the uterine stimulation effect may be decreased.
2. Turn the laboring woman on her side. The position change may increase the quantity of uteroplacental exchange.
3. Administer 5 to 10 liters of oxygen by mask or nasal cannula. The uteroplacental oxygen concentration will be improved.
4. Apply heat to lower abdomen via a towel or blanket. Heat promotes localized circulation and comfort.
5. Give terbutaline 0.25 mg s.c., [2,3] ritodrine 6 mg IV bolus,[4] morphine 8 to 12 mg IM or 1 to 2 mg IV, or meperidine 25 to 100 mg IM or 25 to 50 mg IV. Terbutaline, ritodrine, morphine, and meperidine are likely to temporarily decrease uterine activity. Morphine and meperidine also provide some pain relief.

Occasionally, contractions originate in the mid- or lower uterine segment (i.e., without fundal dominance). They are *incoordinate.* Evidence of such is seen in the lack of cervical dilation or effacement, poor application of the presenting part against the cervix, and/or lack of fetal descent especially during the transitional phase of labor despite very painful contractions. Interventions similar to those for tetanic contractions are likely to be utilized.

A final abnormal uterine contraction pattern is the presence of less than 30 seconds relaxation between the end of one contraction and the beginning of the next and/or a lack of return to normal tonus of 5 to 15 mm Hg. The term given to two consecutive contractions with little or no rest interval is *coupling* (Fig. 3–8,*E*). Oxytocin often precipitates coupling and must be decreased or ceased if infusing. Morphine or meperidine may also be used to stop coupling.

Nurses need to be alert for these nonproductive, painful, hypertonic contractions, that is, tetanic, incoordinate, coupling. Such contractions may cause poor labor progress, lack of control, dehydration and exhaustion in the laboring woman, and fetal distress. These problems can be stated as the following nursing diagnoses:

1. **Coping, ineffective individual related to painful hypertonic contractions.**
2. **Fluid volume deficit related to exertion involved in abnormal labor.**
3. **Activity intolerance related to nonproductive labor.**
4. **Injury, potential for; trauma (to the fetus) related to abnormal contractions.**

The nurse may need to seek medical intervention in the form of medications just mentioned. The given interventions are often effective if other complications, such as fetopelvic disproportion, are not present.

• •

Review Questions

To demonstrate your correct use of the terms for abnormal uterine contraction patterns, place the letter of each term in front of its description:

DESCRIPTION	TERM
1._____Well-established contractions become weak or cease	a. coupling
2._____Contractions lasting 90 seconds or more	b. hypertonic contractions
3._____Contractions that are not fundal dominant	c. hypotonic contractions
4._____Consecutive contractions with little or no rest interval	d. incoordinate contractions
	e. primary uterine dysfunction
	f. secondary uterine dysfunction
	g. tetanic contractions

Provide the correct term for the remaining questions:

5. Primary uterine dysfunction involves nonprogressive contractions from the ____________________ of labor.
6. Hypotonic contractions are __________ ineffective contractions.
7. An excessively intense contraction is (hypotonic, hypertonic).

Answers

(1) f, (2) g, (3) d, (4) a

5. Primary uterine dysfunction involves nonprogressive contractions from the *onset* of labor.
6. Hypotonic contractions are *weak*, ineffective contractions.
7. An excessively intense contraction is *hypertonic*.

• •

The labor nurse is responsible for carefully assessing and charting the uterine activity of a woman in labor. Included should be:

1. subjective and objective findings,
2. nursing interventions taken to relieve discomfort from the monitoring methods,

3. use of a more precise assessment method in the presence of abnormal UC, and
4. reporting any abnormal findings to the physician.

Often UC become more effective if the anxiety level of the woman is decreased; sensitivity and responsiveness to the individual's needs may facilitate improved UC. The relaxation techniques discussed in Chapter 7 are usually very helpful.

Assessing Pain of Uterine Contractions

Often an appropriate nursing diagnosis for the pain of uterine contractions is **comfort, alteration in: pain, acute related to ineffective management of UC pain.** The scientific rationale and nursing interventions for labor pain are discussed in Chapters 6 and 7. Several defining characteristics indicate that discomfort is present. Verbal communication is one. The woman's narrow, usually self-focusing, behavior is another. Her physical actions in the form of verbal utterances and facial gestures and listless or rigid muscle tone further indicate pain. Although uterine contractions are the etiology of the nursing diagnosis, alteration in comfort is the woman's response to the stressor. Sometimes nurses avoid using the term "pain" as they acknowledge the discomfort of the contractions, because that word is likely to heighten any preexisting fears the woman has. At other times, the woman appreciates the nurses' recognition of the contraction pain and the woman is prepared to deal with it.

• •

Review Questions

1. List defining characteristics that you might observe that indicate alterations of comfort related to UC:
   Subjective:____
   Objective:____
2. Give an example of how you would respond to the laboring woman's verbalized concerns about pain:____

Answers

1. Subjective responses to UC discomfort:
   "Those contractions hurt."
   "Will they get worse and when will they stop?"
   (to her support person) "I don't want to talk about your problems."

Objective responses to UC discomfort:
Laboring woman groans throughout UC.
Her eyes appear fearful.
She thrashes when contracting.
She tenses her fists with UC.

2. The response should be oriented to the individual. Use (a) or (b).
   (a) "I am aware that you are experiencing discomfort with your uterine contractions. There are several ways I can help you and your support person to work with them. . . ."
   (b) "I know you are in pain. Let me help you use the techniques you learned in class."

• •

FETAL RESPONSE

UC are regarded as stressful to the fetus even under normal circumstances because at the acme of the contraction there is a reduction in the oxygen supply from the uterus to the fetus. The nurse must rely on objective data for determining fetal oxygen status. Depending on whether a reassuring or nonreassuring FHR pattern is present, the following nursing diagnosis is appropriate: **Tissue perfusion, alteration in relation to interruption in placental blood flow.** Normally the fetus has enough reserve to compensate. However, this is not always true. The FHR is significant because it is the primary indicator of fetal well-being or fetal distress during labor. The nurse is primarily responsible for: (1) assessing characteristics of the FHR, (2) interpreting FHR data as reassuring or nonreassuring, (3) if nonreassuring, taking appropriate action, and (4) documenting the findings, interventions (including notification of the physician, if done), and response (positive or negative) of the FHR pattern if interventions were taken.

Intermittent Fetal Heart Rate Assessment

Intermittent FHR assessment by fetoscope, Doppler unit, or electronic monitor is most meaningful if it is done during the contraction and continued for 30 seconds beyond the end of the contraction. Because the rate is rapid and assessment is often interrupted by environmental distractions (e.g., fetal movement), counting the FHR is best done in two or four 15-second periods. The rate is then determined as beats per minute (BPM).

EXAMPLES:

Getting 30 and 32 for two 15-second periods, multiply 62 by 2 for BPM.

Getting 30, 32, 35, and 31 for four 15-second periods, add them together for BPM.

The FHR is heard loudest over the fetal back. In the normal head down presentation, the FHR is therefore most audible in a lower abdominal quadrant. The second Leopold maneuver (see Fig. 1–4) is useful in determining the location of the fetal back. If the rate is not clearly audible, the assessment apparatus should be repositioned. *Funic souffle,* a soft blowing sound created by the blood flowing through the umbilical vessels, should not be confused with the FHR although the rate is the same. *Uterine bruit*[5] is the sound of blood passing through the uterine blood vessels. It is synchronous with (same as) the FHR.

• •

Review Questions

1. In relation to a UC, when is the best time to assess the FHR?______

2. What counting technique is recommended for determining the FHR?

3. Over what fetal part is the FHR most audible?______

4. What is the term for the blowing sound that occurs as blood flows through the umbilical vessels?______

Answers

1. The best time to intermittently assess the FHR is during the UC and within 30 seconds of the end of the UC.

2. The recommended technique for counting FHR is to count in 15-second segments, obtain at least two 15-second segments, and determine BPM.

3. The FHR is heard best over the *fetal* back.

4. *Funic souffle* is the term for the soft blowing sound that occurs as blood flows through the umbilical vessels.

• •

Several kinds of apparatus can be used for intermittent FHR assessment. A *stethoscope* is the least effective. A *fetoscope* is a modified stethoscope with a head piece (Fig. 3–9, *A* and *B*) that permits bone conduction from the listener's skull and, therefore, increases the audibility of the FHR. This inexpensive apparatus is convenient for FHR auscultation in normal situations. However, the woman should be in a supine position. Gross abnormalities of the FHR may be detected with a fetoscope, but it is difficult to detect FHR changes during UC and through an obese abdomen. A Leffscope, or weighted fetoscope (Fig. 3–9, *C*), may be used in place of a fetoscope. It is especially useful when assessing FHR under sterile drapes during the delivery. A *Doppler unit* (e.g., Doptone, Fetone) is a portable rechargeable electronic instrument that amplifies the sound of the FHR (Fig. 3–9, *D* and *E*). With the volume turned down (to prevent static noise), a gel or mineral oil is applied to the bell to assist with

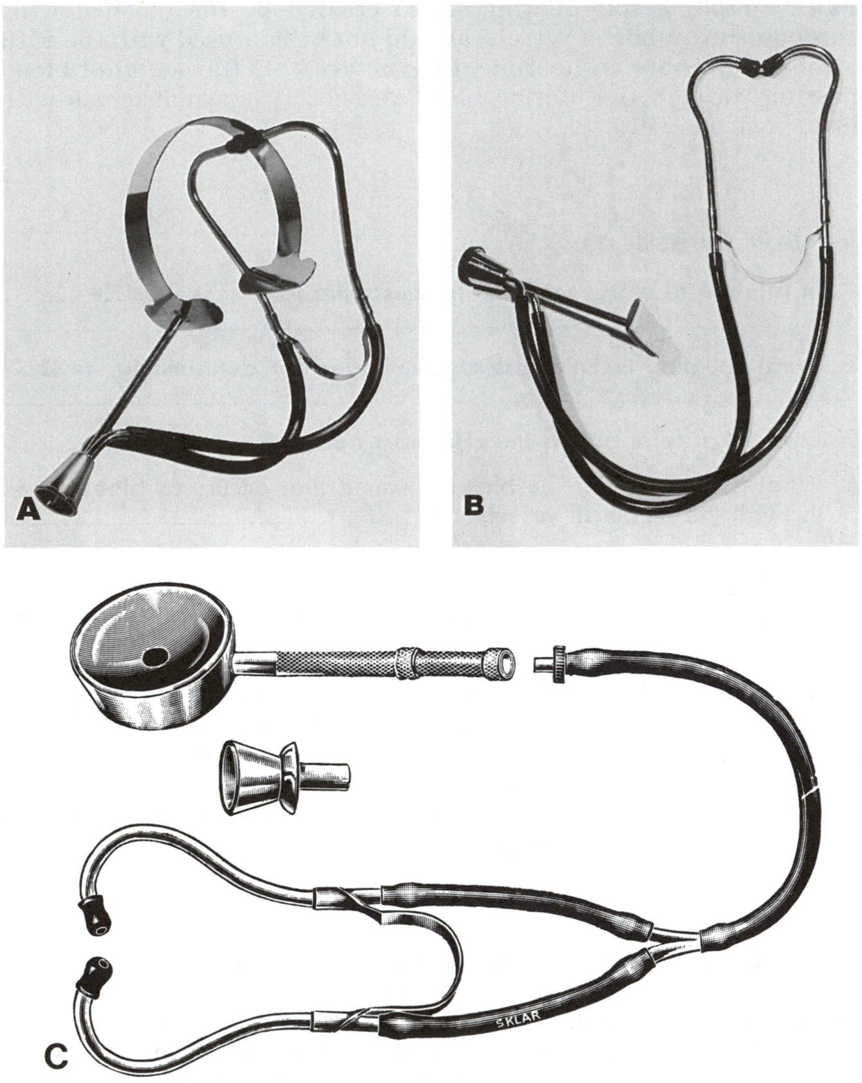

Figure 3–9. Fetoscopes. DeLee-Hillis stethoscopes: (*A* and *B*) head scope model, forehead rest model; (*C*) Leff stethoscope with weighted bells. (DeLee-Hillis photos courtesy of Graham-Field Surgical Company, Inc., New Hyde Park, NY 11040; Leff stethoscope photo courtesy of J. Sklar Manufacturing Company, Inc., Long Island City, NY 11101, with permission.)

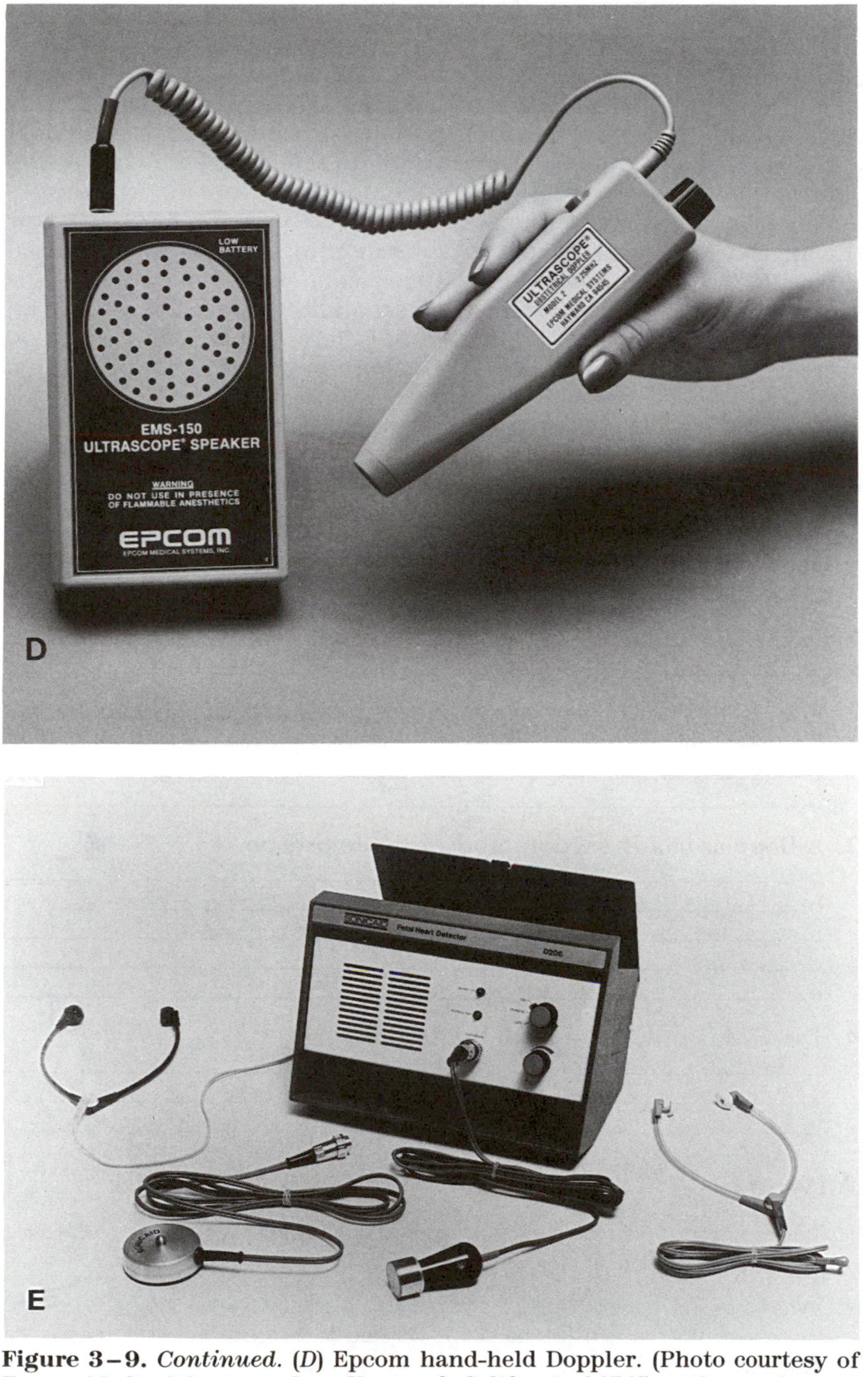

Figure 3–9. *Continued.* (*D*) Epcom hand-held Doppler. (Photo courtesy of Epcom Medical Systems, Inc., Hayward, California 94545, with permission.) (*E*) Sonicaid fetal heart detector. (Photo courtesy of Sonicaid Medical, Inc., Fredericksburg, Va. 22404, with permission.)

the conduction of sound. The gel or oil is removed from the abdomen and the Doppler bell with a dry tissue following every use. The Doppler has several advantages over the fetoscope. It is useful when the FHR is hard to hear, when others such as the parents would also like to hear the rate, when the mother is assuming a sitting, side-lying, or even standing position, when the rate is to be heard during contractions, and when FHR assessment is done under sterile drapes during the delivery. A more stationary *electronic fetal monitor* (EFM), which is used for continuous monitoring, can also be used intermittently. Although this is a very expensive apparatus, if it is already in the unit, it provides the best audio feedback as well as all the advantages of the Doppler. If it is left in place for 15 to 60 seconds, it will also record the FHR both graphically and digitally.

• •

Review Questions

Indicate the rationale for the following nursing interventions during intermittent FHR assessment:

1. The fetoscope is worn on the head.

 ____

 ____

2. Why is (a) the volume turned down and (b) a gel placed on the Doppler bell?
 a. ______________________________________
 b. ______________________________________

3. A Doppler unit is used instead of the fetoscope.
 a. ______________________________________
 b. ______________________________________
 c. ______________________________________
 d. ______________________________________
 e. ______________________________________

4. The EFM is used instead of the Doppler unit.

 ____

 ____

 ____

Answers

1. The fetoscope is worn on the head to permit bone conduction, thereby increasing audibility of the FHR.

2. When using a Doppler unit: (a) the volume is turned down when the gel is applied to prevent static noise; (b) the gel is applied to increase the FHR volume via conduction.

3. A Doppler unit is used instead of the fetoscope because (a) the FHR may be hard to hear with the fetoscope; (b) the parents may want to hear also; (c) the mother's

position might be incompatible with use of the fetoscope; (d) the situation may indicate that the FHR should be heard during UC; and (e) sterile drapes on the mother may prohibit access to the abdomen.

4. The EFM may be used instead of the Doppler unit because it provides better audio feedback and records both graphically and digitally if left in place for 15 to 60 seconds.

Continuous Fetal Heart Rate Assessment

Continuous electronic fetal monitoring (EFM) provides a second-by-second audio and visual FHR recording (Fig. 3–10). EFM is routinely used for the high-risk labor patient, the low-risk woman who develops problems during labor, and the woman whose labor is stimulated by oxytocin. Whether or not continuous monitoring is warranted in the uncomplicated low-risk woman is debatable. Many labor units run a 20-minute "strip" on all newly admitted laboring women as part of the initial assessment process. Twenty minutes presumably is enough evidence of whether or not the FHR is reassuring.[6] Other units run a strip until the fetus demonstrates "reactivity" by the presence of accelerations with movement or UC.

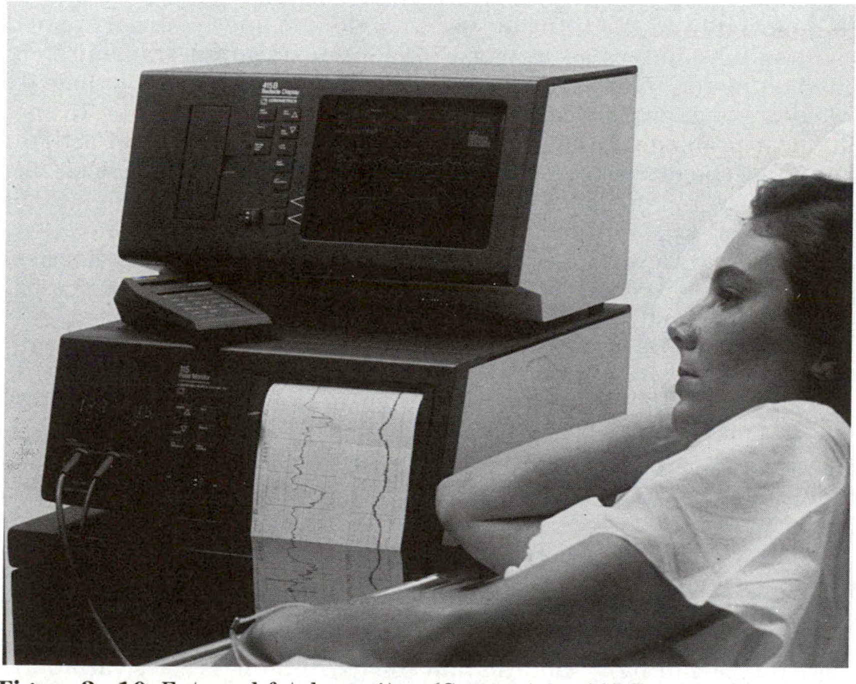

Figure 3–10. External fetal monitor. (Corometrics 115 Fetal Monitor photo courtesy of Corometrics Medical Systems, Inc., Wallingford, Connecticut 06492, with permission.)

Continuous EFM can be done externally or internally. In both cases the FHR is audible via a volume control knob. Depending on the brand of monitor, the heart rate is heard as heart sounds or beeps. The volume should be adjusted so it is not disturbing to the woman and may be increased only during assessment. Some women request that the volume remain audible so they can hear the baby's heart rate during labor. The FHR is displayed digitally or on a circular disk, as well as on a *Z*-fold printout (usually set to move 3 cm per minute), which becomes part of the woman's permanent chart. Because the monitor is very sensitive, the smallest variations in the FHR will be seen. The woman needs to be informed that 1 to 2 seconds of a comparatively low or high FHR are not signs of danger. When in doubt about the accuracy of the monitor's data, the volume can be made audible and the rate compared with the monitor's recording, or the actual FHR can be verified by auscultation with a fetoscope.

The *external EFM* has the advantage of being physiologically noninvasive. A lubricated ultrasound transducer is placed on the mother's (usually lower) abdomen over the site where the FHR is heard best. The transducer is secured by a snug abdominal band (Fig. 3–11). A similar tocotransducer and band may be applied over the fundus to assess UC. The distal end of each transducer is plugged into the monitor. Care must be taken that the monitor cable permits some movement of the mother. Occasionally the dried gel needs to be removed from the transducer and abdomen and fresh gel applied to promote comfort as well as efficient ultrasound transmission. Readjustment of the transducer may be necessary when heavily inked areas appear on the graph; such artifacts can be due to mechanical problems in the monitor. Fig. 3–12 illustrates an artifact caused by the internal electrode hitting the cervix as the mother has a seizure. In the presence of an accurate recording of a normal FHR, the external EFM may be used throughout the labor. For the restless mother or very active fetus, the external monitor may be ineffective. Since the external monitor records an average FHR, for the most precise assessment, internal monitoring is necessary.

An *internal EFM* can be applied once the membranes have ruptured, the cervix is dilated at least 2 to 3 cm, and the fetal presenting part can be reached. During a vaginal exam the physician (or in some hospitals, the nurse), would insert an electrode through a guide about 1 mm into the fetal presenting part, avoiding the face, fontanels, and genitalia (Fig. 3–13). Although it can be applied to the buttocks in a breech presentation, the electrode is often abbreviated SE for scalp electrode or SL for scalp lead. The guide tube surrounding the electrode and wires is removed, the color-coded wires are attached to the posts on the leg plate, electrode paste is applied, and the plate is strapped to the woman's leg. With the leads from the leg plate plugged into the monitor and the current on, precise variations in the FHR are recorded. Occasionally the electrode becomes dis-

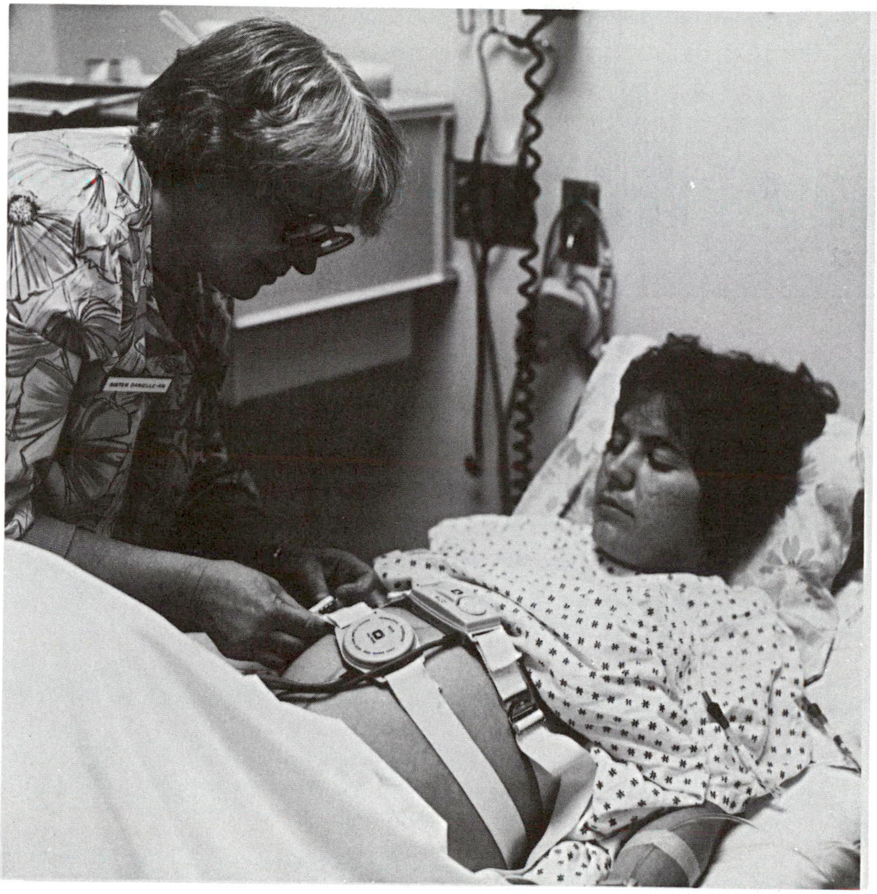

Figure 3–11. External monitor. (From Clark, AL and Affonso, DD: Childbearing: A Nursing Perspective, ed 2. FA Davis, Philadelphia, 1979, p 453, with permission.)

lodged from the fetus, especially during vaginal exams. If this occurs, no FHR would be heard or recorded. On occasion, maternal EKG is picked up especially if the electrode is inadvertantly attached to maternal tissue. In both instances, re-application of the electrode would be necessary.

The slight potential for fetal infection at the site of the electrode insertion can be minimized with the use of sterile technique. The advantages of the internal monitor when indicated outweigh this one disadvantage. Once in place it is more comfortable than the external monitor, allows for more movement by the mother, and provides a very accurate recording.

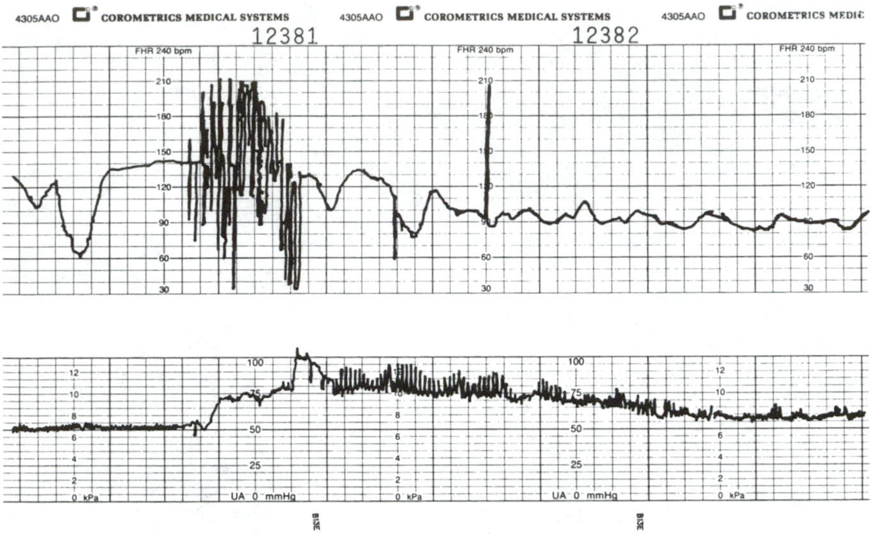

Figure 3–12. Artifact seen in fetal heart rate tracing.

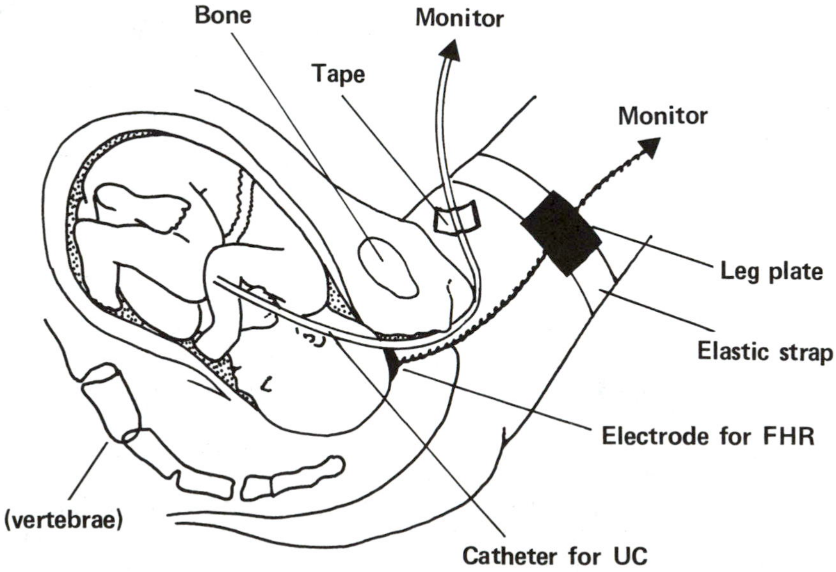

Figure 3–13. Internal monitoring.

Review Questions

1. List three situations in which continuous EFM would more likely be used than intermittent EFM.
   a. ______________________
   b. ______________________
   c. ______________________
2. What advantage does the external EFM have over the internal EFM?
   ____
3. What nursing interventions are specific for the use of an external EFM?
   a. ______________________
   b. ______________________
   c. ______________________
4. What criteria must exist before an internal EFM can be applied?
   a. ______________________
   b. ______________________
   c. ______________________
5. Why would an internal EFM be used in place of an external EFM?
   a. ______________________
   b. ______________________

Answers

1. Continuous EFM would be used instead of intermittent EFM in: (a) high-risk obstetric patients; (b) low-risk women who have problems during labor; and (c) labors augmented by oxytocin.
2. The external EFM is noninvasive, therefore physically nontraumatic, and not a potential source of infection.
3. With the external EFM the nurse needs to: (a) lubricate and secure the transducer on the abdomen where the FHR is heard best; (b) provide for some movement despite the lead cable; and (c) remove and re-apply the conductive gel as needed.
4. The criteria that must exist before an internal EFM can be used are: (a) ruptured membranes; (b) cervix dilated at least 2 to 3 cm; and (c) fetal presenting part can be reached.
5. The internal EFM will be used in place of an external EFM when: (a) there is a poor recording from the external EFM and (b) a more precise assessment is needed than what the external monitor provides.

Fetal Heart Rate Baseline

Each fetus has a unique FHR baseline level. The baseline level decreases with advancing gestational age, namely, it is higher for prematures and lower for postmatures.[7] The *baseline* is the range that exists between contractions for the major portion of a 10-minute period of time. Traditionally the normal range is within 120 to 160 beats per minute (BPM). (There is some variation—110–150, 110–160—among authorities.[7–9]) Table 3–1 identifies the classification of FHR baselines beyond the normal range. During the course of labor the baseline may change. A new baseline exists if the FHR remains within a new range for longer than 10 minutes.

> EXAMPLE: Originally FHR baseline may be 124 to 144 BPM (that is, normal). If the FHR rises to 160 to 170 BPM for longer than 10 minutes, it is relabeled moderate tachycardia. If it falls and remains below 120 for longer than 10 minutes, it is relabeled bradycardia.

The terms tachycardia and bradycardia refer specifically to baseline FHR.

Tachycardia is often associated with maternal fever, reaction to certain maternal drugs, fetal hypoxia, and a premature fetus.[7,9–11] Tachycardia may be an early sign of fetal compromise. LaSala[12] cites several cases in which mild tachycardia occurred before fetal death. In the presence of fetal tachycardia, the nurse should rule out maternal fever (due to chorioamnionitis or dehydration) and drugs like Ritodrine, Isoxsuprine, and Atropine[13] as possible causes. The physician should be informed. Medical intervention is likely if late or variable decelerations or decreased variability also exist. If tachycardia persists, the pediatrician should be informed, because neonatal heart failure is possible[9] and/or a depressed neonate due to hypoxia is likely to be born.

For *bradycardia,* observation alone is prudent when the FHR is 110 or greater, with good variability and no decelerations. (Both variability and periodic decelerations are discussed in the next sections.) Medical intervention is indicated if: (1) the FHR is persistently less than 110,[7] (2) there is poor variability, and/or (3) late or variable decelerations occur.[9] Occasionally the mother's heart rate may be mistakenly identified as the FHR. To avoid this error, the

Table 3–1. CLINICALLY ESTABLISHED FHR CATEGORIES IN BPM

<100	= marked bradycardia
100–119	= moderate bradycardia
120–160	= normal
161–180	= moderate tachycardia
>180	= marked tachycardia

mother's radial pulse should be felt simultaneously while listening to the FHR. If the rates are the same, the muffled sound that is heard is not the FHR but a *uterine souffle.* Persistent bradycardia of usually 50 to 70 BPM is found in a fetus with a congenital heart block.[9]

• •

Review Questions

1. How is FHR baseline determined?
____
____

2. What is the normal FHR baseline range?______________

3. a. An FHR range higher than normal is called______________.
   b. List three causes of this abnormality:
      (1)______________
      (2)______________
      (3)______________

4. What objective data should the nurse collect in the presence of fetal tachycardia? (a)______________
and (b)______________

5. Under what circumstances should a FHR baseline of 160–166 be brought to the attention of the physician?______________
____

6. If persistent fetal tachycardia exists, at or near the time of delivery, the______________ should be informed.

7. An FHR range lower than normal is called______________.
What is a plausible explanation for a range persistently 70 or lower?
____

8. What nursing intervention should be taken when there is (moderate) fetal bradycardia in the presence of good variability and no decelerations?
____
____

Answers

1. The FHR baseline is the range that the FHR assumes between UC during the major portion of a 10-minute period.
2. The normal FHR baseline range is 120 to 160 BPM.
3. *Tachycardia*, a range higher than the normal range for more than 10 minutes, might be due to maternal fever, reaction to certain drugs, fetal hypoxia, and prematurity.
4. The nurse should determine: (a) if the laboring woman is febrile and (b) whether or

not she is receiving a medication like Ritodrine, which might cause fetal tachycardia.

5. In the presence of variable or late decelerations, the physician should be informed of an FHR even slightly above normal.
6. A pediatrician should be made aware of the existence of persistent fetal tachycardia because (1) neonatal heart failure is known to occur and (2) a depressed neonate is likely if other nonreassuring signs are present, that is, late or variable decelerations, decreased variability.
7. *Bradycardia*, a lower than normal FHR range that persists, is found in fetuses with congenital heart block.
8. Observation for nonreassuring FHR patterns is merely continued when there is (moderate) fetal bradycardia in the presence of good variability and no decelerations.

• •

Recognizing Periodic Changes: Decelerations

With each contraction there is a normal decrease of blood flow in the intervillous spaces of the placenta. The normal fetus has enough oxygen reserve so that this decrease causes no apparent change in the FHR. But, in some instances, periodic changes occur in relation to UC. If the FHR rises above the baseline, and then returns, this is called an *acceleration* (see later section on accelerations). When the FHR falls below baseline level, and then returns, this is called a *deceleration*. Authorities vary in their classifications of mild, moderate, and severe.[6,14]

Three types of decelerations are identified: early, late, and variable (Fig. 3–14). *Early decelerations* are traditionally said to be due to head compression, specifically on the fontanel. Schifrin[15] proposes that other mechanisms are also involved, namely: (1) increased intracranial pressure, (2) increased peripheral resistance, (3) increased blood pressure, and (4) vagal reflex deceleration. This deceleration pattern is termed early because its onset is early in (similar with) the UC. Its uniform shape reflects the intrauterine pressure curve, with the maximum amount of FHR deceleration consistently occurring at the acme of the contractions. This benign pattern is not associated with alterations in baseline heart rate or acid-base balance. It is unaffected by position change or oxygen administration and is common during Stage II and with breech presentations. It requires no nursing intervention.

Late deceleration may indicate fetal distress and is due to uteroplacental insufficiency resulting from a decreased blood flow of pO_2 during the UC. Although its uniform shape also reflects the intrauterine pressure curve, it consistently occurs late (greater than 20 seconds) in the contraction. The current practice is to note the nadir (lowest point) of the FHR in relation to the acme of the UC to

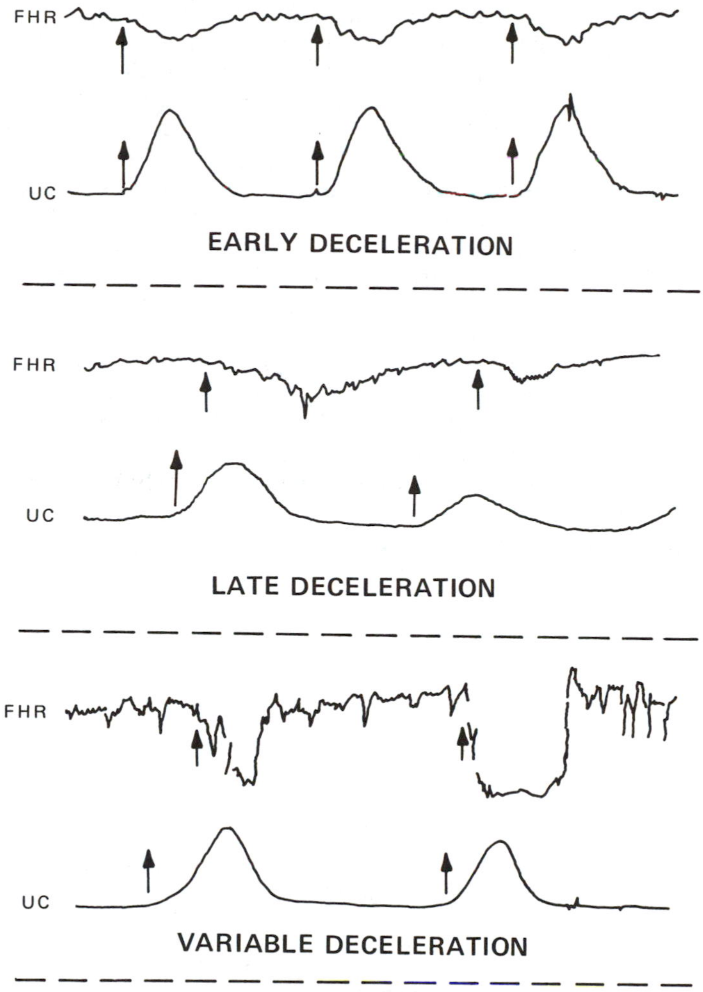

Figure 3–14. Types of fetal heart rate decelerations.

determine the existence of a late deceleration. The size of the late deceleration doesn't indicate the severity of the insult to the fetus. A late deceleration does not return to the baseline until after the end of the UC. There are several potentially *reversible* causes for late decelerations: (1) hyperstimulation with oxytocic agents and (2) maternal hypotension owing to supine position, epidural anesthesia, or hypovolemia. Other causes are usually irreversible: (1) fetal growth retardation, (2) diabetes, (3) hypertension, (4) postmaturity, and (5) placental abruption.[16] Even then the fetal status can be improved with aggressive early nursing intervention. (See next section on intervention.)

Variable deceleration may also be an indication of fetal distress and is the most common periodic change observed in labor (especially in Stage II).[14] Variable deceleration is due to umbilical cord compression or occlusion from clots in the cord. This initially obstructs blood flow through the umbilical vein to the fetus and eventually through the umbilical artery, increasing the fetal blood pressure. If cord compromise is sustained and persistent, hypoxia and metabolic acidosis may result in the fetus. This is indicated by a prolonged deceleration or slow return to the baseline.[14,17]

Variable decelerations are so named because of their variable shape (U, V, or W) and onset (in relation to the UC curve). The variable deceleration varies so that for any single contraction it might mimic an early or late deceleration. It is frequently preceded or followed by "shoulders" (Fig. 3–15,*A*). Normal shoulders last 10 to 12 seconds. "Smoothing out" (Fig. 15,*B*) of the decelerations (i.e., no accelerations following the variable) indicates worsening of the fetal condition.[14,18] Oxorn[19] indicates that a fetal position of occiput posterior may result in variable decelerations without "shoulders." Although mild variables generally result in normal fetal outcome, attempts should be made to relieve them.[14] Criteria that suggest that the variable deceleration is benign and does not require operative intervention are as follows:

1. The FHR deceleration lasts no more than 45 seconds on a repetitive basis.
2. The return of the FHR to the baseline is abrupt. There is no late component manifested by a slow return or a late deceleration after the return to baseline.
3. The baseline rate does not increase.
4. Baseline variability does not decrease.

When any of these criteria are exceeded, it may mean that the fetus is becoming hypoxic and acidotic.[19]

• •

Review Questions

1. List the three FHR deceleration patterns and their causes.
____
____
____

2. Explain the rationale for the naming of each deceleration pattern.
____
____

3. Which two FHR deceleration patterns may indicate fetal distress?
____

4. What is the significance of shoulders?______________________________
____

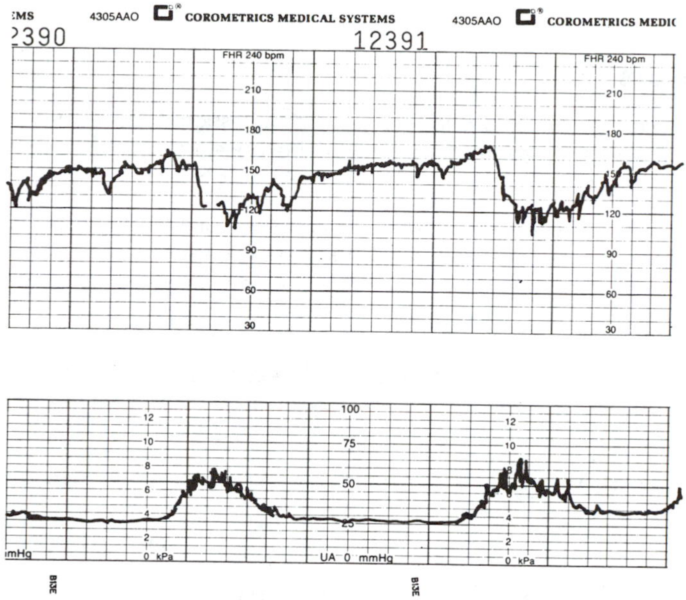

A

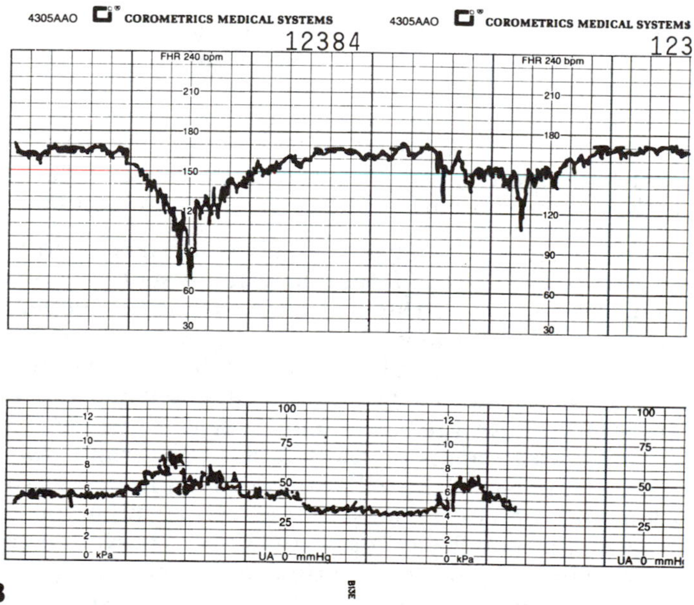

B

Figure 3–15. Variable decelerations with shoulders. (*A*) Reassuring shoulders. (*B*) Smoothing out—condition worsening.

5. What is the significance of prolonged variable deceleration?______

Answers

1. Early deceleration is due to fetal head compression. Late deceleration is due to acute uteroplacental insufficiency. Variable deceleration is due to umbilical cord compression.
2. The names of early and variable deceleration patterns are based on the time of onset of deceleration in relationship to the UC. In late decelerations the lateness of the lowest point of the FHR is noted in relation to the UC acme.
3. Both late and variable decelerations may indicate fetal distress.
4. Shoulders are reassuring accelerations seen just before or just after a variable deceleration. They indicate there is good fetal reserve to overcome the cord compression.
5. A prolonged variable deceleration indicates the fetus is distressed and likely to be hypoxic.

• •

Assessment and Intervention for FHR Decelerations

Routine assessment should be continued in the presence of reassuring patterns, that is, normal variability, early decelerations, mild variable decelerations especially if preceded and followed by shoulders, and uniform accelerations (see next section).

Intervention is necessary when late and (potentially dangerous, that is, other than mild) variable decelerations occur. The interventions for both late and variable decelerations are similar.

1. In order to increase the oxygen supply from the placenta through the umbilical cord to the fetus, the woman should be in a lateral position. The left side is the first choice. If she lies on her left side, pressure is taken off the vena cava and blood flow from the lower extremities increases. Vena cava syndrome or supine hypotension syndrome causes not only maternal hypotension but also FHR deceleration. If the FHR does not increase because the cord is compressed while she is on the left side, then right side position should be assumed. If the FHR still does not increase, knee-chest position, elevation of the legs, or the Trendelenburg position may be necessary although care must be taken to prevent compromise of the woman's respiratory function. (Some states, e.g., California, prohibit knee-chest position in the presence of ruptured membranes.)
2. Hypertonic UC may be the cause of inadequate fetal oxygenation. If oxytocin (which stimulates UC) is being infused, it should be discontinued until further evaluation of fetal status occurs.

3. Oxygen via mask may be given at 5 to 10 liters/minute. Nasal cannula is also permissible.
4. IV fluid should be given to expand the vascular bed volume and increase the blood flow to the fetus unless the woman has fluid restrictions.
5. The physician must be informed of the nursing interventions and outcomes and will need assistance if fetal blood sampling is performed. The nursing supervisor should also be informed of the critical situation.
6. All nursing interventions must be documented on the chart and/ or monitor strip. The maternal-fetal response should also be documented. This indicates that evaluation occurred.

• •

Review Question

List five nursing interventions that would be appropriate in the presence of late or variable FHR deceleration.

a. ____________________
b. ____________________
c. ____________________
d. ____________________
e. ____________________

Answer

In the presence of late or variable FHR decelerations, (a) the woman's position should be altered to facilitate fetal oxygenation; (b) infusion of oxytocin should be stopped; (c) oxygen may be given; (d) IV fluid should be started or the rate increased; and (e) the physician must be informed and assistance should be given if fetal blood sampling is performed. Nursing interventions are to be charted.

• •

Recognizing Periodic Changes: Accelerations

FHR *acceleration* is a periodic increase in the FHR. The acceleration may be *spontaneous*—associated with fetal movement or stimulation but occurring without a contraction. Spontaneous acceleration is indicative of fetal well-being. *Uniform* accelerations occur with and reflect the shape of the contraction. They are common early in labor in the presence of intact membranes, as well as in other than vertex presentations. *Variable* accelerations do not resemble the shape of UC. They appear as increased variability with contractions in the form of "shoulders" on variable decelerations (see Fig. 3–15, *A*). The accelerations mentioned so far (that is, spontaneous, uniform, and variable) are apparently benign responses. Uniform rebound accelerations or "overshoots" occur after variable decelerations and usually last *longer* than 12 seconds. Recurrent overshoots that lack baseline variability appear in a deteriorating fetus and warrant notification of the physician.

• •

Review Questions

1. Accelerations are usually (benign, ominous).
2. A suspicion of overshoots should alert the nurse to____________________________

Answers

1. Accelerations are usually *benign*.
2. Recurrent overshoots with poor variability warrant notification of the physician because of a suspicion of fetal deterioration.

• •

Variability in Fetal Heart Rate

Normally, the FHR baseline varies. You should recall that baseline is the range *between* contractions. The presence of variability suggests normal fetal central nervous system function relative to the FHR.[20] Variability is classified as short-term and long-term. Usually short- and long-term variability increase and decrease together.

Short-term variability refers to FHR changes that occur from one heart beat to the next. For example, beat by beat the rate might be 130, 134, 129, 135. The *presence of short-term variability indicates fetal reserve*—the ability of the fetus to adapt to decreased oxygen exchange during UC. The majority of fetuses with good short-term variability do well even if stressors, such as decelerations, are present. The majority with decreased variability have a good outcome if there are no associated decelerations. Although asphyxia is not the most common cause of decreased variability, almost all fetuses with significant asphyxia, and near death, have decreased or absent variability.[10,20]

There are numerous factors in the etiology of decreased variability.[10,20] (Table 3–2). A decrease may result from fetal reactions to maternal drugs. Probably the least threatening is associated with a 20- to 30-minute fetal (quiet) sleep state. The more serious conditions include fetal prematurity, congenital anomalies, acidosis, and hypoxia. Consideration should be given to the woman's history and current therapy when determining possible reasons for the decreased short-term variability. Good nursing assessment of the mother and documentation are especially important here.

Decreased variability (less than 6 BPM)[10] requires certain nursing interventions. If an external fetal monitor is in use, serious consideration should be given to using an internal fetal monitor.[7]

Table 3–2. ETIOLOGY OF DECREASED VARIABILITY

Fetal sleep state	Prematurity
Drugs	Asphyxia (acidosis, hypoxia)
Atropine—Scopolamine	Anesthesia
Tranquilizers—Diazepam	Tachycardia
Narcotics	Arrhythmias
Barbiturates	Local anesthetics

Although variability usually increases over a period of time, if the decrease is due to fetal sleep or a drug, the decrease could be from other causes. Decreased variability is threatening (ominous) if caused by hypoxia. The physician needs to be informed of the existence of decreased variability that lasts longer than 30 minutes or in combination with late decelerations. When there is no reason to suspect that other than fetal sleep is the cause of a decreased variability to less than 5 BPM, Spencer and Johnson[21] recommend waiting 45 minutes before doing fetal blood sampling (or other tests such as fetal scalp stimulation) to rule out pathologic implications. If the physician chooses to do fetal blood sampling or prepare for immediate delivery, assistance will be needed.

In *long-term variability*, rhythmic changes are assessed over a minimum of one minute to a maximum of ten minutes. For example, during a 9-minute period the FHR may vary between 128 to 140 BPM. The repetitious low FHR and repetitious high FHR during that time interval are termed the *range of long-term variability*. The pattern of 128 to 140 BPM shows a variance or range of 13 BPM (Fig. 3–16). Ignore the occasional decrease to 124 and increase to 144. The figure illustrates a range of 13 BPM and falls within the average, 5 to 15 BPM. This is interpreted as normal range for long-term variability. The following criteria are used to classify the fluctuations of long-term variability:

1. increased = >15 BPM
2. average = 5 to 15 BPM
3. decreased = <5 BPM
4. absent = <2 BPM[20]

Over a 1- to 10-minute period, the fluctuation of long-term variability may consistently appear wavey (Fig. 3–17, *A*). This wavy line is called sinu wave and is characteristic of a *sinusoidal pattern* of long-term variability. It is important to note the range of the long-term variability of the wave because fluctuations of more than 25 BPM (from the bottom of one wave to the top of the next) are an ominous sign of fetal deterioration.[22] In that case the physician must be notified immediately. A sinusoidal pattern of less than 25 BMP also requires physician notification.[10,14,15]

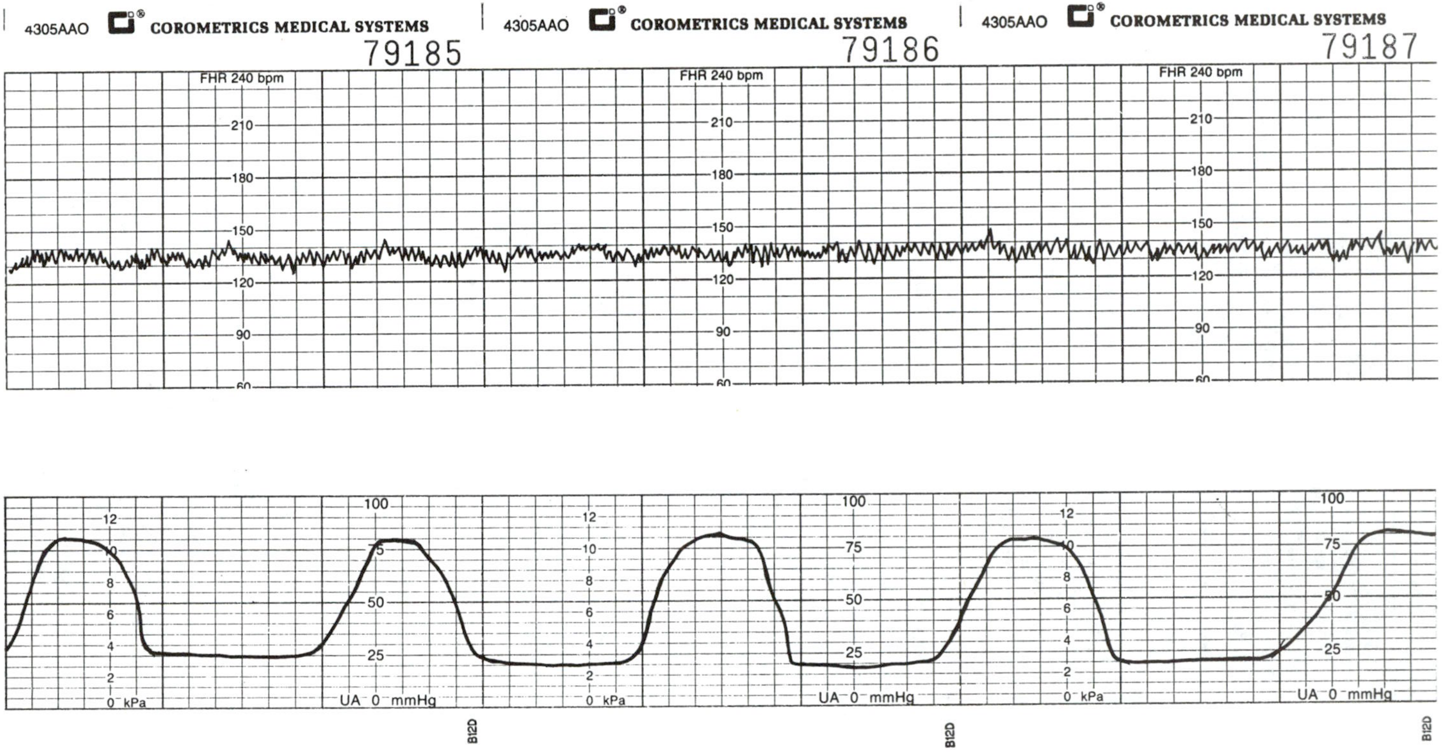

Figure 3–16. Range of long-term variability: 128 to 140 bpm.

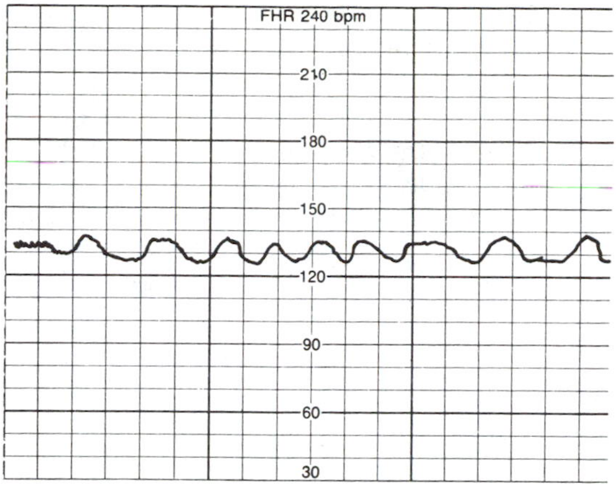

A. Sinusoidal

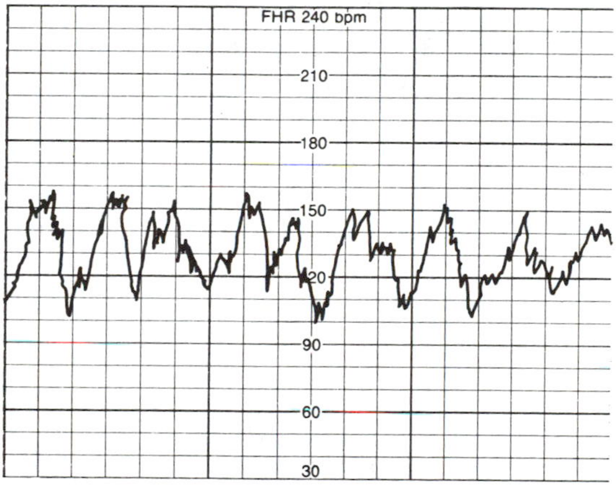

B. Saltatory

Figure 3–17. Variability patterns. (*A*) Sinusoidal. (*B*) Saltatory.

There are two types of sinusoidal patterns: (1) pseudo and (2) true. The pseudosinusoidal is a temporary wavy pattern in which short-term beat-to-beat variability exists. The pseudosinusoidal commonly occurs following the administration of a narcotic or from stress on the fetus, such as from cord compression. True sinusoidal is continuous and lacks beat-to-beat changes. True sinusoidal is due to fetal anemia.

A leaping or *saltatory pattern* is a form of increased variability (Fig. 3–17,*B*). When it occurs alone, no intervention is necessary. The saltatory pattern may have a nonthreatening acceleration with fetal movement or be the response of a highly reactive nervous system. However, the saltatory pattern is usually found following moderate or severe variable decelerations.[20] In this case it probably involves fetal cardiovascular readjustment.

When speaking of good and poor variability (with no indication of long or short term), the reference should be to *only* short-term variability, and then only to baseline variability, not to changes during a deceleration or UC. In most cases, *only internal fetal monitoring provides accurate short-term variability information.* Variability of greater than 5 rarely means other than a normal pH.[21] (See Chapter 9 for more information on fetal pH.)

• •

Review Questions

1. Short-term variability refers to changes in the heart rate from ______________ to ______________.
2. Average long-term variability is ______________ BPM and refers to a period of ______________ minutes.
3. Circle the correct term in the parentheses: When describing variability, the nurse should refer to (short, long) term variability, occurring during (a contraction, a deceleration, neither a contraction nor a deceleration).
4. After administration of a narcotic, a wavy, ______________ pattern may occur. Its presence (should, need not) be communicated to the physician.
5. A saltatory pattern appears as a ______________ and predicts the possible occurrence of ______________ decelerations.

Answers

1. Short-term variability refers to changes in the heart rate from *beat* to *beat*.
2. The average long term variability is *5 to 15* BPM and refers to a *1 to 10*-minute period.
3. Variability means *short*-term variability occurring during *neither a contraction nor deceleration*.
4. A *sinusoidal* pattern is wavy and commonly occurs after giving a narcotic. Its presence *should* be shared with the physician.
5. A saltatory pattern looks like a *leap* and may be associated with *variable* decelerations. This combination is a concern.

• •

CONCLUSION

It is important that nurses and physicians recognize that the laboring woman and her fetus are the primary recipients of health care. Although the assessment of uterine contractions and fetal heart rate are essential, the electronic monitor is only one source of data. Under normal circumstances, the monitor may be unnecessary. Regardless of the assessment methodology used, efforts should be made to maintain the laboring woman's self-esteem, to make her as comfortable as possible, and to provide her with the opportunity for informed consent. The woman and her significant other(s) should be given explanations of what is occurring. They need to be made aware that critical information must be obtained through ongoing assessment and that certain situations warrant specific interventions by the health care team. A trusting relationship with open communication fosters a favorable outcome.

As this chapter indicates, assessment of UC and fetal response is not a simple procedure. Depending on the findings, assessment every 30 minutes during Stage I and every 15 minutes during Stage II may not be frequent enough. A nonreassuring pattern requires that the nurse initiate appropriate nursing interventions, depending on the pattern identified, and notify the physician. In cases where the physician does not respond in a timely fashion and/or manner, hospital policy should provide guidelines for the nurse to follow. The information in this chapter may not be all-inclusive as maternal-fetal monitoring is a continuously developing body of knowledge. Nurses are encouraged to continue to update their skills and knowledge regarding established guidelines and technological advances in maternal-fetal monitoring.

REFERENCES

1. Oxorn, H: Oxorn-Foote: Human Labor and Birth, ed 5. Appleton-Century-Crofts, Norwalk, Connecticut, 1986, p 657.
2. Stephany, T: Terbutaline sulfate for treating tetanic contractions. Matern Child Nurs J 10:394, 1985.
3. Vice, L: Fetal Monitoring Level II. Medical Media Associates Conference, Ann Arbor, Michigan, October 27, 1986.
4. Lipshitz, J and Klose, C: Use of tocolytic drugs to reverse oxytocin-induced uterine hypertonus and fetal distress. Obstet Gynecol 66:165, 1985.
5. Bobak, IM and Jensen, MD: Essentials of Maternity Nursing: The Nurse and the Childbearing Family, CV Mosby, St. Louis, 1987, p G-3.
6. Bracero, LA, et al: Fetal heart rate characteristics that provide confidence in the diagnosis of fetal well-being. Clin Obstet Gynecol 29:3, 1986.
7. Cohen, WR and Yeh, S: The abnormal fetal heart rate baseline. Clin Obstet Gynecol 29:73, 1986.
8. Dudley, DKL: Assessment of the Fetus in Utero. In Oxorn, H: Oxorn-Foote: Human Labor and Birth, ed 5. Appleton-Century-Crofts, Norwalk, Connecticut, 1986, p 617.
9. Schifrin, BS: Exercises in Fetal Monitoring, Vol 1. BPM, Los Angeles, 1985, p 7.
10. Quirk, JG and Miller, FC: FHR tracing characteristics that jeopardize the diagnosis of fetal well-being. Clin Obstet Gynecol 29:12, 1986.

11. Reece, EA, et al: The fetus as the final arbiter of intrauterine stress/distress. Clin Obstet Gynecol 29:23, 1986.
12. LaSala, AP and Strassner, HT: Fetal death. Clin Obstet Gynecol 29:95, 1986.
13. Dudley, DKL: Assessment of the Fetus in Utero. In Oxorn, H: Oxorn-Foote: Human Labor and Birth, ed 5. Appleton-Century-Crofts, Norwalk, Connecticut, 1986, p 618.
14. Schneider EP and Tropper, PJ: The variable deceleration, prolonged deceleration, and sinusoidal fetal heart rate. Clin Obstet Gynecol 29:64, 1986.
15. Schifrin, BS: Exercises in Fetal Monitoring, Vol 1. BPM, Los Angeles, 1985, p 9.
16. Dudley, DKL: Assessment of the Fetus in Utero. In Oxorn, H: Oxorn-Foote: Human Labor and Birth, ed 5. Appleton-Century-Crofts, Norwalk, Connecticut, 1986, p 626.
17. Dudley, DKL: Assessment of the Fetus in Utero. In Oxorn, H: Oxorn-Foote: Human Labor and Birth, ed 5. Appleton-Century-Crofts, Norwalk, Connecticut, 1986, p 627.
18. Schifrin, BS: Exercises in Fetal Monitoring, Vol 1. BPM, Los Angeles, 1985, p 11.
19. Dudley, DKL: Assessment of the Fetus in Utero. In Oxorn, H: Oxorn-Foote: Human Labor and Birth, ed 5. Appleton-Century-Crofts, Norwalk, Connecticut, 1986, p 628.
20. Schifrin, BS: Exercises in Fetal Monitoring, Vol 1. BPM, Los Angeles, 1985, p 8.
21. Spencer, JAD and Johnson, P: Fetal heart rate variability changes and fetal behavioural cycles during labour. Br J Obstet Gynaecol 93:314, 1986.
22. Pritchard, JA, MacDonald, PC, and Gant, NF: Williams Obstetrics, ed 17. Appleton-Century-Crofts, Norwalk, Connecticut, 1985, p 287.

BIBLIOGRAPHY

American College of Obstetricians and Gynecologists: State-of-the-Art Electronic Fetal Monitoring Committee Statement. ACOG, Washington, DC, 1985.

Blank, JJ: Electronic fetal monitoring: Nursing management defined. J Obstet Gynecol Neonatal Nurs 14:463, 1985.

Bracero, LA, et al: Fetal heart rate characteristics that provide confidence in the diagnosis of fetal well-being. Clin Obstet Gynecol 29:3, 1986.

Cohen, WR and Yeh, S: The abnormal fetal heart rate baseline. Clin Obstet Gynecol 29:73, 1986.

Dauphinee, JD: The Basics of Fetal Heart Rate Monitoring Interpretation. National Conference on Obstetric Nursing, Dearborn, Michigan, April 22, 1987.

Dauphinee, JD: Complex and Unusual Fetal Heart Rate Patterns: Challenging Your Skills. National Conferences on Obstetric Nursing, Dearborn, Michigan, April 23, 1987.

Gordon, M: Manual of Nursing Diagnosis, 1986–87. McGraw-Hill, New York, 1987.

LaSala, AP and Strassner, HT: Fetal death. Clin Obstet Gynecol 29:95, 1986.

Lipshitz, J and Klose, C: Use of tocolytic drugs to reverse oxytocin-induced uterine hypertonus and fetal distress. Obstet Gynecol 66:165, 1985.

Low, JA, et al: The relationship between antepartum fetal heart rate, intrapartum fetal heart rate, and fetal acid-base status. Am J Obstet Gynecol 154:769, 1986.

NAACOG: Electronic Fetal Monitoring: Nursing Practice Competencies and Educational Guidelines. NAACOG, Washington, DC, 1986.

NAACOG: Standards for Obstetric, Gynecologic, and Neonatal Nursing, ed 2. NAACOG, Washington, DC, 1981.

NAACOG: Standards for Obstetric, Gynecologic, and Neonatal Nursing, ed 3. NAACOG, Washington, DC, 1986.

Oxorn, H: Oxorn-Foote: Human Labor and Birth, ed 5. Appleton-Century-Crofts, Norwalk, Connecticut, 1986.

Pritchard, JA, MacDonald, PC, and Gant, NF: Williams Obstetrics, ed 17. Appleton-Century-Croft, Norwalk, Connecticut, 1985.

Quirk, JG and Miller, FC: FHR tracing characteristics that jeopardize the diagnosis of fetal well-being. Clin Obstet Gynecol 29:12, 1986.

Reece, EA, et al: The fetus as the final arbiter of intrauterine stress/distress. Clin Obstet Gynecol 29:23, 1986.

Schifrin, BS: Exercises in Fetal Monitoring, Vol I. BPM, Los Angeles, 1985.

Schneider, EP and Tropper, PJ: The variable deceleration, prolonged deceleration, and sinusoidal fetal heart rate. Clin Obstet Gynecol 29:64, 1986.

Spencer, JAD and Johnson, P: Fetal heart rate variability changes and fetal behavioural cycles during labour. Br J Obstet Gynaecol 93:314, 1986.

Stephany, T: Terbutaline sulfate for treating tetanic contractions. Matern Child Nurs J 10:394, 1985.

Vice, L: Fetal Monitoring Level II. Medical Media Associates Conference, Ann Arbor, Michigan, October 27, 1986.

3 POST-TEST

1. Assessment of UC involves determination of activity in the uterine ____________________, since this is where the activity is __________. The parts of the UC include the following: the increasing intensity, called the ________, the strongest part, called the ________; and the decrease in intensity, called the _____.

2. UC are described by the following three terms. Define them.
   a. frequency: ____________________
   b. duration: ____________________
   c. intensity: ____________________

3. In the following situations, designate the correct term for the uterine activity:
   a. palpable band between upper and lower portions of myometrium: ____________________
   b. normally progressing UC become less frequent and less intense: ____________________
   c. UC 90 seconds duration or longer: ____________________
   d. normal uterine activity state between UC: ____________________
   e. UC that begin in the uterine body: ____________________
   f. two consecutive UC that have less than 30 seconds relaxation between them: ____________________
   g. uterine activity that from the start of labor continues to be weak and ineffective: ____________________
   h. extremely forceful UC: ____________________
   i. weak ineffective UC: ____________________

4. Is it acceptable to:
   a. palpate the uterus between UC? _____ Why? ____________________

b. palpate the uterus throughout several UC? ____ Why? ________

c. base your assessment of UC on the mother's description? ____ Why? ________

5. In the presence of which of the following situations would you consider using a continuous UC monitor (C) instead of relying on intermittent assessment by palpation (I):
   a. during suspected primary or secondary uterine dysfunction? ____
   b. during suspected tetanic UC? ________
   c. during suspected coupling of UC? ________
   d. during suspected hypotonic or hypertonic UC? ________
   e. during UC that are subjectively more painful to the mother than they objectively feel to the examiner? ________

6. What criteria must exist before an internal UC and/or FHR monitor can be applied?
   a. ________
   b. ________
   c. ________

7. Using "F" for fetoscope, "D" for Doppler unit or intermittent EFM, "E" for external EFM, and "I" for internal EFM, indicate which FHR assessment apparatus would be best to use in the following situations:
   a. ____ Early uncomplicated labor
   b. ____ Oxytocin induction; membranes intact.
   c. ____ Normal FHR and UC; continuous monitoring preferred.
   d. ____ Occasional variable decelerations following rupture of membranes.
   e. ____ On the delivery table with sterile drapes in place.

8. Use the correct term to describe each of the following FHR?
   a. baseline of 100 to 120 = ________
   b. periodic decrease with contractions = ________
   c. muffled sound consistent with maternal pulse but suspected to be FHR = ________
   d. an increase in FHR briefly before and after variable deceleration = ________
   e. a smooth wavy long-term variability = ________

9. Briefly chart and interpret the following patient data:
   Situation A: Following 20 minutes on the external monitors, the FHR was seen to move frequently between 120 to 145, with a 1- to 2-second 160 BPM, when the mother felt the fetus move. Contractions were starting every 2 to 3 minutes and causing a slight decrease in FHR to 120 at the acme. The contractions were slightly indentable and were 40 to 50 seconds from beginning to end.
   Your charting:
   ____
   ____
   ____
   ____

Your interpretation:

____
____
____
____
____

Situation B: The patient is rocking back and forth in bed, causing the monitors to trace poorly. She says the monitors bother her, and she wants them removed. Furthermore, she is disturbed by the IV infusing oxytocin. Doctor Smith proceeds to replace the external monitors with internal EFM, using standard procedure, while the nurse explains the hows and whys. The monitor tracings give clear patterns with contractions starting every 1½ to 2 minutes, lasting 50 to 75 seconds—some with 20 seconds resting time—reaching 60 mm Hg pressure. FHR ranges from 130 to 134 between contractions with a consistent decrease to 115 beginning after the acme.

Your charting:

____
____
____
____
____

Your interpretation:

____
____
____
____
____

Answers to Post-Test

1. Uterine activity is determined in the *fundus*, since this is where uterine activity is *dominant*. The increasing intensity is the *increment*; the strongest part is the *acme*; the decreasing intensity is the *decrement*.

2. (a) Frequency is from the onset of one UC until the onset of the next. (b) Duration is from the beginning until the end of the UC. (c) Intensity is the strength of the UC at its acme.

3. a. *Bandl's* or *pathologic contraction ring* is a palpable band between the upper and lower portions of the myometrium.
   b. *Secondary uterine dysfunction* occurs when normally progressing UC become less frequent and less intense.
   c. *Tetanic contractions* are of 90 seconds duration or longer.
   d. *Tonus* (or the rested status) is the normal uterine activity state between contractions.
   e. *Incoordinate contractions* are UC that begin in other than the fundus.
   f. *Coupling* is two consecutive contractions that have less than 30 to 60 seconds relaxation between them.

g. *Primary uterine dysfunction* is uterine activity that from the start of labor continues to be weak and ineffective.
h. *Hypertonic* UC are extremely forceful UC.
i. *Hypotonic* UC are weak, ineffective UC.

4. a. Palpation of the uterus between UC is acceptable to determine the tonus and length of rest interval.
   b. Palpating the uterus throughout the UC is acceptable to determine the time of onset, the duration, the intensity (at the acme), and rest interval. Palpating several UC gives a basis of comparison for increase in frequency, duration, and intensity.
   c. Basing your assessment of UC on the mother's description is not acceptable, because her interpretation is not objective.

5. In all of the situations (a through e) continuous assessment is necessary to verify if abnormal UC patterns exist. The external monitor provides a continuous measurement of the UC frequency and durations. More precise information is provided by an intrauterine pressure catheter, including the UC intensity.

6. Before internal UC and/or FHR monitors can be applied, (a) the cervix must be dilated 2 to 3 cm or more, (b) the membranes must be ruptured, and (c) the fetal presenting part must be reachable.

7. a. F— In early uncomplicated labor a fetoscope is used.
   b. E— When membranes are intact but continuous monitoring is needed because of the oxytocin induction, an external EFM is used.
   c. E— When continuous graphing is desirable and the FHR and UC are normal, external EFM is satisfactory.
   d. I— Occasional variable decelerations following rupture of membranes require an internal EFM if the criteria of cervical dilatation and reachable presenting part exist.
   e. D—On the delivery table when the sterile drapes are in place, a Doppler unit is used (or possibly an external EFM).

8. Terms used to describe FHR include:
   a. A baseline of 100 to 120 is *bradycardia.*
   b. Periodic decrease with contractions is *deceleration.*
   c. A muffled sound in the FHR consistent with the maternal pulse is a *uterine souffle.*
   d. A brief FHR increase before and after variable decelerations is *shoulders.*
   e. A smooth wavy long-term variability is a *sinusoidal pattern.*

9. *Situation A:*
   Charting: External EFM in place. FHR 120–145 baseline, accels with fetal activity, early decels noted. UC q 2–3½ mins., 40–60 sec. mod. intensity.
   Interpretation: All normal—baseline, healthy response from fetus, head compression with UC, UC that should eventually cause cervical changes.
   Situation B:
   Charting: Pt. restless. Requesting monitors' removal. Poor tracings. Dr. Smith applied int. EFM and IUC using sterile technique. Procedure and purpose explained by nurse. Good tracings resulted. UC q 1½–2 min., some with 20 sec.

of tonus, 50–75 sec. duration, 60 mm Hg intensity. FHR minimal variability 130–134 with late decels to 115.
Interpretation: Due to patient's intolerance of external monitors and poor tracings, internal monitors were warranted (assuming criteria for such are met). Uterus was hyperactive with strong, too frequent UC and insufficient resting time between contractions. This resulted in uterine-placental insufficiency (late decels), which requires turning the mother to her left, discontinuing or decreasing the oxytocin flow, and constantly monitoring UC and FHR. If late decels continue, the mother should be given oxygen and possibly placed in Trendelenburg or with legs elevated. Keep the doctor informed. Inform the mother of the reasons for these urgent interventions without increasing her anxiety if possible. Cautious measures can be relaxed upon occurrence of q 2–3 minute or less frequent UC with resting interval of at least 30 sec. and FHR varying 6 to approximately 15 BPM between 120–160 with no late or variable decels.

4 GRAPHING LABOR CURVES

Janet S. Malinowski

OBJECTIVES

Upon completing this chapter, you will be able to:

- ▶ Describe Friedman's method of plotting labor patterns.
- ▶ Identify the phases of the S curve seen in a normal cervical dilatation curve.
- ▶ Use a reference that designates the normal time limits for the two dilatation phases.
- ▶ Explain briefly the role of "stress hormones" in prolonging labor.
- ▶ Diagram and state the criteria for, associated factors of, and interventions for the following abnormal dilatation patterns: precipitous labor, prolonged latent phase, slow slope active phase, and arrest of the active phase.
- ▶ Differentiate between normal and abnormal descent patterns in a nullipara and a multipara.
- ▶ State the criteria for protracted descent and arrest of descent.
- ▶ List at least five assessment data the nurse should utilize when evaluating labor curves.
- ▶ Identify five nursing diagnoses that are appropriate for abnormal labor curves.
- ▶ Describe five nursing interventions, with their rationale, pertinent to prolonged labor.
- ▶ Given specific data about a patient in labor, interpret the labor curves and explain the theory that supports the interpretation.
- ▶ Plot all given data on a graph, and draw conclusions about the meaning of the data and the appropriate nursing interventions to be taken.

Graphing the course of a labor is an efficient way to objectively document labor progress as measured by cervical dilatation and fetal descent curves. Although Friedman's labor curves provide guidelines, they are not absolutes. Clinical judgment must always be used in individual situations. The purposes of graphing labor include:

1. assessment of the rate of cervical dilatation and fetal descent,
2. assessment of the effects of nursing interventions, medications and medical procedures,
3. assessment of labor curves to facilitate nursing interventions that *promote* normal labor progress, and
4. provision of legal documentation of labor curves.

By knowing what is normal and what is abnormal on the graph, the nurse can assess labor progress in order to facilitate a safer outcome for the mother and her baby. This chapter presents the basic information that the nurse should know about graphing the curves of Stage I of labor.

METHODOLOGY OF GRAPHING STAGE I LABOR PATTERNS

In 1964, Emanual A. Friedman introduced his analysis of the labor patterns of 500 nulliparous (first labor) and 500 multiparous (other than first labor) women. He graphically recorded their labor patterns and established normal time limits for the various phases of labor. The validity of Friedman's curves is questioned by some because of methodologic flaws, yet hundreds of thousands of labors have been analyzed using his guidelines.

In Friedman's method the labor pattern is plotted on square-ruled paper, with each square being of equal value (Fig. 4–1). The left vertical scale indicates the ascending cervical dilatation (in centimeters from 0 to 10) and is marked with a small circle. The right scale, the descending station (going from minus to plus), is marked with an X. The horizontal axis indicates the time in hours—from onset of labor until complete dilatation. Each time a vaginal exam is performed, the cervical dilatation and station for that time are graphed. It is also helpful to record any other significant interventions (for example, rupture of membranes, administration of medication) at the time they are performed. That way the effects of the interventions can be visualized on the succeeding labor curves.

The time of onset of labor is not clear-cut. A common misconception is that rupture of membranes or occasional contractions indicate the onset. Most authorities say that the *onset of labor* is the time when the woman experiences *regular* uterine contractions that

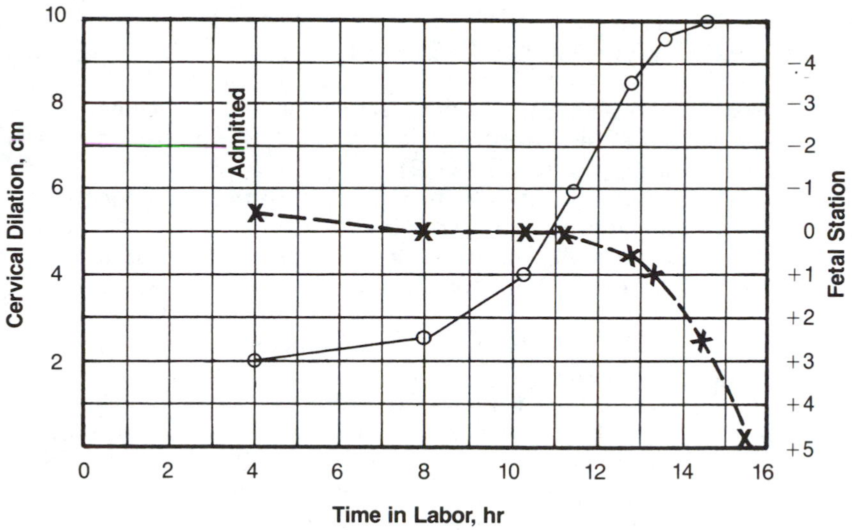

Figure 4–1. Labor pattern plotted using Friedman's method.

lead to progressive cervical changes—dilatation and effacement. Until a regular pattern occurs, true labor has not begun.

• •

Review Questions

1. The two results from each ______________ exam that are routinely plotted on the labor graph are ______________ and ______________.
2. These results are spaced on vertical lines according to the ______________ at which the exams are performed.
3. The onset of labor should be plotted as the time when ______________ ______________.

Answers

1. The two results from each *vaginal* exam that are routinely plotted on the labor graph are *cervical dilatation* and *station*.
2. The results of vaginal exams are recorded according to the *time* at which the exams are performed, with each vertical line being worth an equal amount of time.
3. The onset of labor should be plotted as the time when regular contractions begin, *not* rupture of membranes or occasional contractions.

• •

PHASES OF THE S CURVE IN A NORMAL CERVICAL DILATATION PATTERN

Friedman found that the normal labor pattern of cervical dilatation has an S-shape and that this curve could be divided into two phases: latent and active (Fig. 4–2).

The *latent phase* extends from the onset of regular uterine contractions to the beginning of the increased incline of the active phase—approximately 3-cm dilatation. The nullipara may normally spend up to 20 hours in this phase and the multipara up to 14 hours. As Table 4–1 indicates, the mean time is considerably less. Recall that the mean is the middle between two extremes. The mean number is midway between an equal number of shorter and longer time intervals. During the latent phase the nurse needs to help the laboring woman to relax, both physically and mentally. This is the time to establish rapport, to familiarize the woman with her surroundings, and to discuss the expected occurrences of labor (see Chapter 1).

The latent phase has a barely visible incline. It almost appears flat. During this time the cervix becomes more effaced but only dilates slightly. The duration of the phase is sensitive to extraneous factors. A sedative would prolong it, whereas an enema (stimulant) might shorten it. Although normally more than half the time spent in labor involves the latent phase, its length is no indication of how long the active phase will be.

During the *active phase* the graphic curve begins to incline almost vertically. The phase ends at complete cervical dilatation (10 cm—the end of Stage I). The nurse should anticipate that numerous signs of progress will occur during this phase (see Chapter 1).

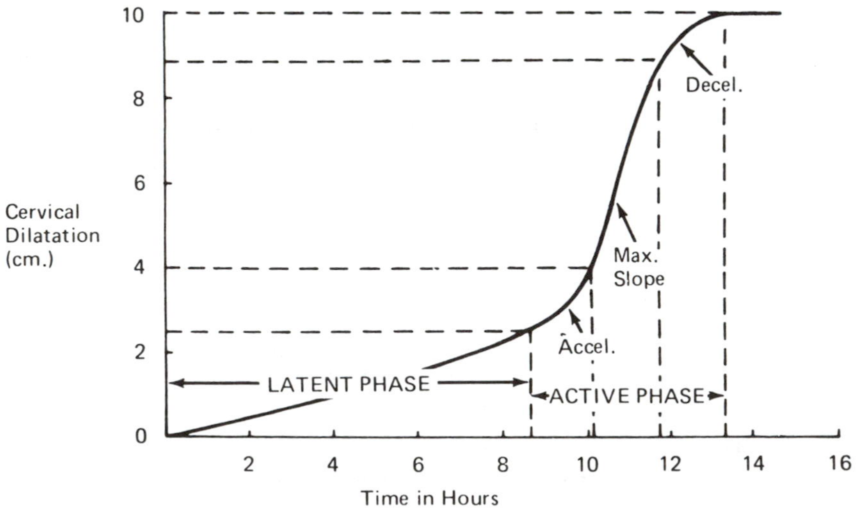

Figure 4–2. Mean labor curve of a nullipara.

Table 4–1. MEANS OF TIME IN STAGE I

	NULLIPARA	MULTIPARA
Latent phase	6.4 hr (20.1)*	4.8 hr (13.6)*
Active phase	4.6 hr (11.7)*	2.4 hr (5.2) *

*Maximum limit of normal

Adapted from Friedman, E: Labor: Clinical Evaluation and Management, ed 2. Appleton-Century-Crofts, New York, 1978, p 49.

Effective labor results in progressive cervical dilatation. Increased pain will require comfort measures, relaxation techniques, and possibly analgesia. The nullipara normally spends up to 12 hours in this phase. Up to 6 hours is normal for the multiparous woman. See Table 4–1 for the mean times.

The active phase is subdivided into three parts. During the *acceleration phase* the cervix begins to dilate more rapidly. During the *phase of maximum slope* (also termed *transition*) the inclination (slope) is steep. The major portion of cervical dilatation occurs here. Last is the *deceleration phase*—a slowing down in the rate of cervical dilatation just prior to complete dilatation. Often this phase is very short. Unless the cervical dilatation is assessed at exactly the right time, a slowing down in the dilatation rate may not be evident.

The S-shaped curve seen in Figure 4–2 is normal for both nulliparous and multiparous women. The length of time that each one spends in each phase differs (refer to Table 4–1). Note that the multipara's times are consistently shorter. The mean length of Stage I for the nullipara is 11 hours, whereas the mean for the multiparous woman is approximately 7 hours. The graph does not enable the nurse to predict the exact time of delivery, but it does document progress, or the lack of progress, in Stage I of labor.

• •

Review Question

Stage I is divided into phases in the following way:

1. ______________________________

2. ______________________________

   a. ______________________________

   b. ______________________________

   c. ______________________________

Answer

Stage I is divided into (1) the *latent phase* and (2) the *active phase*, which is subdivided into (a) *acceleration phase*, (b) *phase of maximum slope* (or *transition*), and (c) *deceleration phase*.

• •

ABNORMAL CERVICAL DILATATION PATTERNS

Friedman identified several abnormal cervical dilatation patterns. *Precipitous labor* involves an extremely short Stage I. On the other hand, the *prolonged latent phase, slow slope* (or *protracted*) *active phase,* and *arrest of the active phase* all involve time beyond the established normal limits for a specific phase. Figure 4–3 presents a graphic view of these abnormal patterns. The primary causes of these prolonged labors are fetopelvic disproportion, malpresentation and malposition, and inefficient uterine action.

DEFINITIONS, ASSOCIATED FACTORS, AND INTERVENTIONS FOR ABNORMAL DILATATION PATTERNS

Precipitous Labor

Labor in which complete dilatation occurs in less than 2 or 3 hours is generally called *precipitous labor.* Friedman is more specific and defines it as rates of dilatation greater than 5 cm per hour in nulliparas, and 10 cm per hour in multiparas.

Less resistance from the maternal soft tissues makes precipitous labor more likely in the multipara than in the nullipara. Other conditions that predispose to precipitous labor include large pelvis,

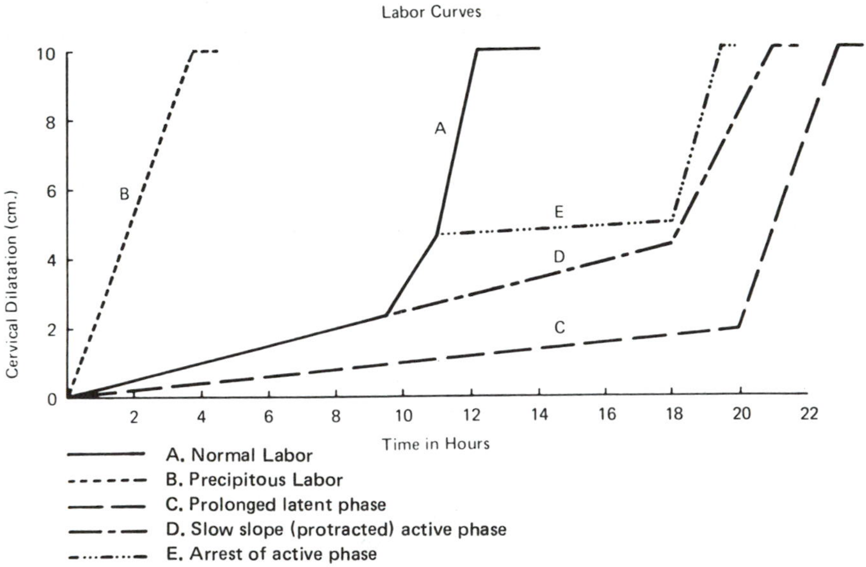

Figure 4–3. Labor curves of nulliparous women.

small baby in favorable position, and very frequent (every 1½ to 2 minutes), long (50 to 60 seconds), intense contractions (increasing 50 mm Hg or more). Upon rupture of membranes and/or oxytocin infusion, labor may also accelerate considerably (see Chapter 5).

Frequent nursing assessment is imperative during precipitous labor. Ideally, the nurse is constantly present. This means calling for help that is needed and not leaving the laboring woman. Careful assessment must be made of the fetal heart rate because there is a significant decrease in oxygen supply when the mother has tumultuous (vigorous) contractions (see tetanic contractions in Chapter 3). Especially when stimulated by oxytocin (see Chapter 5), uterine rupture could result. Evidence of uterine rupture may be severe, abrupt abdominal pain, cessation of contractions, vaginal bleeding, and shock. A decreasing or nonexistent fetal heart rate indicates fetal distress. (See Chapter 8 for more details.) Uterine stimulation with oxytocin is often the cause of precipitous labor. If oxytocin is being used, it must immediately be discontinued. Other interventions rarely slow this fast-moving labor pattern. The nurse should prepare for a supervised, controlled, and preferably sterile delivery and, at the same time, meet the psychologic needs of a woman undergoing a very stressful event.

The following nursing diagnoses may be appropriate for the woman experiencing precipitous labor:

1. **Injury, potential for, trauma (to fetus) related to hypoxia.**
2. **Injury, potential for, trauma (to mother) related to vigorous uterine contractions.**
3. **Comfort, alterations in: pain, acute related to uterine contractions.**
4. **Anxiety [specify] related to unexpected, rapid labor.**

Precipitous labor and *precipitous delivery* are not the same. The latter is a sudden, unexpected birth that is often unattended by the physician or midwife, or necessary equipment. (See Chapter 1 for nursing interventions.) Precipitous delivery may follow an extremely rapid labor or, very rarely, uterine contractions that are not felt by the laboring woman.

• •

Review Questions

1. Precipitous labor involves cervical dilatation at rates of greater than __________ cm per hour in the nullipara and __________ cm per hour in the multipara.

2. Factors that are associated with this very rapid cervical dilatation and fetal descent are:
   a. ____________________
   b. ____________________
   c. ____________________

3. **Identify three potential problems that may occur with precipitous labor: a. ______________, b. ______________, c. ______________.**

4. **List six nursing interventions that should occur during a precipitous labor.**
   a. ______________________________
   b. ______________________________
   c. ______________________________
   d. ______________________________
   e. ______________________________
   f. ______________________________

Answers

1. Precipitous labor involves cervical dilatation at rates of greater than 5 cm per hour in the nullipara and 10 cm per hour in the multipara.

2. Factors that are associated with this very rapid cervical dilatation and fetal descent are: (a) *little resistance from maternal soft tissues*, (b) *large pelvis*, (c) *small baby in favorable position*, (d) *frequent intense uterine contractions*, and (e) *uterine stimulation with rupture of membranes and/or oxytocin*.

3. Potential problems that may occur with precipitous labor include: (a) *fetal injury*, (b) *maternal injury*, (c) *discomfort* and *anxiety*.

4. Nursing interventions during a precipitous labor include:
   a. *constantly stay with the laboring woman*
   b. *assess fetal heart rate for signs of distress*
   c. *observe for signs of uterine rupture*
   d. *stop oxytocin infusion immediately (if oxytocin is being used)*
   e. *facilitate a supervised, controlled, sterile delivery*
   f. *provide psychologic support*

• •

Prolonged Labor

There is no simple explanation for why some labors are prolonged. In the succeeding sections, several possible causes for each type of prolongation are given. The stress phenomenon plays a major role in prolonging labor. When stressed, humans produce (1) catecholamines ("stress hormones"), which include epinephrine and norephinephrine, and (2) cortisol. Labor is a stressful event with physical and psychologic demands. The woman experiences pain, exerts much effort while coping with labor, and may be anxious, fearful, and at times, angry. Excess catecholamine and cortisol production can lead to vasconstriction of the uterine blood vessels, resulting in uterine hypoxia and/or decreased placental perfusion. A uterus with inadequate blood flow does not contract adequately, resulting in prolonged, dysfunctional labor or an arrest of labor. If placental perfusion is decreased, fetal hypoxia can also occur, resulting in fetal distress. By providing the laboring woman with supportive care, including sedatives or anesthesia if necessary, not only is the pain and anxiety decreased, but so is the production of catecholamines and cortisol.

Prolonged Latent Phase. According to Friedman, this abnormal curve occurs when the latent phase is 20 hours or more in a nullipara and 14 hours or more in a multipara. The ambiguous definition of onset of labor makes diagnosis of this abnormality especially difficult.

The most frequent factors associated with prolonged latent phase are as follows:

- Excessive sedation (via narcotic, analgesic or sedative) and anesthesia—the appropriate intervention is to allow time for the effect to wear off.
- False labor—this is treated by rest. Actually the woman is not in the latent phase since true labor has not begun.
- Unripe (thick, uneffaced) cervix—the unripe cervix prolongs only the latent phase. Supportive nursing care is warranted. Once effacement begins, the cervix usually dilates normally. Stimulation via oxytocin and/or amniotomy will be effective only when the cervix is effaced, soft, and dilated 2 to 3 cm.
- Myometrial dysfunction—upon administering oxytocin stimulation, which is highly effective for hypotonic uterine contractions (see Chapter 3), the prolonged latent phase may be terminated. In retrospect the conclusion is that the prolongation was due to myometrial dysfunction.
- Malposition, specifically occiput posterior (OP) and occiput transverse (OT)—this is less frequently associated with prolonged latent phase than those factors previously mentioned. Nursing interventions for malposition are described in Chapter 2.

Supportive nursing care during the prolonged latent phase should promote continuation of the usual activities of daily living. Supportive therapy is warranted in the form of reassurance, nourishment (light eating, oral fluids, or IV glucose solution), and comfort measures to reduce pain and promote sleep (warm bath or shower, massage, ambulation, or medication). Rarely should intravenous therapy and medication be needed except in situations where vomiting or severe pain exist.

The medical management of prolonged latent phase may involve efforts to stop the contractions or stimulate them, or both. An effective terminator of prolonged latent phase is an initial dose of 15 mg morphine subcutaneously, followed 20 minutes later by an additional 10 mg of morphine if needed. The intent is to temporarily stop contractions and provide therapeutic rest. Frequently, several stimulation therapies are tried; for example, ambulation, enema, artificial rupture of membranes (of questionable effectiveness), and, if still necessary, administration of oxytocin. All of these methods may be effective in stimulating uterine contractions and cervical dilatation (see Chapter 5). Cesarean delivery, however, is not a treatment for this abnormality if fetal well-being is apparent.

The prognosis for prolonged latent phase is good. Most labors progress to the active phase. A prolonged latent phase supposedly does not endanger the laboring woman. However, if it goes untreated, maternal exhaustion, low morale, and possibly dehydration and intrauterine infection (if membranes are ruptured) may occur. A prolonged latent phase does slightly increase the risk of fetal/neonatal damage and death.

• •

Review Questions

1. In humans, the stress of labor may produce an excess of ________ and ________. The excess can cause vasoconstriction of ________ blood vessels resulting in decreased ________ perfusion. In turn, there can be prolonged/arrested ________ and/or fetal ________.
2. A prolonged latent phase is one that is greater than ____ hours in a nullipara and greater than ____ hours in a multipara.
3. Prolonged latent phase is closely associated with: (a) ________, (b) ________, (c) ________, (d) ________, and (e) ________.
4. Supportive nursing care during prolonged latent phase includes: (a) ________, (b) ________ and (c) ________.
5. Two general medical approaches to prolonged latent phase are: (a) ________, (b) ________.
6. Possible maternal complications of prolonged latent phase are: (a) ________, (b) ________, (c) ________, and (d) ________.

Answers

1. The stress of labor can produce an excess of *catecholamines* and *cortisol*. The excess can cause vasoconstriction of *uterine* blood vessels resulting in decreased *placental* perfusion. In turn, there can be prolonged/arrested *labor* and/or fetal *hypoxia/distress*.
2. A prolonged latent phase is greater than *20* hours in a nullipara and greater than *14* hours in a multipara.
3. Prolonged latent phase is closely associated with (a) *excessive sedation*, (b) *anesthesia*, (c) *unripe cervix*, (d) *myometrial dysfunction*, and (e) *false labor*.
4. Supportive nursing care during prolonged latent phase includes: (a) *reassurance*, (b) *nourishment*, and (c) *comfort measures*.
5. Two general medical approaches to prolonged latent phase are: (a) *stop contractions and provide rest* (e.g., with morphine), and (b) *stimulate labor with one or more methods*.

6. Possible maternal complications of prolonged latent phase are: (a) *exhaustion*, (b) *low morale/discouragement*, (c) *dehydration*, and (d) *intrauterine infection*.

• •

Prolonged Labor: Active Phase

In a nullipara an active phase of more than 12 hours is abnormal. In a multipara an active phase of more than 6 hours is abnormal. Further characteristics determine what label is assigned to the abnormal active phase.

Slow Slope Active Phase. When the maximum rate of dilatation is 1.2 cm or less per hour in the nullipara or 1.5 cm or less per hour in the multipara, a *slow slope* (or *protracted*) *active phase* exists. (Refer to Fig. 4–3 for a graphic representation.) This is also called primary dysfunctional labor if the slow cervical dilatation is due to insufficient uterine contractions present from the onset of labor.

Frequently, a fetal position of OP or OT is thought to contribute to the poor uterine forces. Malposition, fetopelvic disproportion, and too early amniotomy appear to be the primary causes of this abnormal dilatation pattern. Slow slope active phase occurs more frequently during a first labor because of soft tissue resistance in the pelvis. Usually it does not recur in succeeding labors.

Despite contractions that become stronger and longer, the slowly progressing cervical dilatation curve is difficult to alter, even with uterine stimulation or amniotomy. In some women, the dilatation eventually stops, and a cesarean delivery is required. In others a constant, abnormally slow dilatation continues. The woman finds this prolonged labor to be even more uncomfortable than she anticipated. But as long as she makes some progress and there is no fetal distress, supportive care should be given, along with careful assessments. (See nursing care section at the end of this chapter.)

• •

Review Questions

1. The slow slope active phase is also called the ______________ active phase.

2. The slow slope active phase exists when dilatation is ______________ or less in the nullipara and ______________ or less per hours in the multipara.

3. What are the factors usually associated with slow slope active phase?
   a. ______________ c. ______________
   b. ______________ d. ______________

4. Why would you expect the laboring woman to become frustrated?
   ____

Answers

1. The slow slope active phase is also called the *protracted* active phase.
2. The slow slope active phase exists when dilatation is *1.2 cm* or less in the nullipara and *1.5 cm* or less per hour in a multipara.
3. The primary factors associated with slow slope active phase are: (a) *malposition*, (b) *fetopelvic disproportion*, (c) *too early amniotomy*, and (d) *soft tissue resistance* (in the nullipara).
4. The laboring woman becomes frustrated because the contractions become stronger and longer, but there is little progress and no interventions help to speed up the labor.

• •

Arrest of the Active Phase. In (secondary) *arrest of the active phase,* previously advancing cervical dilatation stops for 2 hours or more. A variation of this abnormality is a prolonged deceleration phase, which is the dilatation from 9 to 10 cm requiring more than 3 hours in the nullipara or more than 1 hour in the multipara. The graph of this arrest is a flattened "curve."

During arrest of the active phase, the uterine contractions do one of two things. They become insufficient to cause progressive cervical dilatation, or, they remain frequent, long, and intense without progressive dilatation.

Fetopelvic disproportion (or bony dystocia) is the major cause of this abnormality. Other associated factors are uterine muscle fatigue (uterine dystocia), excessive sedation and/or anesthesia, and fetal malposition. Attempts may be made to change the fetal position (see Chapter 2), because an undesirable position can result in disproportion. If the fetopelvic disproportion is not resolved in this way, cesarean delivery is necessary. When uterine muscle fatigue occurs, maternal rest and intravenous 5 percent dextrose in Ringer's lactate may be effective. For those women under the influence of sedation or anesthesia, providing time for rest while the effects of the medication wear off usually results in labor progress. If the fetopelvic relationship is favorable, uterine stimulation by amniotomy and/or oxytocin may also be used.

• •

Review Questions

1. Arrest of the active phase is defined as ______________________________
____.
2. Four factors associated with arrest of the active phase are:
   a. ____________________ c. ____________________
   b. ____________________ d. ____________________

3. What are three possible methods of treatment for arrest of the active phase? (a) ______________________, (b) ______________________, and (c) ______________________.

Answers

1. Arrest of the active phase of dilatation is *no progress in dilatation for 2 hours or more during the active phase.*
2. Factors associated with arrest in the active phase are (a) *fetopelvic disproportion,* (b) *uterine dystocia,* (c) *excessive sedation and/or anesthesia,* and (d) *fetal malposition.*
3. Possible methods of treatment are (a) *alteration of fetal position,* (b) *rest and hydration,* (c) *uterine stimulation (amniotomy, oxytocin administration),* and/or *cesarean delivery*

• •

DESCENT PATTERNS

Thus far the focus has been on the graphic pattern of cervical dilatation. Descent of the fetus should also be graphed and analyzed for normal and abnormal patterns.

The normal descent pattern will be considered first. Descent is the first requisite for the birth of the fetus. When the fetal head has descended so that its greatest biparietal diameter is at, or has passed, the pelvic inlet, the head is *engaged.* At this point the occiput is near the spines, almost zero station. Refer to Chapter 2 for additional information. In the nullipara, engagement usually occurs at or before the onset of labor. In the multipara, engagement may not take place until the active phase of dilatation, but once engagement occurs, further descent occurs rapidly. Descent is brought about by four forces: (1) pressure of the uterine contractions and amniotic fluid, (2) direct pressure of the fundus upon the buttocks in a cephalic presentation, (3) contraction of the abdominal muscles during pushing, and (4) flexion of the fetal head, which is eventually followed by extension (see Chapter 2) and straightening of the body.

• •

Review Questions

1. What is the difference between the occurrence of engagement in the nullipara as compared with engagement in the multipara?

____

____

2. Identify the four forces that cause descent:

a. ______________________ c. ______________________

b. ______________________ d. ______________________

Answers

1. In the nullipara engagement occurs at or before the onset of labor. In the multipara engagement may not take place until the active phase of dilatation has begun; thereafter descent occurs rapidly.

2. The forces that bring about descent are *pressure of contractions and amniotic fluid, direct pressure of the fundus upon the buttocks, contraction of the abdominal muscles, and flexion followed by extension of the fetal head and straightening of the body.*

• •

Now look at the normal descent patterns illustrated in Figure 4–4 for the nullipara and in Figure 4–5 for the multipara. Both show the normal S-shaped curve of the cervical dilatation pattern. They also show the descent curve. On the right side the station is calibrated as −1, 0, +1, and so forth. The distance between each point (for example, −1 to 0) is 1 cm. At the top of the graph the descent curve is divided into a latent, an accelerated, and a maximum slope phase. This is not exactly the same as the dilatation curve (at the bottom) because it progresses at a different rate. The shaded area shows that *the maximum slope in dilatation and the onset of acceleration in descent occur at the same time.* The rates at the right of the graphs, determined by Friedman, need not be memorized but are intended to serve as a reference. The rate of descent (like the rate of dilatation) is

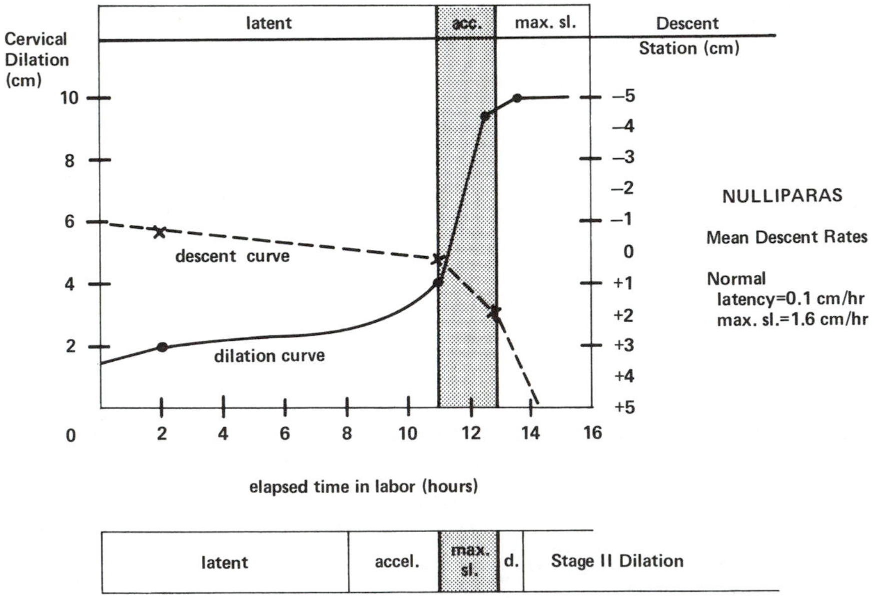

Figure 4–4. Normal pattern in nullipara.

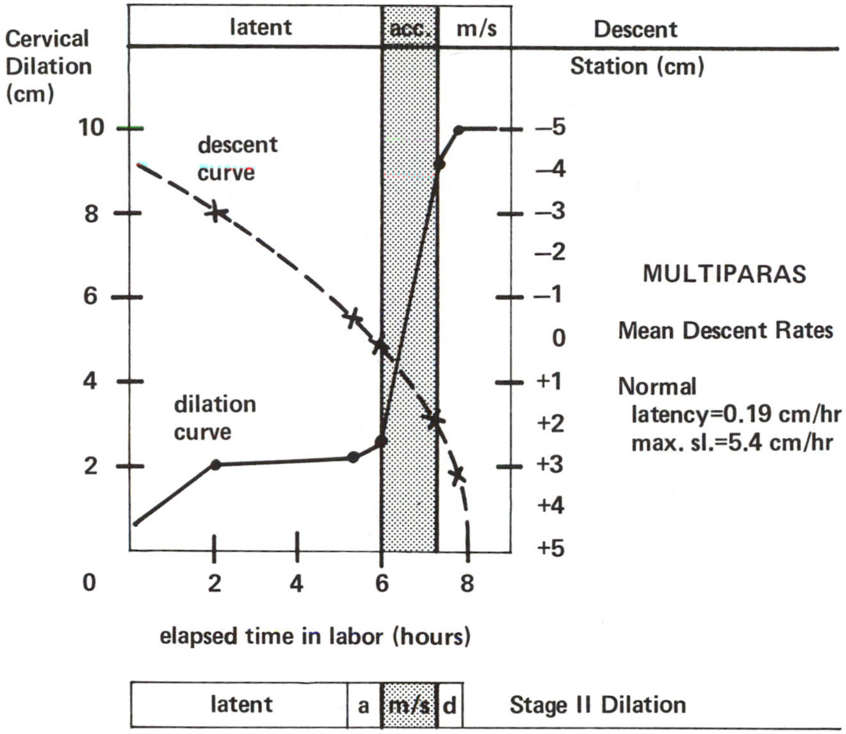

Figure 4–5. Normal pattern in multipara.

normally faster in the multipara than in the nullipara. And, the rate of descent is considerably faster during the maximum slope than in the latent phase. Note the differences in the two descent curves—the initial station, the occurrence of engagement (−1 to 0 station), and the rate of descent.

Abnormal Descent Patterns. Abnormalities in the descent pattern occur twice as often in the nullipara. Two abnormal rates are worth knowing:

A *protracted descent pattern* exists when the rate of descent in the active phase of descent is less than 1.0 cm per hour in the nullipara, and less than 2.0 cm per hour in the multipara. This does not refer to the normally flat latent phase of descent but only the normally descending active phase, which is composed of both the accelerated and maximum slope phases.

An *arrest of descent* during the active phase of descent—no linear advancement of station—exists when there is no progress for 1 hour or more.

There are two major factors associated with abnormal descent patterns: fetopelvic disproportion and malposition (OP and OT being the most common). Both causes make it difficult, if not impossible, for the fetus to fit through the pelvis. Excessive sedation or anesthesia is another possible cause because they make contractions less effective and reduce the tone of the maternal pelvic floor.

Minor fetopelvic disproportion may be spontaneously resolved by molding (overriding of the bones) of the fetal head. Rotation of the malpositioned head to OA may be encouraged by proper positioning of the mother (see Chapter 2), or manual rotation by hand or forceps. Given time, the effects of excessive sedation or anesthesia will decrease and normal descent forces may begin to work again. Conversely, epidural anesthesia may be used to relieve pain and promote relaxation, and thereby promote descent of the fetus in the desired OA position. Oxytocin may be necessary to stimulate efficient contractions. The nurse can be instrumental in facilitating these interventions and explaining their purposes. If descent beyond zero station does not occur, cesarean delivery will be necessary.

• •

Review Questions

1. In a normal labor pattern, the onset of the acceleration of descent occurs at the same time as ____________________.
2. In a nullipara the descent rate is (faster than, same as, slower than) that in a multipara. (Choose one.)
3. Abnormalities in descent patterns occur (more often, less often) in nulliparas than in multiparas. (Choose one.)
4. Complete the following statements for both the nullipara and multipara:
   a. A protracted descent pattern exists when the rate of descent in the active phase of descent is __________ in a nullipara and __________ in a multipara.
   b. An arrest of descent during the active phase of descent exists when there is ____________________.
5. Considering the major causes of abnormal descent patterns, list four ways a nurse can facilitate descent:
   a. ____________________
   b. ____________________
   c. ____________________
   d. ____________________

Answers

1. The onset of the acceleration of descent occurs at the same time as *the maximum slope in cervical dilatation*.
2. A nullipara has a *slower* descent rate than a multipara.
3. Abnormalities in descent patterns occur *more often* in the nullipara.
4. a. A protracted descent pattern in a nullipara is *less than 1 cm per hour*; in a multipara a protracted descent pattern is *less than 2 cm per hour*.

b. An arrest of descent is *no progress for one hour or more.*

5. Ways a nurse can facilitate descent include:
   a. *Allow time for molding of the fetal head to occur.*
   b. *Allow time for the inhibiting effects of sedatives/anesthesia to wear off.*
   c. *Position the mother to facilitate fetal rotation to OA.*
   d. *Explain rationale for interventions and give supportive care.*

• •

CARE IN THE PRESENCE OF PROLONGED LABOR

No matter what the cause of prolongation, the nurse as caretaker is primary assessor and legally responsible (see Chapter 10) for recording her findings and interventions. Periodically assessing the uterine contractions and other signs of progress, she compares these findings with the normal labor graph. Inconsistencies require nursing interventions, including communication with the physician. Astute noninvasive observations by the nurse can often minimize the number of vaginal exams.

Analysis of the data gathered during the assessment process should result in several nursing diagnoses. The following might be applicable:

- **Anxiety [specify] related to changes in expected pattern of labor.** Anxiety, fear, and stress increase catecholamines and cortisol, which in turn may cause dysfunctional labor and fetal distress. Anxiety can be decreased if both emotional and physical needs of the woman are met. Numerous ways are discussed throughout this book.
- **Diversional activity, deficit related to prolonged labor.** Often women need assistance to help pass the time. During latency, walking, TV, games, and so on may be helpful. It is a good time to discuss expectations and preparation for labor. During the active phase, relaxation technique during contractions serves as a distraction from pain.
- **Knowledge deficit [of normal labor/delivery process] related to lack of information (or inadequate preparation, or lack of previous experience).** Lack of knowledge about normal labor occurrences may increase anxiety. In the presence of prolonged labor, the events of the existing labor need to be assessed and realistic expectations presented to the laboring woman. She must be sufficiently informed to make decisions about procedures to be done to her body.
- **Infection, potential for, related to invasive procedures.** Vaginal exams should be done for a definite purpose. They are invasive, cause discomfort, and have a potential risk of infection especially following rupture of membranes.
- **Fluid volume deficit, potential related to excessive fluid loss.** Fluid losses exceed oral replacement at this time. To prevent dehy-

dration, at least 2500 ml of fluid is needed in a 24-hour period. To meet this requirement, during prolonged labor IV infusions are needed. Solutions (e.g., 5 percent dextrose in Ringer's lactate) provide both sugar and electrolytes. This is usually desirable because oral intake is limited during labor, as food is not readily digested, and there is danger of vomiting and aspiration. Light eating may be permitted in early labor in the low risk woman but not if narcotics are used, because then food digestion is further decreased. Clear fluids and ice chips may also be permitted. Oral hygiene should be provided. Since dehydration may cause increases in temperature, BP, pulse, respiration, and FHR, these must be routinely assessed. Intake and output must be monitored. Urine specific gravity may be required.

- **Coping, ineffective individual related to prolonged painful labor.** Past experiences, cultural background, coping techniques, antepartal preparation, and fatigue influence a woman's response to labor. Pain over a prolonged period of time taxes anyone's morale and is likely to result in loss of control. Verbal and nonverbal behavior must be assessed. Supportive care is needed in the form of realistic encouragement and promotion of physical comfort. The support person must be involved when possible. Remarks that may worry the laboring woman should be avoided. Rest may be enhanced by sedation. Judicious pain relief, usually with analgesics or epidural anesthesia, is desirable.
- **Urinary retention [acute]** (or **Bowel elimination, alteration in: constipation) related to pressure of fetal presenting part.** If the bladder or bowel are full, they can cause discomfort and impede labor progress. They are more liable to injury when not empty. Bladder assessment and emptying as necessary should occur every 2 to 3 hours. Catheterization may be needed. An enema may be used to empty the bowel.
- **Injury, potential for; trauma (to the fetus) related to prolonged labor.** The potential for fetal hypoxia, infection, and physical injury are greater in prolonged labor than in normal labor. Frequent if not continuous FHR monitoring is needed (see Chapter 3). Fetal distress may result in passage of meconium. The presence of caput, excessive molding, and malposition should be noted. X-ray may be employed to determine fetal station and position, as well as pelvic size and shape.
- **Injury, potential for; trauma (to mother) related to prolonged labor.** Exhaustion, along with dehydration, tend to result from prolonged labor. By monitoring urinary ketones, acidosis from deficient glucose metabolism can be detected. Both mental and physical rest are needed. Poor aseptic technique, frequent vaginal exams, and fetal monitoring (internal), especially following rupture of membranes, contribute to infection. Postpartal hemorrhage due to uterine atony should be anticipated.

Numerous nursing interventions have been suggested in the

above section. The nurse must evaluate the effectiveness of the nursing interventions and revise them as necessary.

• •

Review Question

Reread the previous section. By underlining or highlighting in some other way, indicate the problems identified in the nursing diagnoses and the nursing interventions recommended.

Answer

1. Anxiety: Meet emotional and physical needs.
2. Deficit in diversional activity: Help pass the time by providing social activities, discuss expectations and preparation for labor, use relaxation techniques during contractions.
3. Knowledge deficit: Assess existing labor and present realistic expectations.
4. Potential infection: Do vaginal exams only for a definite reason.
5. Fluid volume deficit: Give at least 2500 ml fluid intake in 24-hour period using IV as needed and provide for oral hygiene.
6. Ineffective individual coping: Assess verbal and nonverbal behavior, provide realistic encouragement and promote physical comfort. Give pain relief medications judiciously.
7. Urinary/Bowel retention: Empty bladder and bowel every 2 to 3 hours either spontaneously or by way of catheterization or enema.
8. Potential fetal injury: Monitor FHR. Note meconium staining, caput, excessive molding, and malposition.
9. Potential maternal injury: Monitor urinary ketones, use aseptic technique, and anticipate uterine atony during postpartal period.

• •

CONCLUSION

With basic knowledge of normal and abnormal patterns of dilatation and descent, the nurse should be able to function more efficiently in a labor area. If labor graphs are not used, the nurse may want to introduce them as a clinical tool. The nurse should at least be able to draw a mental picture of what is occurring. Based on this image, a determination can be made of whether the pattern is normal or abnormal and if intervention is necessary.

BIBLIOGRAPHY

Bobak, IM and Jensen, MD: Essentials of Maternity Nursing: The Nurse and the Childbearing Family. CV Mosby, St. Louis, 1987.

Dick-Read, G: Childbirth Without Fear, ed 2. Harper and Row, New York, 1959.

Doenges, ME, Kenty, JR, and Moorhouse, MF: Maternal/Newborn Care Plans: Guidelines for Client Care. FA Davis, Philadelphia, 1988.

Friedman, EA: Labor: Clinical Evaluation and Management, ed 2. Appleton-Century-Crofts, New York, 1978.

Knuppel, RA and Drukker, JE: High-Risk Pregnancy: A Team Approach. WB Saunders, Philadelphia, 1986.

Lederman, RP, et al: Relationship of psychological factors in pregnancy in progress in labor. Nurs Res 28:94, 1979.

Lederman, RP, et al: The relationship of maternal anxiety, plasma catecholamines, and plasma cortisol to progress in labor. Am J Obstet Gynecol 132(5):495, 1978.

Oxorn, H: Oxorn-Foote: Human Labor and Birth, ed 5. Appleton-Century-Crofts, Norwalk, 1986.

Sehgal, NN: Early detection of abnormal labor using the Friedman labor graph. Postgrad Med 68(13):189, 1980.

Simkin, P: Stress, pain, and catecholamines in labor: Part 1. A review. Birth 13(4):227, 1986.

Varney, H: Nurse-Midwifery, ed 2. Blackwell Scientific Publications, Boston, 1987.

Whitley, N: A Manual of Clinical Obstetrics. JB Lippincott, Philadelphia, 1985.

POST-TEST 4

1. Fill in the blanks, identifying the various phases in this labor graph.

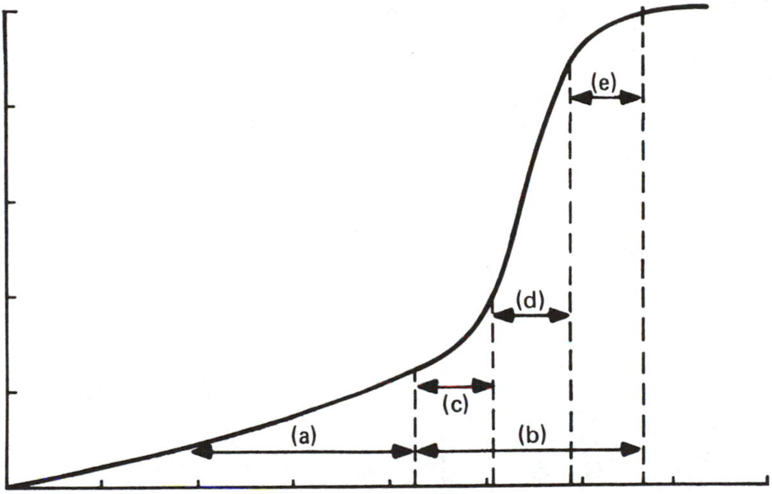

a. ______________________________

b. ______________________________

c. ______________________________

d. ______________________________

e. ______________________________

2. Diagram on the graphs provided and describe in words the following patterns. Place your drawings on top of the normal curves already drawn.

a. Prolonged latent phase:

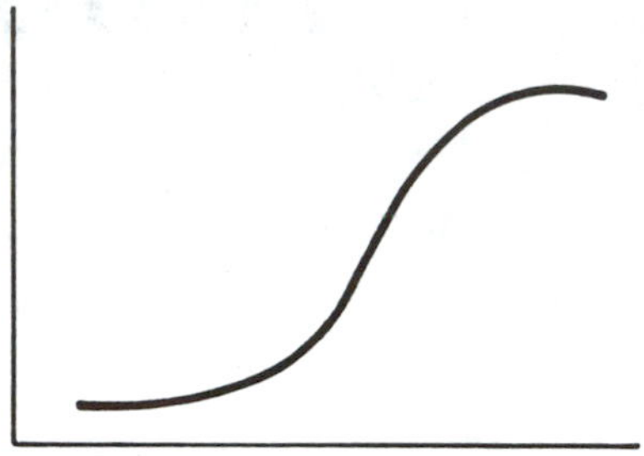

b. Protracted active phase:

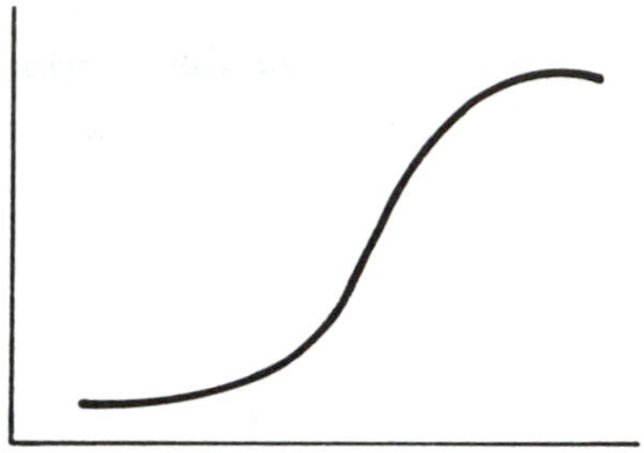

c. Arrest of the active phase:

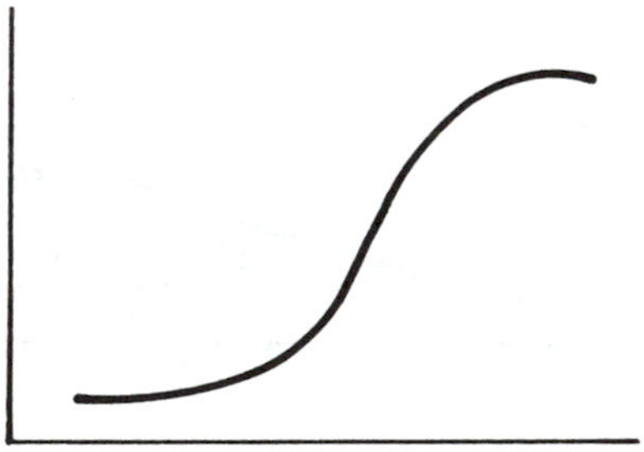

3. Put a check mark (✓) in front of those statements that indicate an abnormal pattern. Following those checked statements, briefly explain why the pattern is abnormal.

_____ a. A nullipara whose total Stage I of labor is 13 hours in length.

____

____

_____ b. A nullipara whose latent phase is 21 hours.

____

____

_____ c. A nullipara who is at zero station 2 weeks before the onset of labor.

____

____

_____ d. A labor that is 3 hours in length.

_____ e. A multipara who is in the active phase for 8 hours.

_____ f. A nullipara who remains at 6 cm for 5 hours.

_____ g. A descent pattern that begins active deceleration as the cervix dilates the most rapidly.

_____ h. A dilatation pattern that does not show a deceleration phase.

4. Describe the following as they apply to both the nullipara and multipara.
   a. Protracted descent pattern:
   b. Arrest of descent:

5. List at least five assessment data the nurse should utilize when evaluating labor curves.
   a.
   b.
   c.
   d.
   e.

6. State five nursing diagnoses that are appropriate for abnormal labor curves.
   a.
   b.
   c.
   d.
   e.

7. Describe five nursing interventions and their rationale that are appropriate for prolonged labor:
   a.
   b.
   c.

d. ______________________________

____

e. ______________________________

____

8. Below you will find the data from two labor records. Time, cervical dilatation, and station are provided. Draw these data on graphs. Analyze the graphs for their patterns. Then summarize your interpretations in writing. Include nursing interventions if they are other than routine care.

Patient A: A multipara

TIME	CERVICAL DILATATION	STATION
12:00 MN	2	−2
5:30 AM	2	−1
6:00 AM	2−3	0
7:00 AM	7	+1
7:30 AM	9	+2
7:45 AM	complete	+4, caput showing

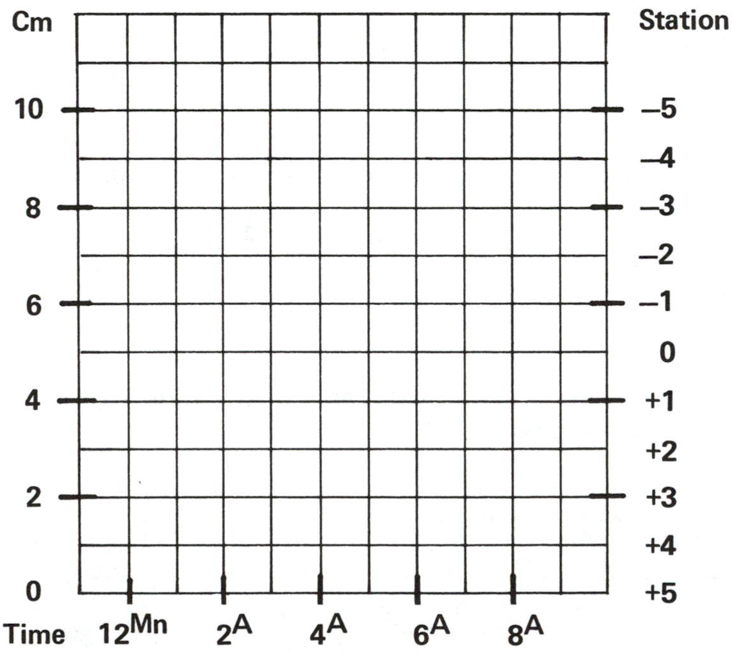

Interpretation: ____

____

____

____

____

Patient B: A nullipara

TIME	CERVICAL DILATATION	STATION
12:00 MN	1–2	−1 to 0
4:00 AM	2	0
8:00 AM	2–3	0 to +1
11:00 AM	4	0 to +1
12:00 noon	5	0 to +1
2:00 PM	6	0 to +1
3:00 PM	7	+1
4:00 PM	7	+1
4:30 PM	8	+2
5:30 PM	10	+2

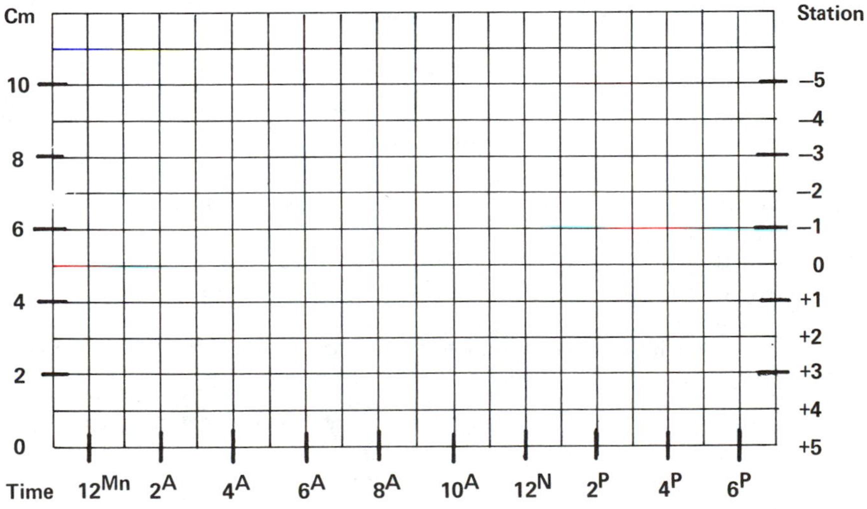

Interpretation: ____

____

____

____

____

Answers to Post-Test

1. The phases in a cervical dilatation graph are: (a) latent phase, (b) active phase, (c) accelerated phase, (d) phase of maximum slope (or transition), (e) deceleration phase.

2. For the drawings refer back to Figure 4–3. The *prolonged latent phase* is

generally flat with 20 or more hours for the nullipara and 14 or more hours for the multipara. The *protracted active phase* involves slow movement through the active phase with 1.2 cm or less per hour cervical dilatation for the nullipara and 1.5 cm or less per hour cervical dilatation for the multipara. *Arrest of the active phase* of labor is indicated by no progress for at least 2 hours.

3. The following statements should be checked and explanations given:
   b. A latent phase that is 21 hours is prolonged.
   d. A labor that is 3 hours is a precipitous labor.
   e. Cervical dilatation in the active phase is from 4 to 10 cm (or is equal to 6 cm). Less than 1.5 cm per hour in the active phase for a multipara is a slow slope. Six divided by 1.5 = 4 hours; greater than 4 hours in the active phase is a slow slope active phase.
   f. Remaining at 6 cm for 2 hours or more indicates an arrest.

4. a. A protracted descent pattern exists when the rate in the active phase of descent is less than 1 cm per hour in the nullipara and less than 2 cm per hour in the multipara.
   b. An arrest of descent during the active phase of descent exists when there is no progress for 1 hour or more.

5. Assessment data the nurse should utilize when evaluating labor curves include:
   a. laboring woman's parity: nullip vs. multip
   b. cervical dilatation curve
   c. fetal descent curve
   d. time interval since previous change in dilatation and descent
   e. total time of labor so far in relation to the maximum norm
   f. characteristics of contractions in relation to rate of labor progress
   g. medications administered (especially oxytocin, sedatives, analgesia, anesthesia)
   h. labor stimulants used (e.g., rupture of membranes)
   i. coping behavior (realizing fear increases catecholamines and cortisol)
   j. fetal heart rate response
   k. a reference that provides guidelines for normal time limits for dilatation phases and descent.

6. The following is a list of nursing diagnoses (not all inclusive) that are appropriate for abnormal labor curves:
   - Anxiety (mild, moderate, severe) related to
     unexpected rapid labor
     changes in expected pattern of labor
   - Coping, ineffective individual related to
     prolonged painful labor
   - Comfort, alterations in: pain, acute related to
     uterine contractions
   - Diversional activity, deficit related to
     prolonged labor
   - Knowledge deficit of normal labor/delivery process related to
     lack of information
     inadequate preparation
     lack of previous experience

- Infection, potential for related to
  invasive procedures
- Fluid volume deficit, potential related to
  excessive fluid loss
- Urinary retention [acute] related to
  pressure of fetal presenting part
- Bowel elimination, alteration in: constipation related to
  pressure of fetal presenting part
- Injury, potential for: trauma to mother related to
  vigorous uterine contractions
  prolonged labor
- Injury, potential for: trauma to fetus related to
  hypoxia
  prolonged labor

7. The following is a list of appropriate nursing interventions and their rationale during specific prolonged labor patterns:

   Prolonged latent phase:

   a. Promote rest and relaxation to avoid exhaustion.
   b. Provide appropriate encouragement to avoid low morale.
   c. Hydrate to avoid dehydration.
   d. Administer ordered medications to temporarily stop contractions and promote rest.
   e. Provide ordered stimulation to stimulate effective contractions and promote cervical dilatation.
   f. Perform vaginal exams infrequently to avoid intrauterine infection.
   g. Monitor fetal status since the fetus is at risk for damage or death.

   Slow slope active phase:

   a. Provide mental and physical support since this labor involves much discomfort but few positive results.
   b. Promote fetal rotation if OP or OT are present since rotation to OA facilitates labor progress.
   c. Monitor for fetal distress recognizing that supportive care alone is justified as long as fetal well-being exists.

   Arrest of the active phase:

   a. Monitor contractions for decreased activity vs. continued activity without progressive dilatation since the treatment to be used is, in part, dependent on this activity.
   b. Assess for indication of fetopelvic disproportion since it is a major cause of arrest.
   c. Provide rest and IV glucose fluids as needed to discourage uterine muscle fatigue.
   d. Seek AROM or oxytocin stimulation as needed to improve contraction activity if fetopelvic relationship is favorable.
   e. Avoid overmedication with sedatives or analgesics since they often slow labor progress and require wearing-off time.

   Abnormal descent:

   a. Promote fetal rotation in the presence of OP or OT, because OA is desired for fetal descent.

b. Assess for indications of fetopelvic disproportion because it is a major cause of abnormal descent.
c. Avoid overmedication with sedatives or anesthesia because they decrease the sensation of the need to push.
d. Promote pain relief and relaxation because pain and tension may inhibit fetal descent.
e. Seek oxytocin order if conditions warrant because without contractions descent will not occur.
f. Empty bowel and bladder since, if full, they cause discomfort and impede fetal descent.

8.

Patient A:

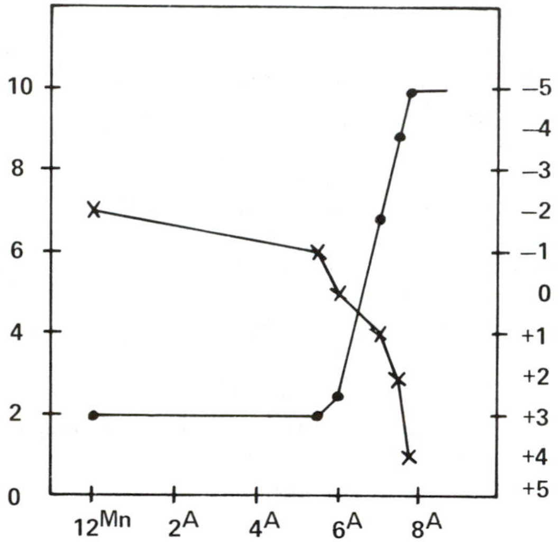

Patient B:

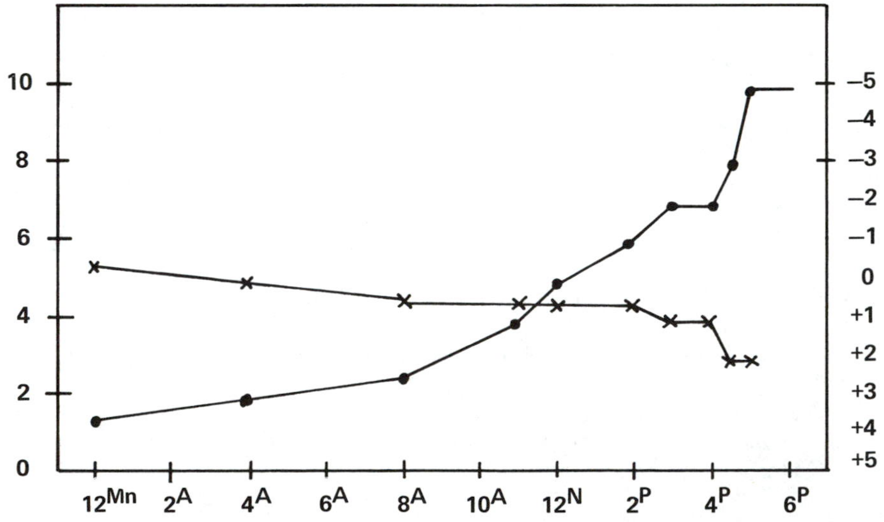

Patient A: This is a normal labor pattern for multipara. Stage I is almost 8 hours long: a normal length is approximately 6½ to 8 hours. The latent phase of dilatation is 6 hours compared with a normal mean of 4.8, but 13.6 hours is the maximum limit. The active phase of dilatation is almost 2 hours compared with a normal mean of 2.4 hours. A normal **S**-curve is shown in the graph.

The descent pattern indicates a normal lack of engagement (about −1 to 0 station) before there is active labor. During the maximum slope of dilatation, the descent rate accelerates slowly and then very rapidly, bringing the presenting part to a visible point at the introitus. This is also indicative of a normal progression of labor.

Nothing in this graph indicates that other than routine labor care is warranted.

Patient B: Since the mean for Stage I of a nullipara is 11 hours, this 17-hour labor is slightly long. The mean of the latent phase of cervical dilatation is 6.4 hours (20.1 maximum); this latent phase is approximately 8 hours (12 MN to 8 AM) and therefore normal in length. The mean for the active phase of cervical dilatation is 4.6 hours (11.7 maximum); because the patient's active phase is 9 hours (8 AM to 5 PM), it is slightly longer than the mean. Two abnormalities in the active phase should be considered: the slow slope and arrest.

Owing to soft tissue resistance in the pelvis, a slow slope frequently occurs in the nullipara. X-ray might be done if malposition or fetopelvic disproportion is suspected. Vaginal exams should be done as infrequently as possible. A stimulant is usually not helpful at this time. The best nursing intervention would be to provide comfort, relaxation, and support to the patient, because she is likely to become frustrated by the slow progress. Normal nursing observations of maternal and fetal conditions would be appropriate. Intravenous fluids should be given and the bladder frequently emptied. Analgesia/anesthesia could be given once in the active dilatation phase (following 4 cm dilatation).

Although there is no progress in cervical dilatation from 3 to 4 PM, this does not meet the requirement of 2 hours for arrest in the active phase.

When analyzing the descent pattern of Patient B, it is apparent that the fetus is engaged (−1 to 0 station) at the onset of labor, which is normal for a nullipara. Little or no progression in descent until well into the active phase is normal. Acceleration in descent should take place during the maximum slope of dilatation, which it does. No special nursing interventions are therefore required.

5 LABOR STIMULATION

Janet S. Malinowski

OBJECTIVES

Upon completing this chapter, you will be able to:

- For the following stimulants—ambulation, breast stimulation, enema, amniotomy, and oxytocin:
  - a. explain the rationale for their stimulation of labor.
  - b. discuss the nursing interventions appropriate before, during, and following stimulation.
  - c. identify contraindications to their use.
- Describe the effects that stripping the membranes and use of laminaria might have on the cervix.
- Differentiate between surgical and medical induction.
- Identify conditions that justify induction.
- Apply the Bishop Scoring System to patient data and interpret the score.
- Discuss the nursing implications of a drug being researched for labor induction.
- Identify a potential problem for each of the specified labor stimulants.

Contractions are needed for labor to progress. The effectiveness of contractions is measured by the rate of cervical dilatation and, eventually, fetal descent. When labor does not progress, stimulation of contractions is often appropriate. This chapter presents the methods of labor stimulation currently used in hospital labor units.

LABOR STIMULANTS

Ambulation

Frequently a woman in false labor or early labor is advised to ambulate (walk) for 30 to 60 minutes or longer. Usually, ambulation causes false labor contractions to stop. These irregular contractions, although uncomfortable, cause minimal cervical changes. For the woman in early true labor, ambulation tends to stimulate uterine contractions. The upright position assumed when walking takes advantage of the principle of gravity and may encourage descent of the fetus. It also brings the fetus into a forward position so that the presenting fetal part is better aligned with the inlet of the pelvis. Pressure on the cervix by the presenting part may stimulate oxytocin production from the posterior pituitary; this in turn increases the frequency of contractions and causes progress in cervical dilatation.

When a woman is instructed to ambulate, she needs to be told where she may go and when she should return. The instructions will depend on the hospital's facilities as well as her psychological and physical condition. If her membranes should rupture or the contractions become considerably more intense and frequent (2 to 3 minutes apart), she should be instructed to return to the unit immediately rather than to wait until the designated time. Providing someone to walk with her and informing her of the advantages of the activity usually result in more active walking. Standing and sitting may provide periodic rest yet continue the positive effect of gravity's pressure. The nurse may need to provide a makeshift bathrobe and slippers so the woman will feel more presentable as she ambulates. Until the uterus is rhythmically contracting, it is not necessary to retake a normal fetal heart rate more than every hour unless membranes are ruptured. When 1 to 3 hours of ambulation does not bring on true labor, discharge instructions should be given, including when to come back to the hospital. Undoubtedly the woman will be disappointed that she is not likely to have her baby that day, and she needs to be reassured that false alarms are not unusual. In this case a nursing diagnosis of **self-concept, disturbance in: self-esteem related to mis-(self)-diagnosed labor** is usually appropriate.

• •

Review Questions

1. What effect does ambulation usually have on false labor?________

____

2. What response should a nurse have for a woman who experiences false labor? ________________________________

____

3. Identify three reasons why the upright position of ambulation may stimulate labor:
   a. ________________________________
   b. ________________________________
   c. ________________________________

4. State four interventions the nurse should take upon receiving the order to ambulate a woman:
   a. ________________________________

b. ______________________________
c. ______________________________
d. ______________________________

Answers

1. Ambulation usually stops false labor.
2. For a woman who experiences false labor, a nurse should provide discharge instructions about when to return to the hospital and provide reassurance that false labor is not uncommon.
3. The upright position (a) encourages the fetus to gravitate (descend) in the pelvis; (b) brings the fetus into a forward position, aligning the fetus better with the inlet of the pelvis; and (c) encourages the presenting part to press on the cervix, which may stimulate oxytocin production and, thereby, increase uterine contractions.
4. Upon receiving the order to ambulate a woman, the nurse should:
   a. Tell her why ambulation is desirable.
   b. Provide her with appropriate clothing, if necessary.
   c. Instruct her about where she can go and when she should return, including conditions that warrant early return.
   d. Provide someone to walk with her.
   e. Retake normal fetal heart rate approximately every hour.

• •

Stripping Membranes

Occasionally a woman will come into the labor unit and say that her membranes were stripped in the doctor's office yesterday. Stripping, or sweeping, the membranes involves inserting a digit (finger) through the uterine cervix and, in a 360 degree sweep, digitally separating the chorioamniotic membrane from the uterine wall in the region of the internal os of the cervix. It is an old method, and the frequency of use is questionable, because many physicians use it casually during an office examination but do not record it as an induction attempt. Stripping the membranes may be appropriate when the uterine cervix is dilated sufficiently to permit entrance of a (doctor's) fingertip, the presenting part is not above −1 station, and the pregnancy is at term with no contractions. This procedure sometimes initiates labor at term, although its effectiveness has not been proven. It often encourages softening and effacement of the cervix. The woman usually experiences **comfort, alteration in: pain, acute** (i.e., cramping and slight vaginal bleeding) **related to stripping of membranes**. The risks include potential infection, bleeding from a previously undiagnosed placenta previa, and accidental rupture of membranes.[1]

• •

Review Questions

1. What is the purpose of stripping the membranes? ______________________________
____

2. What physical symptoms might the woman experience following the procedure?____
____

Answers

1. The purpose of stripping the membranes is to initiate labor and/or encourage softening and effacement of the cervix.
2. The woman might feel cramps and have slight vaginal bleeding.

• •

Enema

Whether or not enemas stimulate labor is controversial. Danforth[2] says there are laboratory studies that support the premise that an enema increases uterine contractility. Intestinal peristalsis produced by the enema is thought to be transferred to the uterus and to start or enhance uterine contractions. More recently, Pritchard[3] states that enemas are not used to stimulate labor.

There continues to be no debate about whether or not an enema, or rectal suppository, empties a full rectum and that a full rectum can impede labor progress. It is for that reason that enema is included here as a labor stimulant. (Likewise, a distended bladder needs to be emptied.) An enema efficiently empties a full rectum, providing more room for fetal descent through the birth canal. Furthermore, a full rectum during Stage II of labor may result in defecation during the fetal expulsion phase. Defecation at this time might inhibit the woman's willingness to push and, therefore, prolong the time in labor. Upon obtaining such assessment data (i.e, full rectum, prolonged fetal descent, and/or inhibition to push due to defecation), the following nursing diagnoses may be appropriate: **bowel elimination, alteration in: constipation related to pressure of fetal presenting part** or **anxiety [specify]** or **self-concept, disturbance in: self-esteem related to exposure during defecation**.

For many years, it was routine to give soapsuds enemas. There are reasons to believe that soapsuds are no longer desirable. Mahan and McKay[4] state that in some instances soapsuds enemas are associated with acute colitis, bowel perforation, gangrene, and anaphylaxis. Instead of soapsuds, warm tap water, normal saline, or commercially prepared Fleet enemas, or glycerine rectal suppositories, could be used. Nurses should follow hospital protocol for evacuation method and solution.

Usually the enema is given shortly after admission to the labor unit. When an enema is ordered, the nurse must first assess for the need, as well as for contraindications. A brief patient history and vital signs, including fetal heart rate, are taken and a vaginal examination is performed. (The fetal heart rate should be re-taken upon completing the expulsion of the enema.) The woman in early labor with none of the contraindications is a potential candidate for an enema. Contraindications to giving an enema include:

1. vaginal bleeding suggestive of abruptio placentae or placenta previa (see Chapter 8), which may potentially cause profuse bleeding and place mother or fetus at risk for increased morbidity or mortality;
2. breech, or other malpresentation, which increases the likelihood of prolapsed cord or spontaneous rupture of membranes due to the uneven fit of the presenting part in the pelvis;
3. premature labor, which decreases the chances of survival of the infant;
4. rupture of membranes (in some institutions), which increases the chances of infection as well as prolapsed cord if the head is not well engaged;
5. advanced labor (cervix dilated 6 cm or more), which stimulates labor to accelerate too rapidly;
6. non-reassuring fetal heart rate (see Chapter 3).

Based on the nursing assessment, the nurse may conclude that the **anxiety [specify] related to the enema procedure** outweighs the advantage of the enema and, therefore, the nurse accepts the woman's refusal. Conversely, the nurse may formulae the following diagnosis: **comfort, alteration in: pain, acute related to a full rectum**. In this case the intervention may be administration of an enema.

Although the principles are similar to that for any adult, the following procedural modifications apply to a laboring woman:

1. the amount may be as much as 1500 to 2000 ml, if tolerated;
2. the tubing is inserted up to 10 to 12 inches (the second mark on most tubes); it may be more difficult to insert the tubing because of the pressure of the fetal presenting part or the presence of hemorrhoids;
3. the air in the tubing does not need to be removed, since it tends to increase peristalsis;
4. during uterine contractions it may be necessary to pinch the tubing, give reassurance, and encourage the woman to concentrate on slow deep breathing techniques;
5. expulsion is immediate and requires approximately 20 minutes to complete;
6. the fetal heart rate is reassessed following the expulsion to assure that no significant changes occurred.

• •

Review Questions

1. State two reasons why an enema stimulates labor:
   a. ______________________________
   b. ______________________________

2. Check (✓) the situations below that are contraindications to an enema:

_____ abnormal or absent fetal heart rate
_____ breech presentation
_____ rupture of membranes
_____ station −2
_____ premature labor
_____ cervix 7 cm dilated
_____ vaginal bleeding (other than bloody show)

3. When administering an enema, what actions should the nurse take regarding the following?
   a. Fetal heart rate:______________________________
   b. Amount of solution:______________________________
   c. Insertion of tubing:______________________________
   d. Complaint of discomfort during a contraction:______________________________
   e. Expulsion of enema:______________________________

Answers

1. Enemas stimulate labor in the following ways:
   a. Intestinal peristalsis is thought to start/enhance uterine contractions.
   b. By emptying the rectum, a nonobstructive pelvis fosters fetal descent.
2. All of the situations given are contraindications to an enema, with the possible exception of rupture of membranes (depending on hospital protocol).
3. When administering an enema to a laboring woman, the nurse should:
   a. Assess for a normal fetal heart rate before giving the enema and immediately following the expulsion.
   b. Fill the bag with 1500 to 2000 ml of solution.
   c. Insert the tubing approximately 12 inches—to the second mark—without removing the air in the tubing. Gently maneuver around the presenting part (the fetal head) and/or hemorrhoids.
   d. To decrease discomfort during a contraction have the woman breathe slowly and deeply, pinch tubing during the contraction, and provide necessary assurance.
   e. Provide for immediate expulsion, allowing at least 20 minutes for its completion.

• •

Nipple Stimulation

Probably the most recent and most convenient labor stimulant is nipple, or breast, stimulation. It is used primarily to initiate uterine contractions in the Contraction Stress Test (see Chapter 9) but can also be used to stimulate true labor. When the nipple is stimulated, nerve impulses leading to the hypothalamus trigger the neurons in the posterior pituitary to release oxytocin into the blood stream, causing uterine contractions.

Stimulation of the nipple should only be done if labor is desired. Contraindications to its use include preterm gestation, placenta previa, and scar tissue in the uterus from cesarean delivery or other uterine surgery.

Hospital protocol may dictate how nipple stimulation should be done. There are several methods, including the following:

- Do intermittent stimulation of one breast by massage or nipple rolling or gently pulling through the gown for two minutes, followed by a five minute rest, and then repeating.
- First apply warm wash cloths on both breasts. Then do continuous nipple rolling to one nipple for ten minutes. If necessary, roll both nipples for ten more minutes.
- Do continuous stimulation until contractions occur.
- Stimulate both nipple and areola.

A&D Ointment or K-Y Lubricating Jelly may be applied to prevent soreness. For some women (and men), nipple stimulation may be a sexually embarrassing activity. This **sexuality pattern(s), altered** or **anxiety [specify] related to labor stimulation by means of nipple stimulation** deserves a private environment. It is necessary to monitor both fetal heart rates and uterine contractions to assess the effects of the stimulation.

• •

Review Questions

1. Explain the rationale for nipple stimulation: ______________________
   ____
2. State three nursing interventions that are necessary during nipple stimulation:
   a. ______________________
   b. ______________________
   c. ______________________
3. Identity three contraindications to the use of nipple stimulation:
   a. ______________________
   b. ______________________
   c. ______________________

Answers

1. Nipple stimulation is a relatively simple method of stimulating oxytocin to be secreted and thereby causing uterine contractions.
2. During nipple stimulation (a) privacy should be provided, (b) fetal heart rate and contractions need to be assessed, and (c) a variety of methods can be used dependent upon hospital protocol.
3. Contraindications to nipple stimulation include (a) preterm gestation, (b) placenta previa, and (c) uterine scar tissue.

• •

INDUCTION—A FORM OF LABOR STIMULATION

Induction means the process of causing or producing.[5] "Induction of labor is labor started by artificial means,"[6] the deliberate initiation of contractions. *Surgical, or mechanical, induction* commonly refers to artificial rupture of the membranes. *Medical induction* usually is limited to the use of oxytocin, although prostaglandin gel is also used. Castor oil, 2 ounces, followed by a soapsuds enema is an infrequently utilized medical induction. The only agent currently approved by the Food and Drug Administration for induction of term labor with a live fetus is oxytocin. PGE_2 is approved for experimental use only.

Surgical Induction of Labor with Rupture of Membranes

A procedure that the physician (and nurse midwife under certain conditions[7]) might perform to improve the efficiency of contractions is an amniotomy (commonly abbreviated AROM or ARM, meaning artificial rupture of the membranes). The procedure stimulates labor for two reasons. One, when membranes are ruptured, a chemical reaction, involving arachidonic acid and prostaglandin, promotes uterine contractions.[8,9] Two, upon rupture of membranes, the fetal head is allowed to be in direct contact with the cervix. This is favorable because the fetal head is thought to be a better cervical dilating wedge than the waters contained in the membranes. In the presence of uncoordinated contractions (see Chapter 3), amniotomy may also improve the contraction pattern and thereby enhance the slow-moving labor.

Many authorities do not advise amniotomy early in labor. Caldeyro-Barcia and associates[10] found that there is an increased incidence of caput succedaneum (swelling of the fetal scalp), out of alignment fetal cranial bones, and early decelerations in the fetal heart rate (not an ominous pattern). They do advocate AROM when internal fetal monitoring is necessary in the presence of suspected fetal hypoxia and acidosis. Lynaugh[11] agrees that AROM should be reserved for occasions when internal monitoring and fetal scalp pH determination are advisable. He states that neonates have a good outcome following AROM despite the increased pressure on the fetal skull. He also found that AROM does not predictably shorten labor. When it does, it is by a maximum of approximately one hour.

Despite the critics, AROM is still done in hopes of shortening labor. The amount of cervical effacement and dilatation seems to be a critical factor in determining the effectiveness of the amniotomy. When an amniotomy is performed, in anticipation of the large amount of amniotic fluid that might be expelled, the nurse should place several absorbent pads under the woman's buttocks and inform her of a possible gush of warm fluid. The woman is placed on her back with her knees flexed. The fetal heart rate is taken just prior to AROM to assure fetal well-being at this time. After a sterile vaginal exam, the physician or nurse midwife ruptures the amniotic sac with a sterile instrument: an amnihook (which resembles a crochet hook), an Allis forceps, or a 25-gauge needle. (Occasionally, the membranes will accidentally be ruptured during the vaginal exam.) No anesthesia is necessary for AROM because there are no nerve endings in the membranes. A small amount of blood from cervical trauma may be evident. If the procedure is explained before it is performed, the woman should be able to relax and experience no trauma. Therefore, the following nursing diagnosis would be appropriate: **anxiety [mild] related to the AROM procedure**.

AROM usually will not be performed if the presenting part of the fetus is high (−2 or above) in the pelvis and not well applied to the cervix, or the presentation is other than vertex since **injury, potential for; (fetal) trauma related to rupture of membranes** may occur. When the amniotic sac is ruptured, the expulsion of fluid causes the presenting part to exert greater pressure on the cervix. If the cord is between the presenting part and the cervix, the cord may be pushed out (prolapsed) through the cervix or compressed between the fetal head and the cervix even though it may not be visible (an occult cord). In either case the fetal heart rate is abnormally slow during and immediately after contractions. That is why it is imperative that the physician or nurse midwife re-examine for cord prolapse. The nurse must take the fetal heart rate immediately after the membranes are ruptured if the physician or nurse-midwife do not.

All the amniotic fluid will not be expelled immediately. The woman should be told to expect to leak fluid, especially during contractions and when changing her position. This will be true until the time of birth when the fluid remaining in the upper portion of the uterus and around the fetus finally is expelled.

• •

Review Questions

1. Fill in the blanks:
   a. Rupture of membranes is called ____________ induction.
   b. The use of oxytocin is called ____________ induction.
2. Give two reasons why ROM might stimulate labor:
   a. ____________
   b. ____________
3. State four reasons why some authorities do not recommend AROM except when internal fetal monitoring is warranted:
   a. ____________
   b. ____________
   c. ____________
   d. ____________

4. What three measures should a nurse take before AROM is performed?
a. ____
b. ____
c. ____

5. What three actions should a nurse perform immediately following AROM?
a. ____
b. ____
c. ____

Answers

1. a. Rupture of membranes is called *surgical* induction.
   b. The use of oxytocin is called *medical* induction.

2. a. Upon ROM a chemical reaction involving arachidonic acid and prostaglandin promotes uterine contractions.
   b. ROM stimulates labor by placing the fetal head in direct contact with the cervix; the head has a better dilating effect than the bag of waters.

3. Some authorities do not recommend AROM unless internal fetal monitoring is necessary, because there is an increased incidence in (a) caput succedaneum, (b) out of alignment fetal cranial bones, and (c) early decelerations of the fetal heart rate. (d) AROM does not predictably shorten labor; when it does, the maximum time is by about one hour.

4. Before AROM is performed, the nurse should:
   a. Be certain that the fetal heart rate is normal.
   b. Physically prepare the woman by placing her on her back with her knees bent and placing protection (padding) under her buttocks.
   c. Explain to the woman what to expect—passage of warm fluid from the vagina until the baby is born.

5. Immediately following AROM the nurse should: (a) assess the fetal heart for a normal pattern and rate, (b) look for a prolapsed cord, and (c) note and record the color and odor (if foul) of the amniotic fluid.

• •

Implications of Rupture of Membranes. Labor may accelerate following AROM, although this is not always the case. The nurse should watch for subtle signs of progress (for example, behavioral changes, and increased body temperature—see Chapter 1), as well as increased effectiveness in uterine contractions. However, once the membranes are ruptured, additional precautions need to be taken. There is increased risk of cord prolapse, adverse changes in fetal presentation, and chorioamnionitis.[1] The intact amniotic sac served as a barrier against bacterial invasion. Now there is **infection, potential for, related to the rupture of membranes** for both mother and fetus. Therefore, vaginal exams should not be as frequent, because the examiner is a possible source of bacteria. Despite the stimulating effects of ambulation, it causes a constant leak and may increase exposure to bacteria. Therefore, the mother is often confined to bed and instructed to use a bedpan for elimination once the membranes are ruptured. Because an increase in body temperature is a sign of infection, her temperature should be taken and recorded every 2 hours (every hour if elevated) following rupture of membranes.

Most authorities believe that the fetus should be born, or that there at least be progressive labor, within 24 hours after rupture of membranes. Some physicians strictly adhere to the 24-hour limit and will stimulate the labor by additional means (for example, oxytocin) if delivery is not imminent. Another alternative is cesarean delivery. Other physicians feel that as long as there is no apparent adverse effect on the woman or fetus, there is no need to deliver the fetus so soon. The woman might even be discharged from the hospital and monitored with daily CBCs or WBCs, or given a prescription for a prophylactic antibiotic. If she is discharged with ruptured membranes before delivery, the woman should be instructed to periodically check her temperature, avoid tub baths and intercourse, not use tampons, and change her perineal pads frequently. The nurse should verify that the woman knows the signs of impending infection (increase in temperature, foul smelling and/or discolored amniotic fluid, rapid pulse) and how and when to get in touch with her physician.

• •

Review Questions

1. Give four nursing measures that should be taken because of the increased likelihood of infection following rupture of membranes:
   a. ______________________________
   b. ______________________________
   c. ______________________________
   d. ______________________________

2. If the woman asked you, "Will I have to deliver my baby within 24 hours, since my membranes are ruptured," how would you answer her? (Choose one.)
   a. "Yes, physicians always deliver the baby within 24 hours after rupture of membranes."
   b. "Yes, because infection may occur now that the barrier to infection—the membranes—has been broken."
   c. "Not necessarily. It is desirable that you deliver within 24 hours, but we will watch you carefully. The status of you and your baby and the progress of your labor will influence the physician's decision if you have not delivered in 24 hours."

Answers

1. Nursing measures to be taken following rupture of membranes include:
   a. Take temperature at least every two hours.
   b. Watch for foul smelling, discolored amniotic fluid.
   c. Check for rapid pulse rate.
   d. Do vaginal exams as seldom as possible; rely on other signs of progress.
   e. Keep the woman in bed; offer bedpan as needed.

2. c is correct.

• •

Medical Induction

There are several advantages to medical induction. It may be planned ahead of time so the woman can enter labor well rested and psychologically prepared. There may be time to make the necessary arrangements for the household. The induction is usually planned for the day shift and on a weekday when the hospital is well staffed and equipped.

Prior to medical induction, the woman should be required to sign a written consent form (see Chapter 10) that lists and explains the most frequent complications and the frequency of their occurrences. These risks include prematurity, increased incidence of infection, postpartum hemorrhage, fetal distress, and failed induction.

For labor to be medically induced there must be a specific indication. These include conditions in which continuation of pregnancy endangers the mother's health or the fetus' well-being. The following is a partial list of conditions warranting medical induction and the rationale for inducing labor:

1. prolonged rupture of membranes — to decrease the likelihood of infection, specifically chorioamnionitis.
2. postmaturity — to prevent further fetal compromise (see Chapter 8).
3. maternal diabetes — to deliver 2 to 3 weeks preterm (based on fetal maturity studies) to prevent fetal demise due to placental insufficiency and to prevent growth beyond the size compatible with vaginal delivery.
4. pre-eclampsia or eclampsia — to reverse progression of the pregnancy-related condition.
5. Rh sensitization — to avert erythroblastosis fetalis (hemolytic disease) in the newborn involving CNS pathology due to high bilirubin level.

Before induction, fetal maturity should be verified, because there is increased risk of fetal prematurity. Amniocentesis provides the L/S ratio and creatinine concentration. X-ray or ultrasound studies indicate several measurements including the biparietal diameter, as well as adequacy of fetopelvic relationships. (See Chapter 8.)

Table 5–1. BISHOP SCORE*

FACTOR	ASSIGNED VALUE			
	0	1	2	3
Cervical dilatation	Closed	1–2 cm	3–4 cm	5 cm or more
Cervical effacement	0–30%	40–50%	60–70%	80% or more
Fetal station	−3	−2	−1,0	+1,+2
Cervical consistency	Firm	Moderate	Soft	
Cervical position	Posterior	Midposition	Anterior	

*Modified from: Bishop, EH: Pelvic scoring for elective induction. Obstet Gynecol 24:266, 1964.

Induction is usually not attempted unless the cervix is favorable—soft and beginning to efface and dilate—and the fetal head is presenting and engaged. The Bishop score is a method of assessing these factors and predicting readiness for induction (Table 5–1). Scores range from 0 to 13. The higher the score is, the greater is the likelihood of successful induction of labor. A score of greater than 4 has an 80 percent success rate.[12] With a low score of 5 or less, 10 to 12 hours of uterine contractions may be necessary.[13]

In a situation in which the cervix is not ripe for induction, one or more *laminaria tents* (sterile dried seaweed) may be placed within the cervix. As they absorb moisture, they swell and may cause softening and dilatation of the cervix. Most of the swelling occurs in the first 4 to 6 hours with the maximum effect achieved in 24 hours.[14] When laminaria is used, oxytocin infusion is frequently necessary to achieve true labor. Often the procedure is the following: the physician places the laminaria in the cervix at night, allowing the cervix to dilate 2 to 3 cm; he removes them in the morning and then starts an oxytocin induction. The nurse's responsibility is no different than it would be for the ordinary woman anticipating labor.

• •

Review Questions

1. What are some advantages of medical induction?
   a. ____________________
   b. ____________________
   c. ____________________
2. What conditions justify medically indicated induction?
   a. ____________________
   b. ____________________
   c. ____________________
3. Why might amniocentesis and x-ray or ultrasound be done before medical induction is begun? ____________________
   ____
   ____

4. What information does a Bishop score of greater than 4 provide?
____
____
____

5. Why would laminaria be placed in the cervix for up to 24 hours?
____
____
____

Answers

1. Advantages of induction include: a. planned time for labor, b. mother rested, c. mother psychologically prepared for labor, d. necessary household arrangements made, and e. hospital usually well staffed and equipped at time of admission.
2. Conditions that justify indicated induction include: a. prolonged rupture of membranes, b. postmaturity, c. maternal diabetes, d. pre-eclampsia/eclampsia, and e. Rh sensitization.
3. Amniocentesis and x-ray or ultrasound may be done before medical induction is begun to verify fetal maturity. X-ray or ultrasound may also be done to ascertain fetopelvic relationships.
4. Based on the status of the cervix and fetal station, a Bishop score of greater than 4 predicts that there is an 80 percent chance of success in induction of labor at this time.
5. Laminaria is dried seaweed that, when placed in the cervix, absorbs moisture and may cause the cervix to soften and dilate. It reaches its maximum effect by 24 hours.

• •

Medical Induction of Labor with Oxytocin

Oxytocin, in the form of Pitocin or Syntocinon, is the drug used most frequently for medical induction of labor. Table 5–2 lists the

TABLE 5–2. COMMON MEDICAL INDICATIONS FOR INDUCTION OF LABOR

MATERNAL	FETAL
Hypertensive disorders	Demise
Diabetes (Class B-R)	Intrauterine growth retardation (IUGR)
Cyanotic cardiac disease	Prolonged pregnancy (42+ weeks)
Rh isoimmunization	+ Contraction Stress Test (CST)
Chorioamnionitis	
Premature rupture of membranes (near term)	

most common maternal and fetal indications for medical induction. Oxytocin is also used for *augmentation*—to improve or reinforce labor. Several hypotonic contraction patterns discussed in Chapter 3 and abnormal cervical dilatation curves discussed in Chapter 4 are augmented with oxytocin. As the Bishop score in Table 5–1 predicts, the more ripe the cervix the less oxytocin is needed. This, in part, explains why an augmented (already started) labor requires less stimulation from oxytocin than an induced (to be started) labor.[13,15] Whether used for induction or augmentation, it is advisable to continue oxytocin infusion for one hour postpartum to avoid uterine atony.[16]

As pregnancy approaches term, the uterus becomes very sensitive to minute amounts of oxytocin. Natural oxytocin is released from the posterior lobe of the pituitary gland and stimulates rhythmic uterine contractions. Synthetic preparations of oxytocin (for example, Pitocin and Syntocinon) likewise act on the smooth muscle of the uterus to stimulate contractions. Oxytocin-stimulated contractions are often more painful than spontaneous contractions due to the comparatively rapid onset of stimulated contractions. Ergots, another classification of oxytocin that includes Methergine, cause sustained uterine contractions that are incompatible with adequate fetal oxygenation and therefore should not be used until following delivery.

Contraindications to Induction with Oxytoxin. The pregnant woman has a right to refuse induction but ordinarily, when the physician explains the rationale for the induction in the presence of no other contraindications (Table 5–3), the woman consents to the procedure. Induction should not be done in the presence of abnormal fetopelvic relationships. These include fetopelvic disproportion, malpresentation, and malposition. Nor should labor be induced when the fetal status is already in jeopardy. Examples include the presence of fetal distress or prematurity. In the presence of uterine scar tissue or hypertonic uterine contractions, induction increases the likelihood of uterine rupture, although many vaginal births after cesarean (see Chapter 7) are stimulated without difficulty. Another contraindication to induction with oxytocin is an overdistended uterus found in a multiple gestation pregnancy, hydramnios, and

Table 5–3. GENERALLY CONSIDERED CONTRAINDICATIONS TO OXYTOCIN INDUCTION

Fetopelvic disproportion	Multiple gestation
Malpresentation	Hydramnios
Malposition	Multiparity greater than 5
Fetal distress	Severe pre-eclampsia
Prematurity	Placenta previa
Hypertonic uterine contractions	

multiparity greater than five. Induction with oxytocin would cause increased risk to mother and fetus in the presence of severe preeclampsia and placenta previa. The nurse as well as the physician in charge are responsible for noting the presence of any of these contraindications.

The benefits of oxytocin must outweigh the risks. Oxytocin requires careful and frequent assessments and necessitates the use of continuous electronic fetal monitoring. (See Chapter 3.) When oxytocin is administered injudiciously, hypertonic uterine contractions are likely to result. In turn, they may cause fetal hypoxia and distress, precipitous labor, placental abruption, uterine rupture, cervical laceration, and/or amniotic fluid embolism. To state these risks in nursing diagnosis format, there is **injury, potential for; (maternal and/or fetal) trauma related to injudicious administration of oxytocin**.

In the event that uterine hyperactivity or fetal distress occur, the oxytocin must be stopped immediately and the mother turned to her left side. This movement will increase oxygen to the fetus, thereby improving the fetal heart rate and decreasing the frequency of uterine contractions, although their intensity increases. The circulatory half-life of oxytocin is 3 to 4 minutes although the uterine effects last 20 to 30 minutes.[15] If fetal distress is evident, the rate of the main line IV should be increased and nasal oxygen administered at 5 to 10 liters per minute to the mother. The responsible physician must be informed and come to evaluate both mother and fetus. All nursing observations and interventions should be documented in the order that they occurred. A flowsheet, including all pertinent information, is effective for the medical record.

Administration of Oxytocin Induction. The obstetric department of each institution should establish a written protocol for the preparation and administration of oxytocin.[13] Therefore, the following will vary depending on the institution. In many cases, the "should" will be a "must" and the assessments will differ. The nurse is responsible for having adequate knowledge of the patient, the specific protocol for induction, and the effects of the drug.

Oxytocin is always administered intravenously and as a rule by a controlled infusion pump device, such as an IVAC, Harvard pump, Imed, or Auto-syringe. This precisely controls the amount of medicine administered. (Oxorn[17] states that a Murphy drip is also acceptable.) Dosages are calculated and documented in milliunits per minute (mU/min) to guarantee a standardized approach. A piggyback setup — two IVs of the same solution, one without oxytocin (primary line) and one with oxytocin (secondary line) — makes it possible to discontinue the oxytocin immediately, if necessary, without disturbing the intravenous infusion. It also decreases the possibility of giving a bolus of oxytocin when administering other medications. The junction of the Y adapter in the tubing should be as close as possible to the laboring woman's arm so that a change from one solution to the other will be immediate. Ten units (10,000 mU) of oxytocin are placed in 1000 ml of 5 percent dextrose in water, normal saline, or lactated Ringer's solution. (In the diabetic, dextrose may need to be omitted, depending on serum glucose levels.) The initial dose may be as low as 0.5 but no more than 1 mU per minute.

For the first 20 minutes it is recommended that the nurse remain at the bedside to evaluate the effect of oxytocin on maternal contractions and fetal heart rate. At 15- to 20-minute intervals (a few authorities say not greater than 30 minutes[18–21]), the rate is increased by no more than 1 to 2 mU per minute until a normal uterine contraction pattern begins. Oxytocin must be administered with extreme caution because its effect is unpredictable. In general, the minimum dose should be used to foster effective uterine response. Ideally, the contractions will attain a frequency of 3 to 4 minutes, a duration of 50 to 60 seconds, and an intensity of moderate to strong with at least a 30-second resting period. (Some authorities[16] recommend a frequency of 2 to 3 minutes and a duration of 40 to 50 seconds.) Care must be taken to maintain sufficient contraction quality, that is, duration and intensity. If the frequency of the contractions becomes too close, Steer and Beard's study[22] shows that the contraction quality decreases. Most term labors establish an adequate labor pattern at 4 to 8 mU per min.[22–24] Seldom is more than 20–40 mU needed to achieve progressive dilatation.[13] The current trend is to achieve a contraction pattern that promotes the latent phase of dilatation, not a rapid movement into the active phase (see Chapter 4). Therefore, once the desired contraction pattern is achieved and the cervix dilated 5 to 6 cm, the oxytocin rate can be reduced at 1 to 2 mU increments.[13]

A physician who has privileges to perform cesarean deliveries must be available to the labor unit whenever oxytocin is being administered, and be present when the infusion is started.[13,25] The physician or nurse must assess the uterine contractions and fetal response at least every 15 minutes. Whenever possible, a continuous electronic monitor should be used. Following rupture of membranes, an internal fetal monitor is desirable. The oxytocin dose in mU/min should be recorded on the monitor's graph paper each time the dose is altered. The laboring woman should maintain a lateral recumbent or sitting position. This avoids vena cava syndrome and increases placental perfusion.

Tetanic contractions (lasting longer than 90 seconds) and tumultuous (violently agitated) labor may result and cause: (1) fetal distress due to impaired placental and fetal circulation during the contractions; (2) abruptio placentae (premature separation of the placenta); (3) amniotic fluid emboli; (4) lacerations to the cervix and neonatal injuries; and (5) rupture of the uterus. In the presence of any of these complications, the oxytocin must be discontinued immediately and the doctor must be informed.

When oxytocin is infusing, it is the nurse's responsibility to assess and document not only the uterine and fetal heart rate response but also the blood pressure and urine output. Preferably, the blood pressure and pulse are monitored every 30 minutes or with each increase in dosage, whichever is more frequent. Initially the blood pressure is slightly decreased due to the oxytocin infusion. As much as a 30 percent sustained increase in blood pressure is predictable.[15] A high concentration of oxytocin may cause hypertension accompanied by a frontal headache. Both of these side effects disappear when the drug is stopped. Prolonged use of oxytocin can cause water intoxication. In order to prevent this, an electrolyte solution (e.g., lactated Ringer's) and an increased concentration of oxytocin should be used to limit the volume of the fluid infused in doses exceeding 20 mU per minute.[15] At the same time, efforts must be made to maintain adequate hydration. To avoid dehydration and exhaustion, as well as to enhance effective uterine contractions, there should be an intake of 125 ml per hour.

Throughout the oxytocin induction, which can occur over a period as long as three days with overnight periods providing for rest, it is advantageous to have a well-informed laboring woman and support person. **Knowledge deficit [about the induction of labor] related to lack of exposure** is a problem that the nurse, and physician, must deal with. Likewise, the **anxiety [specify] related to interruption in the normal labor process** can further prolong the laboring period. The anxious woman needs to know that her **comfort, alteration in: pain, acute** (abrupt onset of uterine contractions) **related to oxytocin-induced contractions** is an expected outcome but that measures can and will be used to help the woman to cope with her laboring process. Far too often, nurses get so involved in the oxytocin procedure that they overlook the human aspect of it. Nurses are equally responsible for meeting the psychological needs of the laboring woman. Several ways to do this are identified in Chapters 1 and 7.

• •

Review Questions

1. What are the actions of oxytocin? ______________________________
____

2. Name two oxytocics used to stimulate labor: a. ______________ and b. ____

3. Summarize the nursing interventions appropriate during the administration of oxytocin by filling in the blanks:
   a. Set up piggyback IV of: ______________________________
   ____
   b. Give initial dose of: ______________________________
   c. Increase dose every __________ by (what amount?) __________ ______________________ depending on ______________________
   ____
   d. Assess and record uterine contractions and fetal heart rate every:
   ____

e. Maintain rate that causes ideal contractions, which are: ________
____

f. Stop the induction immediately in the presence of ________ contractions or ________ distress.

g. Monitor vital signs for ________ and I&O for ________
____

h. If the first day of induction is not successful, prepare mother for:
____

Answers

1. Oxytocin initiates (induces) or reinforces (augments) uterine contractions.
2. *Pitocin* and *Syntocinon* are oxytocics used to stimulate labor.
3. Nursing interventions appropriate during administration of oxytocin:
   a. Set up piggyback IV of *one bottle with 1000 ml of 5% D/W, NS, or RL and a second bottle with the same solution but with 10 U oxytocin added.*
   b. Give initial dose of *0.5 to 1 mU per minute.*
   c. Increase rate every *15 to 20 minutes* by *1 to 2 mU intervals,* depending on *uterine response and fetal heart rate.*
   d. Assess and record uterine contractions and fetal heart rate every *15 minutes.*
   e. Maintain rate that causes ideal contractions, which are *a frequency of 3 to 4 minutes and duration of 50 to 60 seconds.*
   f. Stop the induction immediately in the presence of *hypertonic* contractions and *fetal* distress.
   g. Monitor vitals signs for *hypotension* and for *signs of water intoxication.*
   h. If the first day of induction is not successful, prepare mother for *a possible second or third day of induction.*

• •

Medical Induction of Labor with Prostaglandin Gel

Prostaglandin is a hormone that comes in several forms. Intravenous E_2 and F_2 are very effective in inducing uterine contractions early in pregnancy for medically induced abortions. They are usually not used for term labor because they frequently cause nausea, vomiting, and diarrhea, although they may be preferred for women with renal or cardiac disease, because they do not have the antidiuretic effects of oxytocin.[26]

Intravaginal prostaglandins, preferably PGE_2 as a vaginal suppository, is currently used as an effective labor stimulant. The dose of PGE_2 is 0.2 mg in 10 ml hydroxyethylcellulose gel. Contractions usually begin within a few minutes following insertion.[27] PGE_2 has several advantages over intravenous oxytocin and amniotomy because usually the success of an induction is dependent upon the status of the cervix. PGE_2 is known to work effectively on an unripe cervix[28,29] with a high rate of success. Compared to oxytocin, there is the same risk of uterine hypertonicity, and the same uterine stimulating effects when the cervix is ripe. PGE_2 does not have the side effects found in the intravenous prostaglandins. An advantage over amniotomy is that there is no problem of infection and thus no "24-hour limit for delivery."

Prostaglandin gel is approved by the FDA for experimental use only. Prior to administering PGE_2, assessment of the uterine activity and fetal heart rates should be done for 20 minutes using a continuous monitor, and a vaginal examination should be performed to determine the status of the cervix. A physician inserts the PGE_2 suppository or viscous gel using either a plastic catheter, which is then removed, or a diaphragm, into the posterior vaginal fornix. For at least 30 minutes the woman should assume a side lying position to increase placental perfusion, and continuous monitoring should be done. Then, some institutions permit ambulation or even discharge until the onset of labor. The temperature should be assessed every hour because there is potential **hyperthermia related to prostaglandin's effect on the hypothalamus**. An increase of 2 degrees F (1 degree C) is likely to occur without suspecting other causes. The nurse must also watch for nausea, vomiting, and diarrhea, because electrolyte imbalance may result.

• •

Review Question

Identify three areas that the nurse should assess when a woman at term is given prostaglandin gel:

a. ____

b. ____

c. ____

Answer

When a woman at term is given prostaglandin gel, the nurse is responsible for assessing:

a. uterine activity and fetal heart rate prior to insertion of gel and for at least 30 minutes after,
b. temperature every hour anticipating an elevation of no more that two degrees F above normal,
c. nausea, vomiting, and diarrhea that may cause electrolyte imbalance.

• •

CONCLUSION

Throughout this chapter several labor stimulants were identified, along with the nurse's role as assessor and intervenor. Several examples of appropriate nursing diagnoses were included. As clinical experiences occur that warrant the use of these stimulants, it is wise for the nurse to periodically refer to this information to evaluate how well the nurse has applied this knowledge. Hospital protocol should also reflect principles similar to those expressed in this chapter. By being well informed the nurse is more likely to be a safe practitioner, protecting the patient(s), oneself, and the employer.

REFERENCES

1. ACOG: Induction of labor. ACOG Technical Bulletin, No 49, Washington, DC, 1978.
2. Danforth, DN (ed): Obstetrics and Gynecology, ed 4. Harper & Row, Philadelphia, 1982, p 721.
3. Pritchard, JA, MacDonald, PC, and Gant, NF: Williams Obstetrics, ed 17. Appleton-Century-Crofts, Norwalk, Connecticut, 1985, p 333.
4. Mahan, CS and McKay, S: Preps and enemas: Keep or discard? Contemp Obstet Gynecol 22:129, 1983.
5. Thomas, CL (ed): Taber's Cyclopedic Medical Dictionary. FA Davis, Philadelphia, 1981, 1–16.
6. Oxorn, H: Oxorn-Foote: Human Labor and Birth, ed 5. Appleton-Century-Crofts, Norwalk, Connecticut, 1986, p 685.
7. Varney, H: Nurse-Midwifery, ed 2. Blackwell Scientific Publications, Boston, 1987, pp 259–260.
8. Gilbert, ES and Harmon, JS: High-Risk Pregnancy and Delivery: Nursing Perspectives. CV Mosby, St. Louis, 1986, p 435.
9. Knuppel, RA and Drukker, JE: High-Risk Pregnancy: A Team Approach. WB Saunders, Philadelphia, 1986, p 225.
10. Caldeyro-Barcia, R, et al: Adverse perinatal effects of early amniotomy during labor. In Gluck, B (ed): Modern Perinatal Medicine. Year Book Medical Publishers, Chicago, 1974, pp 431–449.
11. Lynaugh, KH: The effects of early elective amniotomy on the length of labor and the condition of the fetus. J Nurs-Midw 25:3, 1980.
12. Friedman, EA: Labor: Clinical Evaluation and Management, ed 2. Appleton-Century-Crofts, New York, 1978, p 334.
13. NAACOG: The Nurse's Role in the Induction/Augmentation of Labor. NAACOG OGN Nursing Practice Resource, January 1988.
14. Oxorn, H: Oxorn-Foote: Human Labor and Birth, ed 5. Appleton-Century-Crofts, Norwalk, Connecticut, 1986, p 690.
15. Marshall, C: The art of induction/augmentation of labor. J Obstet Gynecol Neonatal Nurs 14:25, 1985.
16. Oxorn, H: Oxorn-Foote: Human Labor and Birth, ed 5. Appleton-Century-Crofts, Norwalk, Connecticut, 1986, p 676.
17. Oxorn, H: Oxorn-Foote: Human Labor and Birth, ed 5. Appleton-Century-Crofts, Norwalk, Connecticut, 1986, p 675.
18. Seitchik, J and Castillo, M: Oxytocin augmentation of dysfunctional labor. I. Clinical data. Am J Obstet Gynecol 144:899, 1982.
19. Seitchik, J and Castillo, M: Oxytocin augmentation of dysfunctional labor. II. Uterine activity data. Am J Obstet Gynecol 145:526, 1983a.
20. Seitchik, J and Castillo, M: Oxytocin augmentation of dysfunctional labor. III. Multiparous patients. Am J Obstet Gynecol 145:777, 1983b.
21. Thomford, PJ, Fields, LB, and Miller, FC: Low dose oxytocin infusion at term alters endogenous oxytocin pulses. Scientific Program and Ab-

stracts, 34th Meeting of the Society for Gynecologic Investigations, March 18–21, 1987. Abstract No. 151, p 102.
22. Steer, PJ and Beard, RS: Bettering control of oxytocin infusions. Contemp Obstet Gynecol 19:117, 1982.
23. Cibils, L: Enhancement and induction of labor. In Aledjm, S (ed): Risks in the Practice of Modern Obstetrics. CV Mosby, St. Louis, 1975, pp. 182–209.
24. Petrie, RH: The pharmacology and use of oxytocin. Clin Perinat 8:35, 1981.
25. Oxorn, H: Oxorn-Foote: Human Labor and Birth, ed 5. Appleton-Century-Crofts, Norwalk, Connecticut, 1986, p 679.
26. Gilbert, ES and Harmon, JS: High-Risk Pregnancy and Delivery: Nursing Perspectives. CV Mosby, St. Louis, 1986, p 440.
27. Prins, R, et al: Cervical ripening with intravaginal prostaglandin E_2 gel. Obstet Gynecol 61:459, 1983.
28. Hefni, MA and Lewis, GA: Induction of labour with vaginal prostaglandin E_2 pessaries. Br J Obstet and Gynaecol 87:199, 1980.
29. O'Herlihy, C and MacDonald, HN: Influence of prostaglandin E_2 vaginal gel on cervical ripening and labor. Obstet Gynecol 54:708, 1979.

BIBLIOGRAPHY

ACOG: Conduct of labor. In Precis III: An Update in Obstetrics and Gynecology. ACOG, Washington, DC, 1986, p 133.

ACOG: Induction of Labor. ACOG Technical Bulletin #49, 1978.

———: A "natural" oxytocin contraction stress test. Am J Nurs 84(6):707.

Bobak, IM and Jensen, MD: Essentials of Maternity Nursing: The Nurse and the Childbearing Family, ed 2. CV Mosby, St. Louis, 1987.

Danforth, DN (ed): Obstetrics and Gynecology, ed 4. Harper & Row, Philadelphia, 1982.

Elliot, JP and Flaherty, JF: The use of breast stimulation to ripen the cervix in term pregnancies. Am J Obstet Gynecol 145:553, 1982.

Gantes, M, Krichhoff, KT, and Work, BA: Breast massage to obtain contraction stress test. Nurs Res 34(6):338, 1985.

Gilbert, ES and Harmon, JS: High-Risk Pregnancy and Delivery: Nursing Perspectives. CV Mosby, St. Louis, 1986.

Jhirad, A and Vago, T: Induction of labor by breast stimulation: Obstet Gynecol 41:347, 1973.

Knuppel, RA and Drukker, JE: High-Risk Pregnancy: A Team Approach. WB Saunders, Philadelphia, 1986.

Marshall, C: The art of induction/augmentation of labor. J Obstet Gynecol Neonatal Nurs 14(1):22, 1985.

Marshall, C: The nipple stimulation contraction stress test. J Obstet Gynecol Neonatal Nurs 15(6):459, 1986.

Murray ML, Canfield, S and Harmon, J: Nipple stimulation-contraction stress test for the high-risk patient. Matern Child Nurs J 11(5):331, 1986

NAACOG: Induction of Labor. NAACOG Technical Bulletin #4, 1979.

NAACOG: The Nurse's Role in the Induction/Augmentation of Labor. NAACOG OGN Nursing Practice Resource, January 1988.

Oxorn, H: Oxorn-Foote: Human Labor and Birth, ed. 5. Appleton-Century-Crofts, Norwalk, Connecticut, 1986.

Pritchard, JA, MacDonald, PC and Gant, NF: Williams Obstetrics, ed. 17. Appleton-Century-Crofts, Norwalk, Connecticut, 1985.

Reeder, SJ and Martin, LL: Maternity Nursing: Family, Newborn, and Women's Health Care, ed. 16. JB Lippincott, Philadelphia, 1987.

Vice, L: Fetal Monitoring Level II. Medical Media Associates Conference, Ann Arbor, October 27, 1986.

Varney, H: Nurse-Midwifery, ed. 2. Blackwell Scientific Publications, Boston, 1987.

Whitley, N: A Manual of Clinical Obstetrics. JB Lippincott, Philadelphia, 1985.

POST-TEST 5

1. (Circle True or False) An enema is given on the labor unit because:
   a. T F It might stimulate uterine contractions.
   b. T F It empties the lower intestinal tract.
   c. T F It prevents the likelihood of fecal contamination during delivery.
   d. T F It may cause less inhibition to push following complete cervical dilatation.

2. (Circle Yes or No) In which of the following situations should a nurse question the order for an enema for a laboring woman?
   a. Y N Woman is bleeding in excess of bloody show.
   b. Y N A primigravida's cervix is 3 cm dilated and station is −2.
   c. Y N A multipara's cervix is 3 cm dilated and station is 0.
   d. Y N The fetus is in breech presentation.
   e. Y N The fetus is post-term.

3. When giving an enema to a tense woman in early labor, what information about the procedure can you give the woman that might ease this situation? (Include at least 4 suggestions.)
   ____
   ____
   ____
   ____

4. Circle True or False and explain your answer.
   a. T F Stripping the membranes and rupture of membranes are the same thing. ______________________________
   ____
   b. T F Ambulation is contraindicated once labor begins.
   ____
   c. T F Nipple stimulation may require privacy in the woman's labor unit. ______________________________
   ____
   d. T F As the laminaria swells it may cause progress in cervical changes. ______________________________
   ____

5. Explain why:
   a. Fetal heart rate should be taken immediately following AROM.
   ____
   ____
   ____
   b. The presence of dark-colored, foul-smelling fluid is significant in a vertex presentation. ______________________________
   ____
   ____
   c. A woman with ruptured membranes is usually confined to bed.
   ____
   ____
   ____

6. Circle True or False for the following statements about Pitocin and Syntocinon:

   a. T F They are forms of oxytocin.
   b. T F They stimulate labor if the cervix is ripe.
   c. T F They may cause water intoxication (antidiuresis).
   d. T F They may alter the fetal heart rate and the maternal blood pressure.
   e. T F They require observation for uterine hyperactivity.

7. Circle True or False regarding which of the following principles should be observed in the use of oxytocin to stimulate labor?
   a. T F The condition of the fetus must be satisfactory.
   b. T F Oxytocin should be used only in cases of uterine dysfunction.
   c. T F There should be no predisposition to uterine rupture.
   d. T F Oxytocin should be used in cases in which it is important to terminate the pregnancy quickly, for example, in abruptio placentae.
   e. T F A responsible physician should be constantly available while the mother is receiving oxytocin.

8. Mrs. Adam, a G3P2, is 41 weeks pregnant. Her cervix is dilated 2 cm, soft, 20 percent effaced, anterior. The fetal station is −2. Using the Bishop scoring system, interpret her chances for being successfully induced.
   ____
   ____
   ____
   ____

9. The name of the drug used only experimentally to induce labor is
   ____

10. Match the potential problems in Column I with the specific labor stimulants listed in Column II. Each item should be used only once.

COLUMN I	COLUMN II
a. Self-esteem disturbance	_____ Stripping membranes
b. Discomfort (cramping, slight vaginal bleeding)	_____ Rupture of membranes
c. Alterations in bowel elimination	_____ Oxytocin
d. Potential fetal infection	_____ Ambulation during questionable false labor
e. Altered sexuality pattern	_____ Prostaglandin
f. Alteration in comfort (abrupt onset of contractions)	_____ Nipple stimulation
g. Potential hyperthermia	_____ Enema

Answers to Post-Test

1. (a) True, (b) True, (c) True, and (d) True. (Refer back to question.)
2. (a) Yes, (b) Yes, (c) No, (d) Yes, and (e) No. (Refer to question.)
3. To ease the situation while giving a tense woman an enema:
   a. Familiarize the woman with the equipment, inform her of the length of time she will need to retain the solution, and tell her that she will be allowed to completely evacuate the contents on the toilet.
   b. Inform her that the procedure should not hurt, the tube will be lubricated, and if resistance is met, progression of the tube will be stopped and the tube repositioned; the procedure can be stopped during contractions.
   c. Inform her that the flow of solution can be stopped when she feels enough pressure and/or uterine contractions occur.
   d. Tell the woman to try slow deep breathing during the procedure.
   e. Explain the purposes for the enema (see Question 1).
4. a. False. Stripping of membranes is a digital loosening of the membranes from the uterus and is done to encourage cervical softening and effacement. Rupture of membranes involves breaking the membranes.
   b. False. Ambulation may be encouraged during early labor, since it may stimulate labor. (There are some instances when it is contraindicated, for example, following ROM or sedation.)
   c. True. Many women feel uncomfortable performing sexually related activities (e.g., nipple stimulation) in other than a private setting.
   d. True. Laminaria absorbs moisture from the cervix, causing the laminaria to swell and possibly causing the cervix to soften and dilate.
5. a. An abnormal fetal heart rate pattern may indicate abnormal pressure on the cord. This may occur following AROM.
   b. Dark-colored amniotic fluid indicates meconium, which is abnormal in vertex presentation. A foul smell indicates possible infection.
   c. The woman is confined to bed to reduce the chance of introducing infection.
6. All of the responses about Pitocin and Syntocinon are True. Pitocin and Syntocinon: (a) are forms of oxytocin, (b) stimulate labor if the cervix is ripe, (c) may

cause water intoxication (antidiuresis), (d) may alter the fetal heart rate and the maternal blood pressure, and (e) require observation for uterine hyperactivity.

7. a, c, and e are True. The following principles should be observed in the use of oxytocin to stimulate labor: a. The fetal condition must be satisfactory, c. There should be no predisposition to uterine rupture, and e. A responsible physician should be constantly available while the mother is receiving oxytocin.
b and d are False. b. Although oxytocin is used in cases of uterine dysfunction (i.e., augmentation), it is also used to induce labor. d. Oxytocin should not be used in the presence of abruptio placentae because of the danger of hemorrhage.

8. The Bishop scoring system gives Mrs. Adam a total of 6 points: 1 point for 2 cm, 2 for soft, 0 for 20 percent, 1 for −2 station, 2 for anterior. A score greater than 4 gives her a success rate of 80 percent. (She also has in her favor a term pregnancy and probably nonresistent pelvic soft tissue because she is a multipara.)

9. Prostaglandin E_2 (PGE_2 gel) is an experimental drug used to induce labor.

10. The correct answers are b, d, f, a, g, e, c. This is how they match:

POTENTIAL PROBLEM	LABOR STIMULANT
a. Self-esteem disturbance	a. Ambulation during questionable false labor
b. Discomfort (cramping, slight vaginal bleeding)	b. Stripping membranes
c. Alterations in bowel elimination	c. Enema
d. Potential fetal infection	d. Rupture of membranes
e. Altered sexuality pattern	e. Nipple stimulation
f. Alteration in comfort (abrupt onset of contractions)	f. Oxytocin
g. Potential hyperthermia	g. Prostaglandins

6 MANAGEMENT OF PAIN WITH DRUGS

Carolyn G. Pedigo

OBJECTIVES

Upon completing this chapter, you will be able to:

- ▶ Discuss psycho-physiological responses to pain in labor.
- ▶ Identify four theories regarding the cause of pain in labor.
- ▶ Discuss five supportive nursing interventions that may be used in conjunction with drugs to decrease pain perception.
- ▶ Define the terms analgesia and anesthesia as they apply to labor and delivery.
- ▶ Describe how anesthesia is used to block pain impulses during labor and delivery.
- ▶ Identify three considerations that may influence the decision of whether or not to use drugs for pain relief.
- ▶ List three side effects of pain relief with drugs that may be considered undesirable for the mother, and the resulting effects of the maternal side effects on the fetus and newborn.
- ▶ Discuss the action and side effects of the following: narcotic agonists, narcotic antagonists, mixed agonists/antagonists, and sedatives used during labor: meperidine, alphaprodine, oxymorphone, naloxone, levallorphan, butorphanol, nalbuphine, pentazocine, secobarbital, pentobarbital, promethazine, and hydroxyzine.
- ▶ Differentiate among the following types of anesthesia used during labor and delivery: epidural, caudal, saddle, spinal, paracervical, and pudendal blocks; local perineal infiltration; inhalation and intravenous anesthesia.
- ▶ Discuss the use of epidural analgesia.
- ▶ Describe emergency nursing interventions that may be carried out as a result of complications following the administration of anesthesia.
- ▶ Discuss advantages, disadvantages and potential complications of general (inhalation and intravenous) anesthesia.

This chapter has been prepared to help the reader understand the importance of the proper use of drugs for relief of pain, tension, and anxiety during labor and delivery as a supplement to nonpharmacologic nursing interventions for pain. Nonpharmacologic pain intervention by the nurse may provide all the support necessary to a laboring woman, allowing her to progress relatively comfortably through the process of labor and delivery. If additional intervention with drugs becomes necessary, then as little medication as possible should be used.

The major focus of this chapter is pain relief through drugs. Psychophysiologic responses to pain are included to help the reader assess the presence and degree of pain experienced by a woman in labor in order to determine the need for drug intervention. Partial or full relief of pain may be achieved with drugs at various times. Safety is the main focus whenever drugs are administered during labor and delivery. The degree of safety is determined by assessing the effects of drugs upon the mother and how these may indirectly affect the fetus or newborn. A pharmacology book should be consulted for additional information about the drugs mentioned throughout this chapter.

A suggested prerequisite to this chapter is a basic understanding of the normal anatomy and physiology of the reproductive system in relation to the labor and delivery process.

PSYCHO-PHYSIOLOGIC RESPONSES TO PAIN

Labor and delivery can be a fascinating and exciting time for the expectant family. It is the culmination of pregnancy and also the beginning of the long-awaited birth of the child. The term *labor* means work, and yet, that term has many other associations. Unfortunately, the major association in our society is negative—pain. Pain should be viewed as a positive signal since in the absence of pain, labor and consequently delivery might occur without warning thus depriving the woman and her baby of appropriate medical/nursing care. Pain is a normal physiological process that is a natural part of labor and delivery. (See Chapter 7 for a discussion of the following theories of pain: Fear, Tension, Pain Cycle; Psychophysical Pathway [Lamaze]; Gate Control Theory; and Endogenous Pain Control Theory.)

Pain is a subjective phenomenon that exists when an individual experiences a sensation, interprets the sensation as discomfort, and exhibits a psychological and physiologic reaction to the sensation. Perception of pain during labor may be intensified by progressive uterine contractions, fatigue, lack of sleep, tension, anxiety, and fear. Previous experience with pain, personal expectations of pain in labor, and one's own cultural concept of pain will affect the perception of pain and the individual's response to pain.

Pain as Stress

Pain during labor causes maternal stress, however, a certain amount of stress can be beneficial since it triggers a physiologic compensatory response in which catecholamines (epinephrine and norepinephrine) are released to prepare the body for action. As a result of this response, heart rate, blood pressure and oxygen uptake increase. Blood is shunted to the vital organs (brain, liver, heart). These responses are regarded as a coping response.[1] The stress of labor also affects the fetus, triggering the release of fetal catecholamines. This is an adaptive fetal response to decreased oxygen that occurs during regular rhythmic uterine contractions. Energy stores are mobilized and oxygen expenditure is decreased.[2] The fetus is prepared for extrauterine life by the "normal" stress of labor.

Pain as Distress

Excess or uncontrolled pain causes normal maternal *stress* to become *distress*. Maternal reactions can trigger an excessive release of catecholamines and cortisol causing constriction of uterine arteries. When uterine arteries constrict, blood flow to the uterus is decreased, causing uterine hypoxia that may lead to dysfunctional or prolonged labor. Blood flow to the placenta is also decreased, causing fetal hypoxia resulting in fetal distress. Constriction of uterine arteries combined with shunting of blood away from the uterus and placenta can prolong fetal hypoxia.[3] Maternal hyperventilation (a possible response to distress) causes a rise in maternal pH resulting in decreased release of oxygen from maternal hemoglobin, thus further compromising the fetus.[4] The fetus may respond to the distress of hypoxia by producing excess catecholamines which may cause fetal heart rate abnormalities and/or neonatal respiratory distress, cold stress, and metabolic acidosis.[5]

Unfortunately, there is no definitive line between stress and distress caused by pain in labor. Assessment is critical. Nurses must assess for physiological reactions to pain which may include increases in blood pressure, heart rate, respirations, perspiration, pupil diameter, muscle tension (fisted hands, rigidity, grimacing, facial tension), muscle activity (twisting, turning, pacing), and inefficient contractions that prolong labor. Nurses must be responsive to verbal expressions of pain which can include statements about pain, cries for help, and moaning and groaning. Nonverbal expressions of pain can include depression, withdrawal, hostility, and fear.

CAUSE OF PAIN IN LABOR

No *one* cause of pain in labor has been determined. Numerous theories about the causes of pain in labor have been hypothesized. Some theories are the following:

1. *anoxia* of compressed muscle cells of the uterus brought about with each contraction
2. *compression* of the nerve ganglia in the cervix and lower uterine segments during contractions
3. *stretching* of the cervix during dilatation and effacement
4. *stretching* and displacement of the perineum as the fetus descends through the birth canal
5. *pressure* on the urethra, bladder, and rectum as the fetus descends
6. *fear* resulting in tension that causes pain and more fear as a spontaneous occurrence (see Chapter 7 for discussion of the Fear-Tension-Pain Cycle)

• •

Review Questions

1. Pain is a subjective phenomenon that exists when an individual:
   a. experiences ______
   b. interprets ______
   c. exhibits ______
2. Identify six factors that may intensify a woman's perception of pain during labor.
   a. ______
   b. ______
   c. ______
   d. ______
   e. ______
   f. ______
3. Explain the difference between *stress* and *distress* caused by pain in labor.
   ______
   ______
   ______
   ______
4. Identify three physiologic and three behavioral indications of pain perception.

Physiological:	Behavioral (verbal or nonverbal):
a. ______	a. ______
b. ______	b. ______
c. ______	c. ______

5. List four theories of the cause of pain in labor.
   a. ______
   b. ______
   c. ______
   d. ______

Answers

1. Pain exists when an individual: (a) experiences a sensation, (b) interprets the sensation as painful, and (c) exhibits a psychological and physiologic reaction to the sensation.

2. Factors that may intensify a woman's perception of pain during labor include: (a) progressive uterine contractions, (b) fatigue, (c) lack of sleep, (d) tension, (e) anxiety, (f) fear, (g) previous experience with pain, (h) personal expectations of pain in labor, and (i) cultural concept of pain.

3. Pain during labor causes maternal stress which triggers the release of catecholamines as a coping response. Catecholamines prepare the laboring woman for action and assist the fetus to adapt to decreased oxygen. Excessive pain can cause maternal distress which triggers the release of excess amounts of catecholamines in the mother and the fetus. The mother may experience prolonged labor and the fetus may experience prolonged hypoxia.

4. Indications of pain perception. Physiologic reactions include increased: (a) blood pressure, (b) heart rate, (c) respirations, (d) pupil diameter, (e) muscle tension, (f) muscle activity, and (g) inefficient contractions causing prolonged labor. Behavioral reactions may be verbal or nonverbal, including: (a) statements about pain, (b) cries for help, (c) moaning and groaning, (d) depression, (e) withdrawal, (f) hostility, and (g) fear.

5. Current theories of the cause of pain in labor are:
   a. hypoxia of compressed muscle cells of the uterus brought about with each contraction
   b. compression of the nerve ganglia in the cervix and lower uterine segments during contractions
   c. stretching of the cervix during dilatation and effacement
   d. stretching and displacement of the perineum as the fetus descends through the birth canal
   e. pressure on the urethra, bladder, and rectum as the fetus descends
   f. fear resulting in tension that causes pain and more fear as a spontaneous occurrence.

• •

NONPHARMACOLOGIC NURSING INTERVENTIONS FOR PAIN RELIEF DURING LABOR AND DELIVERY

If labor and delivery are believed to be a painful experience and if drugs can be given to alleviate that pain, then how can the nurse be important in providing pain relief during the labor and delivery experience? The nurse can be successful or ineffective depending on the interventions' consistency with the physiologic and psychological aspects of labor and delivery. The nurse should first focus on nonpharmacologic methods of pain relief. Nursing interventions can provide relief from discomfort and help the laboring woman to feel cared for. This can contribute to a decreased perception of pain thus decreasing the need for and amount of drug intervention. (See Chapter 7 for a discussion of several nonpharmacologic nursing interventions for pain relief.) If the use of drugs becomes necessary, they should only be used to enhance the effectiveness of nonpharmacologic measures. *Drugs alone are not the answer.*

In order to help a laboring woman cope with pain the nurse needs to first determine the woman's perception of the experience. Nursing assessment should include acknowledgment of whether or not pain is present, the woman's description of the characteristics of the pain, and the meaning of the pain experience to the woman. According to McCaffery, "Pain is whatever the experiencing person says it is and exists whenever he says it does."[6] The nurse should explore how much the woman knows about pain. How does she feel about the pain experience? Does she know what she can do to help reduce the pain? Does she expect to be given drugs to alleviate the pain?

Effective nursing interventions that might be employed prior to, or in conjunction with, drugs to facilitate maternal coping and decrease the amount of drugs needed include the following:

1. Alleviate fear. Providing information can decrease fear of the unknown. It can also assist the laboring woman to establish realistic expectations. The woman may experience **comfort, alteration in: pain, acute related to lack of knowledge about the labor process.**
2. Praise positive efforts made by the couple. Feedback is an important component in encouraging the continuation of coping behaviors. There is **coping, ineffective individual related to inadequate or ineffective support during labor.**
3. Promote rest between contractions. Rest will conserve energy needed to cope with each contraction. Create a restful environment free from unnecessary distractions. There is potential **activity intolerance related to inadequate rest during labor.**
4. Provide distraction. This provides an alternative focus during contractions thus decreasing awareness and perception of pain. Visual concentration combined with effleurage (rhythmic massage) and comfortable appropriate breathing patterns may significantly decrease the need for pain relief via drugs. There is **comfort, alteration in: pain, acute related to inadequate use of distraction techniques.**
5. Provide cutaneous stimulation. This may provide pain relief or a decrease in the degree of pain perception. Cutaneous stimulation may be achieved with massage, pressure, vibration, bathing, and hot or cold applications. There is **comfort, alteration in: pain, acute related to ineffective application of cutaneous stimulation.**
6. Promote relaxation. Relaxation decreases muscle tension and is usually combined with other interventions such as drugs and/or

distraction to promote pain relief. There is **comfort, alteration in: pain, acute related to generalized muscle tension during labor.**

7. Use guided imagery. This can effectively decrease the level of pain as well as promote relaxation and decrease anxiety. There is **comfort, alteration in: pain, acute related to inadequate support with guided imagery.**
8. Accurately assess reactions to pain, response to nonpharmacologic nursing interventions and *need* for drugs. Continuous assessment of the effectiveness of nonpharmacologic methods of pain relief will allow the nurse to determine if pain relief measures need to be supplemented with drugs and when. Continue promoting the use of alternative methods after drug administration to decrease the frequency and amount of drugs needed. There is **comfort, alteration in: pain, acute related to continued perception of uterine contractions.**
9. Assess the effectiveness of drugs while observing for potential side effects. Safety for both mother and baby is critical whenever drugs are employed. Know the recommended dose, route of administration, action and side effects of any drug you administer. There is **injury, potential for;** (maternal/fetal/newborn) **related to drugs received during labor.**

• •

Review Question

List five nonpharmacologic measures the nurse can use or suggest in giving support.

a. ______________________________
b. ______________________________
c. ______________________________
d. ______________________________
e. ______________________________

Answer

The nurse can use or suggest the following nonpharmacologic measures: (a) alleviate fear, (b) praise positive efforts, (c) promote rest, (d) provide distraction, (e) provide cutaneous stimulation, (f) promote relaxation, (g) use guided imagery, (h) assess need for drugs, and (i) assess effectiveness of drugs.

• •

ANALGESIA AND ANESTHESIA

At times, nonpharmacologic nursing interventions for pain may need to be supplemented with analgesia and anesthesia during labor and delivery. The purpose of analgesia and anesthesia during labor and delivery is to provide as much relief from pain as necessary through *minimal* pharmacologic intervention thus minimizing undesirable side effects of drugs on the fetus, the newborn, and the mother. Most medications received by the woman in labor can cross the placenta and affect the fetus. Once the decision to use drugs has been made, the selection and timing of analgesia and anesthesia is crucial. Choice of analgesia and anesthesia varies widely depending on geographic location.

What is meant by analgesia and anesthesia? *Analgesia* refers to the absence or decreased awareness of a normal sensation of pain. Analgesia is brought about most often by the use of drugs and when used during labor is usually employed during Stage I. *Anesthesia* refers to a partial or complete loss of sensation with or without loss of consciousness. Anesthesia is also brought about most often by the use of drugs and is usually employed toward the end of Stage I and during Stages II and III of labor.

During Stage I of labor, pain impulses (Fig. 6–1) due to uterine contractions and cervical dilatation are transmitted by nerve fibers from the cervix and uterus via the pelvic nerve plexus, the superior hypogastric and lumbar sympathetic chains to T–10, T–11, and T–12 (thoracic nerves), and L–1 (lumbar nerve). Pain relief during Stage I interferes with pain impulses reaching the spinal canal or provides systemic relief of pain. During Stage II, perineal pain impulses are transmitted by the pudendal nerve plexus to S–2, S–3, and S–4 (sacral nerves).[7] Pain relief for delivery blocks pain at the level of S–2 through S–4.

• •

Review Questions

1. Analgesia refers to: ____
____
____

2. Anesthesia refers to: ____
____
____

3. Pain relief during stage I may be accomplished by blocking pain impulses from the pelvic nerve plexus and superior hypogastric and lumbar sympathetic chains at the spinal levels of ______________.

4. Pain relief during delivery may be achieved by blocking pain impulses from the pudendal nerve plexus at the spinal level of ____________.

Answers

1. *Analgesia* refers to the absence or decreased awareness of a normal sensation of pain.

2. *Anesthesia* refers to a partial or complete loss of sensation.

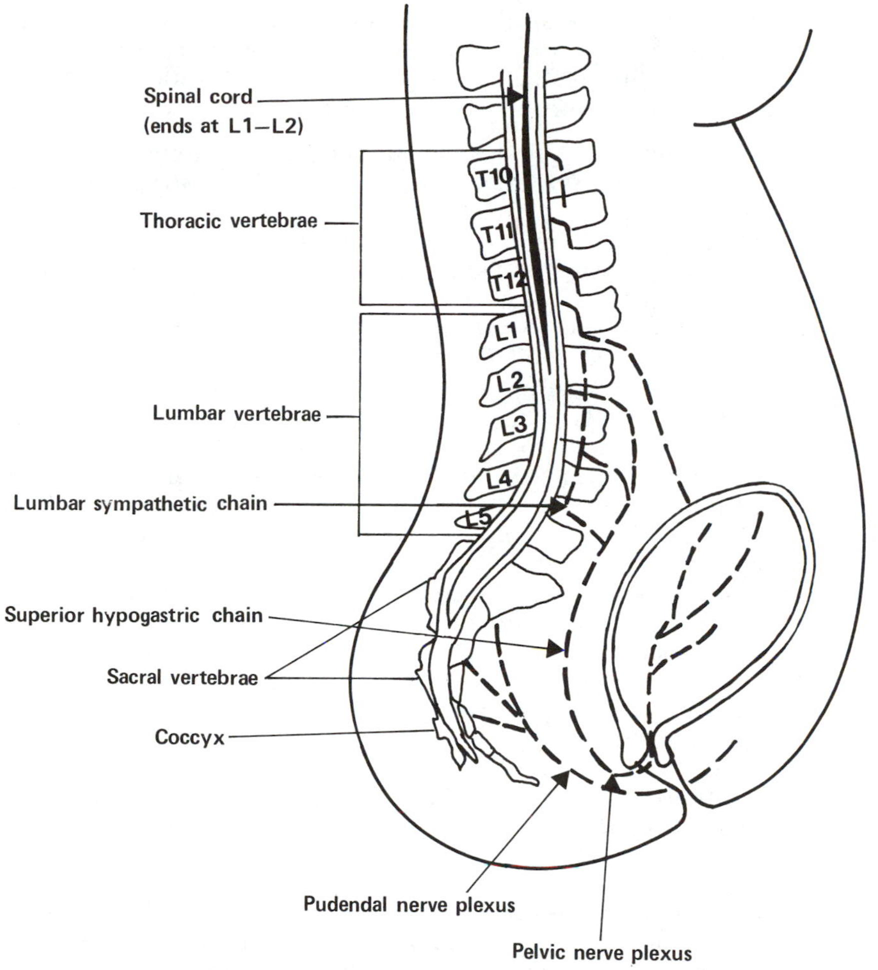

Figure 6–1. Uterine impulse (pain) pathway to the spinal canal.

3. Pain relief during the first stage of labor may be accomplished by blocking pain impulses from the pelvic nerve plexus and superior hypogastric and lumbar sympathetic chains at the spinal levels of *T–10 through L–1*.

4. Pain relief during delivery may be achieved by blocking pain impulses from the pudendal nerve plexus at the spinal level of S–2, S–3, and S–4.

• •

CONSIDERATIONS THAT INFLUENCE THE DECISION TO USE DRUGS

Since excessive pain perception can be detrimental, it is evident that decreasing the sensation of pain with analgesics is often desirable and necessary, and/or preferred by the laboring woman. In choosing a method of pain relief, the nurse should keep in mind the objective of providing as much relief from pain as possible without causing undesirable medication side effects on the mother, fetus, and newborn. The following considerations must be carefully made:

1. Potency of the drug: the drug should be potent enough to relieve pain yet have only minimal side effects on the mother, fetus, or newborn.
2. Possible side effects on the mother, fetus, and newborn: direct effects on the mother cause indirect effects on the fetus and/or newborn in the following ways:
   a. impaired maternal ventilation or arterial hypotension can cause decreased fetal oxygenation resulting in initial fetal heart rate tachycardia with loss of variability and eventually leading to bradycardia
   b. maternal arterial hypertension can cause abruption of the placenta resulting in fetal anoxia and possible death
   c. alteration in the forces of labor can cause fetal trauma due to prolonged labor or rapid labor and delivery that may be unattended
3. Phase of labor: if analgesic intervention is employed
   a. too early (before 4 cm dilatation—latent phase), analgesia may temporarily interfere with the progress of labor, stopping or slowing down the frequency, intensity, and duration of the contractions and possibly necessitating the use of Pitocin augmentation
   b. in the active laboring woman (usually between 4 to 6 cm dilatation—acceleration phase) analgesia can decrease the experienced pain so that the woman is able to relax and labor may progress at an optimal rate (see Chapter 4 for labor graphs)
   c. late in labor (within 30 to 60 minutes of delivery—transition and for stage II), analgesia may lead to the delivery of a sedated newborn who may need resuscitative measures; this is usually seen in a newborn with low Apgar scores

• •

Review Questions

1. List three considerations that must be made before initiating analgesia or anesthesia.
   a. ______________________________
   b. ______________________________
   c. ______________________________

2. List 3 possible side effects of analgesia as they appear in the mother, and the resulting effect on the fetus/newborn.

MATERNAL EFFECT	FETAL/NEWBORN EFFECT
a. ______	a. ______
b. ______	b. ______
c. ______	c. ______

Answers

1. Before initiating analgesia or anesthesia to provide pain relief without undesirable side effects, the following considerations must be made:
   a. potency of the drug
   b. side effects on the mother and fetus/newborn
   c. stage of labor and progress made

2. Direct effects on the mother that indirectly cause effects on the fetus/newborn include:

MATERNAL EFFECTS	FETAL/NEWBORN EFFECTS
a. impaired ventilation or arterial hypotension	a. decreased fetal oxygenation, decreased fetal heart rate
b. arterial hypertension and placental abruption	b. fetal anoxia and death
c. alteration in forces of labor	c. fetal trauma

• •

THE ACTION AND SIDE EFFECTS OF DRUGS USED DURING LABOR

Systemic drugs most commonly used during labor may be classified as: (1) narcotic agonists, (2) narcotic antagonists, (3) mixed narcotic agonists/antagonists, and (4) sedatives. Table 6-1 shows the drugs most commonly administered and when they are given during labor.

Narcotic Agonists

Narcotic agonists (analgesics) are narcotic or synthetic narcotic (opium-based) drugs that are effective in reducing pain without causing loss of consciousness. Narcotic agonists provide analgesia by binding to and activating central and peripheral nervous system opiate receptor sites. (See Chapter 7 for discussion of the endogenous theory of pain relief.) In addition to providing analgesia, narcotic agonists also produce sedation, antispasmodic action, euphoria, and decreased anxiety.

Narcotic agonists depress two vital centers. In the respiratory center, they initially depress the brain's response to carbon dioxide. This response, called the hypercapnic drive of respirations, is dimin-

Table 6–1. DRUGS COMMONLY USED DURING LABOR*

PHASE I LATENT (1–3 cm)	PHASE II ACCELERATION (4–7 cm)	PHASE III MAXIMUM SLOPE (8–10 cm)
	Narcotic agonists- - - - (meperidine, alphaprodine, oxymorphone)	- - - - - - - - - - - - - - - - - ->
	Narcotic agonists + - - - Narcotic antagonists (meperidine, alphaprodine, oxymorphone + naloxone)	- - - - - - - - - - - - - - - - - ->
		Narcotic - - - - - - - - - -> antagonists alone (naloxone)
	Mixed agonists/ antagonists - - - - - - - - (butorphanol, nalbuphine, pentazocine)	- - - - - - - - - - - - - - - - - ->
Sedatives alone- - - - - - (secobarbital, pentobarbital, promethazine, hydroxyzine)	- - - - - - - - - - - - - - - - - - - -	- - - - - - - - - - - - - - - - - ->
	Narcotic agonists + - - - Sedatives (meperidine + promethazine, hydroxyzine)	- - - - - - - - - - - - - - - - - ->

*The arrows denote the desired length of action of each drug.

ished or eliminated resulting in slow, labored respirations.[8] Depression of the cough center deprives the body of an important protective mechanism for maintaining airway clearance. The resulting nursing diagnosis is **breathing pattern, ineffective related to narcotic agonists**.

Histamine release is stimulated by many narcotic agonists causing vasodilatation that results in orthostatic hypotension. Visible flushing and warming of the skin is evident and the woman may complain of dizziness and lightheadedness when changing positions.

Stimulation of the medulla by many narcotic agonists causes nausea, vomiting, and dizziness. Other side effects of narcotic agonists include delayed gastrointestinal action, biliary spasms, and urinary retention.

Nursing implications for administration of narcotic agonists include careful assessment of maternal BP, pulse rate, and respirations (rate, rhythm, depth, and quality), and bladder status. Ongoing assessment of FHR pattern and variability with electronic monitoring is important. (See Chapter 3 for evaluation of FHR.) Oxygen and narcotic antagonists should be readily available.

Neonatal neurobehavior may be affected by all narcotic agonists. Narcotics given to the mother 1 to 3 hours prior to delivery may produce neonatal respiratory depression, because the narcotic is synthesized by the fetal liver and activated within the fetal system during that period of time.[9] A good rule of thumb is to *refrain from administering narcotic agonists after* complete dilatation in the primigravida and after 7 to 8 cm dilatation in the multigravida. Narcotic agonists that provide analgesia during labor include: meperidine hydrochloride (Demerol), alphaprodine hydrochloride (Nisentil), and oxymorphone hydrochloride (Numorphone). Epidural morphine is discussed later in the chapter.

Meperidine Hydrochloride. Meperidine (Demerol) is the most common synthetic narcotic agonist used during labor. It is administered IM, 50 to 100 mg every 3 to 4 hours or slow IV push, 25 to 50 mg every 3 to 4 hours. Meperidine, IM, provides peak analgesia in 40 to 60 minutes, and IV, in 5 to 7 minutes with a duration of 2 to 4 hours. When administering IV meperidine, injection during the peak (acme) of a contraction is thought to decrease placental transfer of the drug to the fetus. *Give slowly—during the acme of several contractions.* The major side effect of meperidine is respiratory depression. When administered with other narcotics, sedatives or general anesthetics, meperidine potentiates the central nervous system (CNS) depressant effects (respiratory and circulatory depression) of these agents. Meperidine frequently causes nausea and vomiting, sweating and dizziness. Other potential side effects include tremors, palpitations, tachycardia, and delirium.

Meperidine, if administered at the appropriate time, may promote cervical relaxation producing increased progress of labor. If given too early in labor, it may temporarily disrupt the labor pattern and prolong labor. DeVoe and colleagues[10] and later, Reffel and colleagues,[11] however, found a slight increase in uterine activity following meperidine administration, not a decrease. In practice, it is generally recommended that meperidine *not* be administered before 5 to 6 cm dilatation in the primigravida and *not* before 3 to 4 cm in the multigravida. This is only a guide. The character and progression of the woman's labor must be carefully evaluated to determine the most appropriate time for administration of meperidine.

Recent research with meperidine revealed that infant tissue levels of meperidine were higher in infants born 2 to 3 hours after maternal drug administration than those born 1 to 2, or greater than 3 hours after a single dose.[12,13] Meperidine administered during labor may also cause subtle neurobehavioral changes in the newborn during the first 24 hours of life and possibly longer. These newborns tend to be less alert and generally demonstrate sluggish behavior. They exhibit a decreased response to maternal stimuli such as startling, cuddling, and consoling.[14–16] It may be difficult to help the new mother understand that her baby will become more alert and responsive with time. The new mother has a need to feel adequate in her ability to care for her baby particularly through her ability to feed him. She may feel quite frustrated and sometimes inadequate when he is too sluggish to eat. Supportive nursing intervention is of particular importance at this time.

Alphaprodine. Alphaprodine (Nisentil) is a synthetic narcotic agonist that is similar to morphine and meperidine. During labor, the initial IV dose is 0.4 to 0.6 mg per kg of body weight. Onset of action is 1 to 2 minutes with a duration of 30 to 90 minutes. Alphaprodine may also be given SC, 0.4 to 1.2 mg per kg of body weight. The onset of action SC is 2 to 30 minutes with a duration of 1 to 2 hours. Alphaprodine should never be administered IM because the absorption rate is unpredictable with this route.

Alphaprodine frequently causes drowsiness, sweating, dizziness, and urticaria. When administered with other narcotics, sedatives, or general anesthetics, alphaprodine potentiates the CNS depressant effects (respiratory and circulatory depression) of these agents.

Sinusoidal fetal heart rate patterns have been identified following the administration of alphaprodine to the laboring woman, but subsequent morbidity/mortality rates in these neonates have not increased.[17]

Oxymorphone Hydrochloride. Oxymorphone (Numorphone) is a potent semisynthetic narcotic agonist. It may be used during labor, however its use is not common because of its great potential for causing respiratory depression and emesis. It may be given IV—0.5 mg, or IM/SC—0.5 to 1.0 mg every 4 to 6 hours.

Oxymorphone frequently causes dizziness, nausea and vomiting, and euphoria. When combined with other narcotics, sedatives or general anesthetics, oxymorphone can cause increased respiratory depression, hypotension, and coma.

Narcotic Antagonists

Narcotic antagonists bind to central and peripheral opiate receptor sites in the nervous system. They counteract the respiratory depression caused by narcotic agonists by displacing agonists from opiate receptor sites. Narcotic antagonists must be used with caution in cases of known or suspected maternal narcotic addiction as they may produce abrupt withdrawal symptoms. Narcotic antagonists used during labor include naloxone (Narcan) and levallorphan (Lorfan).

Naloxone. Naloxone (Narcan) is a pure antagonist that is used for complete or partial reversal of neonatal respiratory depression. It is the drug of choice for **gas exchange, impaired related to maternal narcotic agonists received during labor**. Naloxone is also the drug of choice when the cause of depression is unknown because it will not cause further depression.[17] Naloxone may be administered IM, but is usually administered IV because it has a rapid onset of action and is very short acting, only 2 to 3 minutes.[18] Since the respiratory depression caused by narcotic agonists may outlast the antagonist effect, careful monitoring of the need for repeated doses of naloxone is crucial. Neonatal administration of Naloxone is 0.01 mg per kg of body weight, IV, via the umbilical vein immediately after birth. The dose may be repeated in 5 minutes and again as needed if the initial dose produces a reversal of respiratory depression. If no reversal occurs after 2 to 3 doses, the drug should be discontinued.[17]

Naloxone may also be administered to the *mother*, 0.4 mg IM or IV, 5 to 15 minutes prior to delivery. Hodgkinson and associates[19] found that naloxone administered to the mother 15 minutes prior to delivery does reverse the narcotic depression in the neonate at 2 hours of age. However, at 4 and 24 hours of age, these newborns displayed almost as much depressed neurobehavior as newborns exposed to meperidine alone. Therefore, Hodgkinson and associates recommended reversing narcotic respiratory and neurobehavioral depression of the neonate by administering naloxone to the newborn immediately after birth.

When naloxone is administered to reverse respiratory depression, the nurse must maintain an open airway and be prepared for the possibility of initiating CPR. Assess vital signs frequently since hyperventilation may occur following the administration of naloxone. Naloxone administered to the laboring woman may cause a reversal of narcotic analgesia and postpartum bleeding.

Levallorphan. Levallorphan (Lorfan) is a narcotic antagonist with weak agonist properties. It is effective in partial or complete reversal of respiratory depression caused *only* by narcotics. If respiratory depression is caused by other drugs, levallorphan will only enhance that depression because of its agonist properties. Therefore, it is indicated for neonatal narcotic depression only if naloxone is not available. Levallorphan, 1 mg IV, may be given to the mother just prior to delivery, or immediately after birth, to the neonate: 0.05 to 0.1 mg IM, SC, or preferably IV via the umbilical vein. The duration of action is 2 to 5 hours.

• •

Review Questions

1. __________ is the most common narcotic agonist used during labor.
2. List three actions of narcotic agonists.
   a. __________
   b. __________
   c. __________
3. The major fetal or neonatal side effect of maternal narcotic agonist administration during labor is __________
   __________.

4. **Narcotic antagonists used to reverse the major side effect of narcotic agonists are _________ and _________, but _________ is considered to be the drug of choice.**

Answers

1. *Meperidine hydrochloride (Demerol)* is the most common narcotic agonist used during labor.
2. Narcotic agonists used during labor produce (a) pain relief, (b) sedation, (c) antispasmodic action, (d) euphoria, and (e) decreased anxiety.
3. The major fetal or neonatal side effect of narcotic agonists is *respiratory depression of the fetus/newborn*.
4. *Naloxone (Narcan)* and *levallorphan (Lorfan)* are narcotic antagonists used to reverse the respiratory depression caused by narcotic agonists. *Naloxone* is the drug of choice.

• •

Mixed Narcotic Agonists/Antagonists

Mixed narcotic agonists/antagonists are drugs that contain both agonist and antagonist properties. They occupy the same receptor sites as agonists although the exact mechanism of action has not been established. They are metabolized by the liver and are excreted primarily by the kidneys. Although they may be used during labor, they are not recommended during pregnancy or lactation.[18]

Adverse reactions to mixed agonists/antagonists usually affect the central nervous system and the gastrointestinal tract: respiratory depression, nausea, vomiting, lightheadedness, sedation and euphoria. Dry mouth and urinary retention are common. Other adverse effects are visual hallucinations, confusion, disorientation, and hypertension. Thus **thought processes, alteration in** and **sensory-perceptual alteration: visual, auditory, gustatory, olfactory** are **related to the use of mixed agonists/antagonists**.

Mixed agonists/antagonists should be used with caution in the presence of other central nervous system depressants such as barbiturates because they will enhance the respiratory depressant effects of those drugs. Mixed agonists/antagonists are contraindicated in suspected or known cases of narcotic dependence because they will almost always precipitate withdrawal symptoms.

Nursing interventions with administration of mixed agonists/antagonists include frequent assessment of maternal vital signs and level of consciousness along with continuous electronic fetal heart rate monitoring.

Mixed agonist/antagonist drugs used during labor include butorphanol tartrate (Stadol), nalbuphine hydrochloride (Nubain), and pentazocine hydrochloride (Talwin).

Butorphanol Tartrate. Butorphanol (Stadol) is a potent mixed agonist/antagonist analgesic. The onset of action is 10 to 30 minutes with a duration of 2 to 4 hours. It is given IV—1 mg, or IM—2 mg every 3 to 4 hours. Specific side effects include respiratory depression, sedation, nausea, dizziness and clamminess. If respiratory depression occurs, it can be reversed with naloxone.

Nalbuphine Hydrochloride. Nalbuphine (Nubain) is a partial synthetic mixed agonist/antagonist opiate. Nalbuphine is pharmacologically similar to butorphanol and produces analgesia that is equal to morphine. The onset of action is less than 15 minutes lasting 3 to 6 hours. The recommended dose during labor is 10 mg per 70 kg of body weight IV, IM, or SC every 3 to 6 hours. The initial IV dose is 5 mg.

Nalbuphine can cause respiratory depression equal to that of morphine;[18] however, the depression does not increase with cumulative doses of nalbuphine.[17] Naloxone is the drug of choice for reversing the respiratory depressant effects of nalbuphine.

Pentazocine Hydrochloride. Pentazocine (Talwin) is a synthetic mixed agonist/antagonist analgesic. The onset of action is 15 to 30 minutes with a duration of 3 to 4 hours. The recommended dose during labor is 20 mg IV every 2 to 3 hours or 30 mg IM every 3 to 4 hours. The SC route should be avoided since pentazocine can cause severe tissue damage. Side effects include respiratory depression and dysphoria. Naloxone is the specific drug for reversal of respiratory depression.

• •

Review Questions

1. Adverse reactions to mixed agonists/antagonists usually involve two systems: ________________ and ________________.

2. The most significant side effect of mixed agonists/antagonists is ________________.

3. Describe nursing interventions employed with administration of mixed agonists/antagonists. ________________

Answers

1. Adverse reactions to mixed agonists/antagonists usually involve the *central nervous system* and the *gastrointestinal tract.*

2. *Respiratory depression* is the most significant side effect of mixed agonists/antagonists.

3. Nursing interventions with the administration of mixed agonists/antagonists include frequent assessment of maternal vital signs and level of consciousness along with continuous electronic fetal heart rate monitoring.

• •

Sedatives

Sedatives are drugs that may be used during false labor or early prodromal labor to promote emotional well-being by decreasing apprehension, fear and anxiety. Sedatives cause sedation, relaxation, some hypnosis and no amnesia. However, recollection may be confused or distorted. Restlessness or **activity intolerance related to the use of sedatives** may occur when used alone in the presence of moderate to severe pain. Sedative drugs most commonly used are *barbiturates* such as *secobarbital sodium (Seconal)* and *pentobarbital sodium (Nembutal)*. The usual dosage is 100 to 200 mg PO, or 50 to 100 mg IM as a one-time dose.

Barbiturates rapidly cross the placenta and accumulate in the fetal liver and central nervous system causing respiratory depression in the neonate. In addition, significant neonatal behavioral changes have been identified in newborns whose mothers received barbiturates during labor. During the first four days of life, these infants exhibit a poor sucking reflex, fewer sucks per minute, lower sucking pressure, and decreased formula intake as compared with infants whose mothers had not received barbiturates during labor.[20] Barbiturates are contraindicated during pregnancy and lactation.[18] For these reasons, current practice supports only minimal use of sedatives during early labor.

Other sedatives used during labor are *promethazine (Phenergan)* which is a sedative/antihistamine and *hydroxyzine pamoate (Vistaril)* which is a sedative/hypnotic. Both drugs may be used alone in early labor (1 to 3 cm) or during active labor combined with narcotic agonists to promote sedation, relieve anxiety and decrease nausea and vomiting. The recommended dosage during labor for promethazine is 12.5 to 25 mg, IM or IV every 4 to 6 hours, and for hydroxyzine is 25 to 50 mg IM every 4 to 6 hours.

When combined with narcotic agonists, promethazine and hydroxyzine potentiate the analgesic action, thus reducing the total amount of agonist needed. They also cause additive central nervous system depression when combined with other depressants such as narcotics and sedatives.

The most common adverse effects of promethazine are excess sedation, confusion, and disorientation. Other adverse effects include hypotension, dizziness, tachycardia, dry mouth, blurred vision, headache, restlessness, weakness, and urinary retention.

The most common adverse effects of hydroxyine are drowsiness and dry mouth. Other side effects include dizziness, headache, blurred vision, lassitude, dysuria, urinary retention, and constipation.

Both promethazine and hydroxyzine are contraindicated during lactation.[8]

• •

Review Questions

1. Barbiturates may be used in false or early prodromal labor to decrease:
   a. ____________________ b. ____________________
   c. ____________________

2. List three behavioral changes observed in the newborn during the first four days of life following barbiturate administration to the mother during labor.
   a. ____________________
   b. ____________________
   c. ____________________

3. List three expected actions of promethazine or hydroxyzine during labor.
   a. ____________________ b. ____________________
   c. ____________________

Answers

1. Barbiturates may be used in false or early prodromal labor to decrease: (a) apprehension, (b) fear, and (c) anxiety.

2. Newborn behavioral changes associated with barbiturate administration to the mother during labor may include: (a) poor sucking reflex, (b) fewer sucks per minute, (c) lower sucking pressure, and (d) decreased formula intake.

3. Promethazine or hydroxyzine are used during labor to
   a. promote sedation,
   b. relieve anxiety, and
   c. decrease nausea and vomiting.

• •

DRUG-INDUCED ANESTHESIA DURING LABOR AND DELIVERY

Anesthesia is the partial or total loss of sensation with or without loss of consciousness. Most anesthetics are used at the time of delivery, although some are administered during the acceleration phase of labor. There is a wide variation in choice of anesthetic agents according to geographic location.

Local anesthesia blocks sensory nerve pathways at the organ level, producing anesthesia to the organ only.

Regional anesthesia blocks sensory nerve pathways along the large sensory nerves from an organ and its surrounding tissues (lumbar epidural, caudal, saddle, spinal, paracervical, pudendal, and local perineal infiltration blocks). See Figure 6-1 for uterine impulse (pain) pathways to the spinal canal. Regional anesthesia is usually achieved by the injection of a local anesthetic agent such as etidocaine (Duranest), bupivacaine (Marcaine), mepivocaine (Carbocaine), lidocaine (Xylocaine), tetracaine (Pontacaine), procaine (Novocaine), and chloroprocaine (Nesacaine). Local anesthetic agents readily cross the placenta to the fetus. Etidocaine and bupivacaine have high protein-binding capabilities, and therefore, cross the placental barrier in smaller quantities. The amount of anesthetic agent that crosses the placenta to the fetus is thought to be related to the anesthetic's protein-binding ability.[18]

General anesthesia is a progressive depression of the central nervous system, causing loss of sensation in the entire body and loss of consciousness (intravenous and/or inhalation). General anesthesia is not as commonly used in labor and delivery as regional anesthesia.

Research findings about neurobehavioral effects of anesthetic agents on the neonate are controversial. Scanlon and colleagues (1974)[21] found that lidocaine caused a "floppy but alert" neonate with decreased neurobehavioral responses. In a later study (1976) on the same population, there were no adverse effects with bupivacaine.[22] Murray and coworkers (1981)[23] found that bupivacaine caused neonates at one day of age to perform poorly on motor and physiologic responses. Rosenblatt and colleagues (1981)[24] found that epidural bupivacaine caused cyanosis and unresponsiveness to surroundings at birth. As late as six weeks of age, these infants had decreased visual skills and alertness, however, they exhibited increased muscle tone. Abboud and associates (1982–1984)[25–28] found no effects with lidocaine, bupivacaine, or chloroprocaine. Lester, Als, and Brazelton (1982)[29] hypothesized that research comparing specific agents is not valid since there were too many drug potentiating variables omitted and neonatal neurobehavioral effects were too subtle to be defined accurately. Additional research with better control for variables and more subtle measurements of neonatal behavior must be undertaken. In the meantime, judicious use of anesthetic agents can provide pain relief as well as promote safety for the mother and fetus/neonate.

REGIONAL ANESTHESIA DURING LABOR AND DELIVERY

Regional anesthesia is used primarily to achieve anesthesia of the pelvic area (Fig. 6–2). However, varying degrees of temporary loss of sensation to the lower extremities may also occur. The duration of anesthesia to the lower extremities varies according to the drug used, the dosage, and the route of administration. It is important to be aware of these factors in order to prevent damage while positioning the woman on the delivery table and removing her legs from stirrups. In order to avoid **injury, potential for; (maternal) trauma related to regional anesthesia**, ambulation should not be

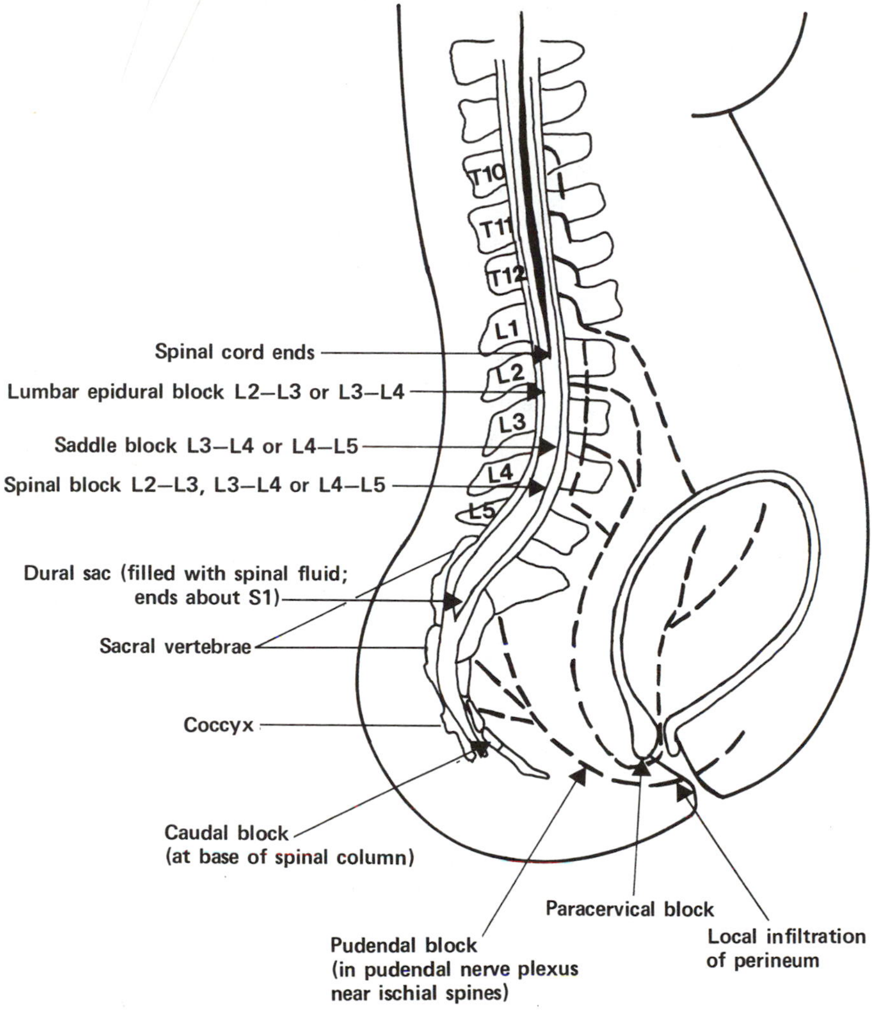

Figure 6–2. Schematic drawing of the sites of anesthetic infiltration.

attempted until full sensation to the lower extremities has returned. Table 6–2 shows when regional anesthesia is most commonly administered during labor and delivery. Refer to this table periodically as you read the remainder of this chapter.

The following advantages, disadvantages, and nursing care apply to all methods of regional anesthesia.

Advantages of regional anesthesia:

1. It provides anesthesia from the end of Stage I (continuous epidurals and caudals may be given earlier) through the repair of the episiotomy.

Table 6–2. REGIONAL ANESTHESIA USED DURING LABOR/DELIVERY*

STAGE I†	STAGE II‡	STAGE III§
Continuous Lumbar Epidural Block (3–6 cm) ------	------------------------	----------->
Continuous Caudal Block (4–5 cm) ------	------------------------	----------->
Paracervical Block (3–4 cm) ------>		
	Lumbar Epidural Block --	----------->
	Saddle Block ---------	----------->
	Caudal Block ---------	----------->
	Spinal Block ---------	----------->
	Pudendal Block --------	----------->
	Local Perineal Block (just prior to delivery) ----	----------->

*The arrows denote the desired duration of action of anesthesia.

†STAGE I—From the beginning of labor to complete dilatation of the cervix.

‡STAGE II—From complete dilatation through delivery of the baby.

§STAGE III—From delivery of the baby through delivery of the placenta.

2. It tends to prevent precipitous delivery because the urge to push is blocked, although the ability to push is present in varying degrees.
3. The mother remains awake and is able to participate in the birth experience.

Disadvantages of regional anesthesia:

1. The most common side effect is maternal hypotension, causing decreased oxygenation to the fetus. Hypotension is a result of vasodilatation with pooling of blood in the major pelvic vessels and compression of the vena cava by the gravid uterus. Prevention of maternal hypotension may be achieved by (a) IV fluid hydration (500 to 1000 ml) of the mother prior to administration of the anesthetic agent, and (b) positioning the mother on her side

during labor or using the left lateral tilt position during labor and delivery. This helps avoid supine hypotension syndrome (see Chapter 1).

2. The mother's decreased urge to push usually decreases pushing effectiveness, necessitating the use of forceps or vacuum extraction to facilitate the delivery. There is an increased incidence of persistent occiput posterior and occiput transverse positions[30] with the use of regional anesthesia.
3. Owing to increased pressure in the epidural and subarachnoid spaces during labor contractions, injection of anesthetic agents must be done between contractions to prevent excessively high anesthesia levels.[31] Accidental high level of anesthesia, resulting in respiratory arrest of the mother, is a rare but serious complication.
4. Some women may develop a postspinal headache due to loss of spinal fluid through a puncture of the dura (spinal block and saddle block). The incidence of postspinal headache is only 2 percent when a small needle is used for the procedure but increases with pregnancy.[4] Bed rest after a dural puncture does not seem to reduce the incidence of spinal headache, however, many physicians still order that the woman be kept flat 4 to 12 hours after delivery. Additional techniques that may be used to prevent postspinal headache include: hyperhydration, blood patch (injecting 5 to 10 ml of the woman's own blood epidurally at the site of spinal puncture), and epidural infusion of Ringer's lactate. Abdominal binders (see Chapter 2) may also prevent headache by decreasing spinal fluid loss.
5. It may cause uterine contractions to decrease in frequency and intensity. If labor fails to progress, oxytocin augmentation may be necessary.
6. It causes decreased sensitivity to the filling urinary bladder (beyond the normal decreased sensitivity) so that some women need to be catheterized after delivery to prevent bladder distention which may cause postpartum hemorrhage, urinary stasis/infection, and so forth.

Nursing care is extremely important before, during, and after the regional administration of an anesthetic agent because of the possible undesirable side effects that may occur to the mother and fetus/newborn. Important nursing measures include:

1. *positioning*, helping the woman maintain the desired position during administration of the anesthetic
2. *providing* emotional support
3. *monitoring*, continually, labor patterns, blood pressure, pulse, and fetal heart rate closely to detect deviations
4. *evaluating* bladder status for distention/retention
5. *being aware* of and assessing for possible side effects of the anesthetic agent

6. *initiating* emergency measures related to maternal hypotension or fetal bradycardia (see Chapter 3)
7. *instructing* and *coaching* for effective pushing during Stage II
8. during the postpartum period, *assessing* bladder status, fundal consistency and placement, and return of sensation to the lower extremities

• •

Review Questions

1. List three advantages of regional anesthesia.
   a. ______________________________
   b. ______________________________
   c. ______________________________
2. List three disadvantages of regional anesthesia.
   a. ______________________________
   b. ______________________________
   c. ______________________________
3. List three nursing responsibilities related to the administration of regional anesthesia.
   a. ______________________________
   b. ______________________________
   c. ______________________________

Answers

1. Advantages of regional anesthesia are: (a) it provides anesthesia during Stages I, II, and III, (b) it tends to prevent precipitous delivery, and (c) the mother is able to participate in the birth experience.
2. Disadvantages of regional anesthesia are: (a) maternal hypotension, causing decreased oxygenation of the fetus, (b) the mother's decreased urge to push causes increased use of forceps for delivery, (c) anesthetic injection into the epidural and subarachnoid spaces must be done between contractions, (d) loss of spinal fluid may cause postspinal headache, (e) labor progression may be interrupted necessitating oxytocin augmentation, and (f) after delivery, bladder catheterization may be necessary to prevent bladder distention.
3. Nursing responsibilities related to the administration of regional anesthesia include: (a) helping the woman maintain the desired position during administration of the anesthetic, (b) providing emotional support, (c) continually monitoring contractions, blood pressure, pulse, and fetal heart rate, (d) evaluating bladder status, (e) assessing for side effects of anesthetic agents, (f) initiating emergency measures related to maternal hypotension and/or fetal bradycardia, (g) instructing and coaching effective pushing, and (h) during the immediate postpartum period, assessing for bladder distention, fundal consistency and placement, and return of sensation to the lower extremities.

• •

Lumbar Epidural Block

The *lumbar epidural block* (see Figs. 6–1 and 6–2) is a regional anesthetic affecting the entire pelvis by blocking nerve impulses at the level of T–12 through S–5. Blockage of T–10 through L–1 provides anesthesia from the umbilicus to midthigh, rendering complete relief of pain for vaginal delivery. Epidural is the most widely used regional anesthetic for labor and delivery. With the woman in a Sims or sitting position, the anesthetic agent is injected into the epidural space (the space surrounding the dura) which lies between the dura mater and the ligamentum flavum. The site of entry is the space between L–2 and L–3 or L–3 and L–4.

Cesarean delivery may be accomplished with an epidural block, however, anesthesia must block nerves from T–8 to L–5. This level provides anesthesia from the midline just below the xiphoid process to the toes. Movement and pressure may be felt in this area but no pain.

The major complication of epidural anesthesia is dural puncture (the needle is inserted beyond the dura mater into the spinal canal) which causes spinal block anesthesia. Depending on the site of insertion and the amount of anesthetic agent, this accidental puncture of the dura with injection of anesthetic agents into the subarachnoid space may cause severe hypotension, coma, and respiratory arrest.

Lumbar epidural block using bupivacaine as the anesthetic agent has been reported to produce undesirable side effects in the newborn which include muscular hypotonia, diminished Moro reflex, occasional behavioral alterations, and decreased motor activity.[24]

The *continuous lumbar epidural block* is the same as the lumbar epidural block except that it provides continuous anesthesia during Stages I through III. It can be introduced at 3 to 4 cm in the multigravida and 4 to 6 cm in the primigravida and maintained through a polyethylene tubing.

Epidural blocks may also be used to administer *analgesia*. Pain relief can be achieved during the first stage of labor by administering morphine through a catheter placed in the epidural space. When given epidurally, morphine inhibits the transmission of painful sensations to the higher brain centers. The dosage needed for pain relief is lower than with more traditional methods because the drug is absorbed and begins acting before being metabolized by the liver. The onset of action is slow (15 to 60 minutes). Therefore, alternative methods of pain relief may need to be used during the waiting period. The most common side effects associated with epidural analgesia are respiratory depression (early—within 1 hour; late—within 6 to 10 hours), urinary retention, pruritus, and nausea and vomiting. The use of an apnea monitor for at least 24 hours postpartum is advisable. Resuscitative equipment should be readily available.[32]

Caudal Block

The *caudal block* (see Figs. 6–1 and 6–2) is a regional anesthetic affecting the entire pelvic area. Therefore, following its administration the woman does not feel uterine contractions or perineal stretching. The amount of anesthetic agent injected will determine the level of anesthesia achieved. For a vaginal delivery, blockage of T–10 to L–1 will provide anesthesia from the umbilicus to mid-thigh. The anesthetic agent is injected into the caudal space of the sacral canal which is level with the last sacral vertebra. This is a potential space surrounding the dura and does not contain cerebrospinal fluid. The caudal block is administered during the second stage of labor just prior to delivery, with the woman in a Sims or knee-chest position. A disadvantage of caudal anesthesia is that accidental injection of the fetus may cause apnea, bradycardia, convulsions, and central nervous system damage. Caudal anesthesia is not commonly used in obstetrics today.

The *continuous caudal block* is the same as the caudal block except that it provides anesthesia during Stages I through III. By inserting a polyethylene tubing into the caudal space when 4 to 5 cm dilatation is reached, the effect of anesthesia may be maintained through repeated injections of the anesthetic agent into the tubing as necessary every 45 to 90 minutes.

Saddle Block

The *saddle block* (see Figs. 6–1 and 6–2) is a regional block that anesthetizes those parts of the body which come in contact with a saddle (perineum, lower pelvis, and upper thighs) by blocking nerves from S–1 to S–4. This block is rarely done. The anesthetic agent is injected into the spinal fluid in the subarachnoid space. The site of injection is the space between L–3 and L–4 or L–4 and L–5. Following injection, the woman remains sitting for 3 to 5 minutes to insure an appropriate level of anesthesia. Pain relief for delivery is not complete, because only the sacral nerves are blocked, however, the woman is able to push more effectively with a saddle block than with a spinal block.

Spinal Block

The *spinal block* or *subarachnoid block* (see Figs. 6–1 and 6–2) is a regional anesthetic used just prior to delivery. The spinal block is not commonly used in obstetrics today. A hyperbaric (heavier than spinal fluid) anesthetic solution is injected into the subarachnoid space between the dura and the spinal canal. This cavity is filled with cerebrospinal fluid. The spinal cord usually ends at L–1. Therefore, the site of injection is the space between L–2 and L–3, L–3 and L–4, or L–4 and L–5. The woman may be in a sitting or side-lying position (Sims) with the head slightly elevated. The back must be arched like an angry cat or a rainbow to permit an easier insertion of the needle between the vertebrae.

Spinal block for cesarean delivery requires blockage of impulses to the level of T–8. This provides anesthesia from the midline just below the xiphoid process to the toes. Anesthesia levels above T–4 will stop respiratory function. In order to achieve the desired level of anesthesia, dosage of the agent and the woman's position are important. The woman is placed in a supine position immediately after administration of the block.

A low spinal block (to the level of T–10) provides complete relief of pain for a vaginal delivery with loss of sensation from the umbilicus to the toes. Compared to a cesarean delivery, a smaller amount of anesthetic is used and the woman remains sitting for 30 to 60 seconds before being placed in a supine position. A low spinal block is sometimes inappropriately called a saddle block.

• •

Review Question

The following are regional block anesthetics that can be used prior to a vaginal delivery. For each type, identify the area of anesthesia desired, position of the patient, stage in labor when used and the most common side effects. You may need to go back and review the appropriate section on the previous pages.

TYPE	AREA OF ANESTHESIA	POSITION	STAGE	MOST COMMON SIDE EFFECTS
Lumbar Epidural Block				
Caudal Block				
Saddle Block				
Spinal Block				

Answer

For a vaginal delivery, each type of regional anesthetic involves the following area of anesthesia, position of the patient, stage in labor when used and the side effects.

TYPE	AREA OF ANESTHESIA	POSITION	STAGE	SIDE EFFECTS
Lumbar Epidural Block (Continuous)	Umbilicus to toes	Sims or sitting	II (I)	Maternal hypotension
Caudal Block (Continuous)	Umbilicus to midthigh	Sims or knee-chest	II (I)	Maternal hypotension
Saddle Block	Perineum, lower pelvis, upper thighs	Sims or sitting	II	Headache; maternal hypotension
Spinal Block	Umbilicus to toes	Sims or sitting	II	Headache; maternal hypotension

• •

Paracervical Block

The *paracervical block* is a regional anesthetic procedure that blocks nerve pathways from the uterus during labor (see Figs. 6–2 and 6–3). It is not commonly used today. The block is effective in relieving pain due to uterine contractions and cervical dilatation. It does not extend to the vagina and vulva. Therefore, it is ineffective

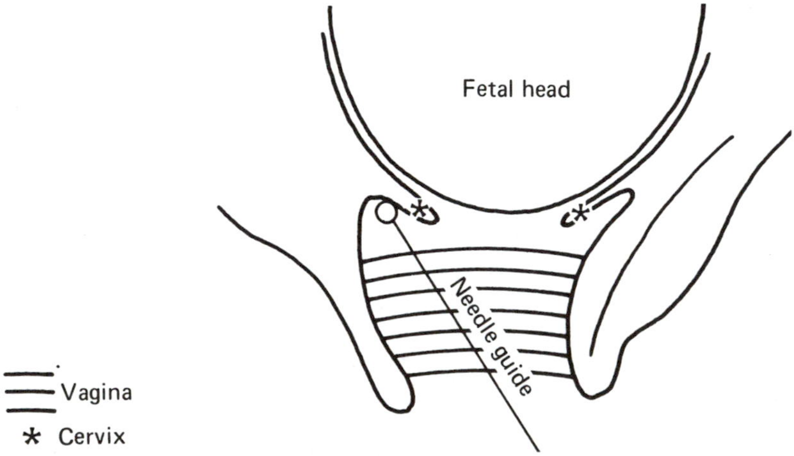

Figure 6–3. Paracervical block injection site.

for pain relief during delivery (stretching of the vagina and vulva, episiotomy/repair). A one percent (1%) solution of an anesthetic such as mepivocaine, lidocaine, or procaine can be used. Mepivocaine seems to provide the longest anesthetic effect. The anesthetic agent (5 to 10 ml) is injected bilaterally into the paracervical nerve endings through the vaginal canal or transperitoneally with the woman in a lithotomy position.

A paracervical block is administered during the first stage of labor when the cervix is dilated at least 3 to 4 cm and gives complete relief of pain 80 percent of the time. The anesthetic effect in the cervical region is dramatic, achieved almost immediately and lasts 45 to 60 minutes, depending on the type and amount of agent used. The procedure may be repeated every 60 to 90 minutes as necessary. It is important to use a fetal monitor in conjunction with paracervical blocks. *Transient fetal bradycardia* may develop within 2 to 10 minutes of paracervical block administration and last 3 to 30 minutes. This side effect is thought to be caused by uterine artery constriction (a local reaction to the anesthetic agent) leading to decreased placental perfusion. Fetal bradycardia could add insult to a fetus experiencing undetected distress from other causes. The procedure should *not* be repeated if fetal bradycardia occurs. The paracervical block should be used *only* with normal labor and an uncompromised fetus in order to avoid **injury, potential for; trauma related to paracervical anesthesia**.

The length of the needle (approximately 12 to 15 inches) may be frightening to the laboring woman. The nurse should explain that the length is necessary in order to reach the cervical area. Transvaginally, the needle is inserted through a guide with only 6 to 12 mm of actual needle inserted into the mucosa.

The paracervical block relieves pain and is easy for an obstetrician to administer. The disadvantages of a paracervical block are:

1. a 10 to 70 percent incidence of fetal bradycardia[4]
2. unpredictable effect on labor progress; labor may be shortened or prolonged
3. when the anesthetic wears off, the return of sensation is abrupt and may be interpreted as quite painful
4. the procedure, owing to its short duration, may need to be repeated several times during a primipara's labor (which is considerably longer than a multipara's)
5. it is not effective for delivery since it can only be used during the first stage of labor when the cervix is still palpable
6. if accidentally injected into the fetus it may cause apnea, bradycardia, convulsions, and central nervous system damage to the fetus

Despite the advantages of the paracervical block, the potential complications are considered to be very hazardous and therefore, some have advocated omitting the use of this block completely from the practice of obstetrics.

• •

Review Questions

1. The paracervical block is a regional anesthetic procedure used during labor to relieve pain by: ____________________
____

2. What nursing action should be taken immediately following administration of a paracervical block?
____
____

3. List three advantages of a paracervical block.
   a. ____________________
   b. ____________________
   c. ____________________

4. List four disadvantages of a paracervical block.
   a. ____________________
   b. ____________________
   c. ____________________
   d. ____________________

Answers

1. Paracervical blocks are used during labor to relieve pain by *blocking nerve pathways from the uterus.*

2. Immediately following the administration of a paracervical block the nurse should closely monitor the *FHR* for at least 30 minutes anticipating transient bradycardia.

3. Advantages of a paracervical block are: (a) it is given during the first stage of labor, (b) it gives complete pain relief 80 percent of the time, (c) anesthesia is achieved almost immediately, (d) it can be repeated when it wears off, and (e) it is easy to administer.

4. Disadvantages of the paracervical block are: (a) transient fetal bradycardia, (b) unpredictable effect on labor progress, (c) abrupt return of pain, (d) short duration of anesthesia, (e) not effective for delivery, and (f) apnea, bradycardia, convulsions, and central nervous system damage to the fetus if accidentally injected.

• •

Pudendal Block

The *pudendal block* (see Figs. 6–1 and 6–2) is a regional anesthetic that provides anesthesia to the perineal area, vulva, and vagina. The block interferes with impulses from S–2 to S–4 by injection of the anesthetic agent into the pudendal nerve endings at the ischial spine level (bilaterally). The block is administered just prior to delivery before the perineum becomes distended by the presenting part. Once distention occurs, it may be too late to achieve *effective* anesthesia. A long needle similar to that used for a paracervical block is inserted through the vaginal wall with the woman in a lithotomy position. The onset of action is immediate, with a duration of 30 minutes. The pudendal block may be the anesthesia of choice for a delivery following labor without analgesia or with the use of paracervical blocks during the first stage of labor. Complications are not common but may include sciatic nerve damage, broad ligament hematoma, and perforation of the rectum.

Advantages of the pudendal block are:

1. It produces marked relaxation of the perineal muscles, facilitating an easier delivery with decreased possibility of perineal tears.
2. The woman is still able to push effectively, although the urge to push is slightly diminished.
3. There are seldom side effects in the fetus or newborn, unless it is accidentally injected with the anesthetic agent.

Disadvantages of the pudendal block are:

1. The woman may still experience pain with contractions and stretching of the vaginal wall during delivery and placental expulsion.
2. The woman may be unable to control her pushing efforts, causing perineal tears during delivery of the baby.

Local Perineal Infiltration

The *local perineal infiltration* (see Figs. 6–1 and 6–2) is a regional anesthetic used alone or sometimes in conjunction with other regional anesthetics, if necessary. Just prior to delivery, medication is injected locally into the perineal body to desensitize the episiotomy site. It can be repeated after delivery if necessary for the repair. Chloroprocaine, lidocaine, and mepivocaine are most commonly used because of their rapid tissue diffusion.

Advantages of local perineal infiltration are:

1. The woman is able to push effectively and cooperate in the delivery of the baby.
2. There are no side effects on the fetus or newborn.
3. It provides effective anesthesia for cutting and repair of the episiotomy/lacerations.

Disadvantages of local perineal infiltration are:

1. It does not eliminate pain or discomfort from perineal distention, contractions, or placental expulsion.
2. Used alone, it is usually only effective for the episiotomy/laceration repair.

• •

Review Questions

1. The pudendal block is used to block nerve endings at the ______ to provide relaxation of ______ and anesthesia of the ______.
2. List two advantages of the pudendal block.
   a. ______
   b. ______
3. List two disadvantages of the pudendal block.
   a. ______
   b. ______
4. Local perineal infiltration is used just prior to delivery to desensitize the ______.
5. List two advantages of local perineal infiltration.
   a. ______
   b. ______

Answers

1. The pudendal block is used to block nerve endings at the *ischial spine level* to provide relaxation of *perineal muscles* and anesthesia of the *perineum.*
2. Advantages of the pudendal block are: (a) it produces marked relaxation of the perineum facilitating an easier delivery with decreased possibility of perineal tears, (b) the mother is still able to push effectively, although the urge is slightly diminished, and (c) there are seldom side effects on the fetus or newborn unless it is accidentally injected with the anesthetic agent.
3. Disadvantages of the pudendal block are: (a) the woman may still experience pain with contractions and stretching of the vaginal wall during delivery and placental expulsion, and (b) perineal tears may occur due to the inability to control pushing efforts.
4. Local perineal infiltration is used just prior to delivery to desensitize the *episiotomy site.*
5. Advantages of local perineal infiltration are: (a) the woman is able to push effectively and cooperate in the delivery of the baby, (b) there are no side effects on the fetus or newborn, and (c) it provides effective anesthesia for cutting and repair of the episiotomy.

• •

EMERGENCY NURSING MEASURES FOR COMPLICATIONS FOLLOWING ANESTHETIC ADMINISTRATION

The most frequently occurring side effects associated with anesthesia are *maternal hypotension* and *fetal bradycardia.* In other words, there is concern about **cardiac output, alterations, in: de-**

creased (maternal and fetal) related to the administration of anesthetics. A sudden episode of severe *nausea* may be the first sign of hypotension. If hypotension occurs, the nurse should:

1. *Turn* the woman to her left side to relieve uterine pressure on iliac veins and inferior vena cava and to promote venous return, thereby increasing oxygen supply to the fetus. If this does not correct the maternal hypotension and fetal bradycardia, then:
2. *Administer* oxygen at 5 or 7 to 10 liters per minute via face mask.
3. *Discontinue* any oxytocic drug if it is being given.
4. *Increase* the intravenous flow rate (if the woman has an IV) to increase circulatory volume.
5. *Elevate* the woman's legs to increase blood volume in the central circulation.
6. *Observe* fetal heart rate pattern for bradycardia and decelerations via electronic fetal monitoring.
7. *Notify* the physician.
8. DO NOT LEAVE THE WOMAN ALONE.

Occasionally a woman may exhibit signs of an allergic or toxic reaction to local anesthetic agents. Although this is rare, it is important for the nurse to be aware of the following signs and symptoms in order to notify the physician immediately. Progressive symptoms include:

1. lightheadedness,
2. dizziness,
3. slurred speech,
4. metallic taste,
5. numbness of tongue and mouth,
6. muscle twitching,
7. loss of consciousness, and
8. generalized convulsions.[33]

Immediate treatment involves establishing an airway, administering oxygen, and controlling convulsions. The physician may order Succinylcholine which enables endotracheal intubation by controlling muscle spasms. Succinylcholine causes the body to become totally flaccid. Although the woman can see and hear, she is unable to move. This is a very frightening experience. The nurse should explain what is happening and provide as much support as possible. Barbiturates or diazepam may be ordered to control convulsions. The nurse must support cardiovascular function with rapid administration of intravenous fluids. Fetal distress may occur as evidenced by persistent bradycardia or late fetal heart rate decelerations. By turning the woman on her left side, there is increased placental perfusion and thereby oxygen to the fetus. Prompt reversal of maternal convulsive state will promote fetal recovery in utero. Fetal recovery in utero (intrauterine resuscitation) is preferred over neonatal resuscitation after an emergency delivery.

• •

Review Questions

1. Following the administration of an anesthetic agent, you note that the fetal heart rate baseline has dropped to 90 to 100 beats per minute, and the woman's blood pressure has decreased significantly. List at least five emergency measures you should carry out:
   a. ______
   b. ______
   c. ______
   d. ______
   e. ______
2. If a woman develops an allergic or toxic reaction to a local anesthetic agent, immediate treatment would involve:
   a. ______
   b. ______
   c. ______

Answers

1. The following emergency nursing measures should be initiated: (a) turn the mother on her left side, (b) give oxygen at 5 or 7 to 10 liters per minute, (c) discontinue oxytocic, (d) increase the intravenous flow rate, (e) elevate the woman's legs, (f) observe fetal heart rate pattern for bradycardia and decelerations, (g) notify the physician, and (h) DO NOT LEAVE THE WOMAN ALONE.
2. The immediate treatment following allergic or toxic reaction to a local anesthetic agent is: (a) establish an airway, (b) administer oxygen, and (c) control convulsions.

• •

GENERAL ANESTHESIA DURING LABOR AND DELIVERY

General anesthesia is a progressive depression of the CNS, causing loss of sensation in the entire body and loss of consciousness. It may be achieved with intravenous anesthesia or inhalation anesthesia or a combination of both. General anesthesia is rarely used today for vaginal deliveries although it is sometimes used in emergencies when rapid delivery is crucial.

A potentially life threatening complication of general anesthesia is **airway clearance, ineffective related to aspiration of stomach contents**. This can be prevented by:

1. maintaining minimal stomach contents by limiting oral intake and administering drugs (cimetidine, metaclopromide) to increase gastric emptying,
2. decreasing the acidity of gastric contents with antacid drugs such as sodium citrate, and

3. preventing regurgitation of gastric contents during induction of general anesthesia by the application of cricoid pressure during intubation.[4]

Inhalation Anesthesia

Inhalation anesthesia is seldom used today for vaginal deliveries although it is sometimes used for emergencies where rapid delivery is important (for example, cesarean births, fetal distress). It is important to deliver the baby within 5 to 7 minutes after administration of the gas, because inhalation anesthesia rapidly crosses the placenta to the fetus resulting in anoxia and respiratory depression of the fetus and newborn. In nursing diagnosis terms, there is **(fetal/newborn) gas exchange, impaired related to inhalation anesthesia**. Inhalation anesthesia produces depression of the central nervous system, therefore, it is important to continually monitor maternal vital signs before, during, and after administration of the anesthetic. Continual fetal heart rate monitoring is essential prior to delivery followed by Apgar scoring and assessment of the newborn immediately after delivery.

Advantages of inhalation anesthesia:

1. It produces greater overall body muscle relaxation (it especially facilitates cesarean births).
2. It causes decreased possibility of convulsions (pregnancy-induced hypertension) because it depresses the central nervous system. This may be the anesthetic of choice for the woman with severe pre-eclampsia.
3. It provides rapid induction, thus making it the preferred choice in some obstetrical emergencies.

Disadvantages of inhalation anesthesia:

1. There is an additive CNS depressant effect when combined with narcotic agonists or sedatives.
2. Rapid placental diffusion of anesthesia causes fetal anesthesia with respiratory depression and anoxia of the newborn.
3. Increased possibility of maternal aspiration of gastric contents may cause pneumonia or even death.
4. The woman is unable to participate in the delivery.
5. The father's presence at the delivery is usually undesirable.
6. A trained anesthetist or anesthesiologist must be present to administer the agent.
7. Recovery period for the woman is longer, with postpartum nausea and vomiting often present.
8. The woman must be assessed carefully for postpartum hemorrhage due to the uterine relaxant effect of nitrous oxide.

Nitrous Oxide. Nitrous oxide is combined with oxygen and inhaled through a mask in gaseous form to produce analgesia and altered consciousness but not true anesthesia. It may be used alone with oxygen as an analgesic during Stage II or as an induction agent. It must be combined with a more potent inhalation anesthetic agent (halothane, enflurene, isoflurane) to provide anesthesia for difficult vaginal deliveries or cesarean births. Because of its low potency, adverse effects occur only with prolonged use.[8]

Halothane (Fluothane). Halothane is a potent general anesthetic which can be administered with oxygen and nitrous oxide. Induction and recovery are rapid with little nausea and vomiting. Halothane is nonirritating to the respiratory tract. Therefore, secretions are minimal. The major side effects are hypotension and decreased cardiac contraction force. With deep levels of anesthesia, hypoxia and acidosis may occur as a result of respiratory depression.[8]

Enflurane (Ethrane). Enflurane is a potent general anesthetic which can be administered with nitrous oxide and oxygen. Induction and recovery are rapid with no significant respiratory depression unless a deep level of anesthesia is achieved. The major side effects are hypotension, hypothermia and shivering. High concentrations of enflurane can cause uterine relaxation with resultant bleeding postpartum.[8]

Isoflurane (Forane). Isoflurane is a potent general anesthetic that is usually combined with nitrous oxide and oxygen to decrease the amount of isoflurane needed. In high concentrations, mechanical support of respiratory function may be necessary because of its respiratory depressant effect. Induction and recovery are rapid with good skeletal muscle relaxation. The two major side effects are respiratory depression and hyperthemia.[8]

Intravenous Anesthesia

Intravenous anesthesia is rarely seen in modern obstetrics. Sodium pentothal (a short-acting barbiturate) is injected into the blood stream, causing a loss of sensation to the entire body and a loss of consciousness. It causes rapid induction of anesthesia (within 30 seconds of administration) and prompt recovery. Sodium pentothal is rarely used alone and is normally used for induction of inhalation anesthesia. Constant monitoring of vital signs is imperative.

Major disadvantages of intravenous anesthesia include:

1. depression of maternal vital centers (respiratory, vasomotor and cardiac) with bronchospasms, laryngospasms and hypotension,
2. fetal depression due to rapid placental transfer, and
3. fetal hypoxia due to maternal hypotension.

• •

Review Questions

1. Maternal regurgitation and aspiration of gastric contents is a potentially life-threatening complication of general anesthesia. Discuss three methods of prevention.

a. ______________________________
b. ______________________________
c. ______________________________

2. **When administering inhalation anesthesia for a delivery, the most important consideration is ______________________________.**

3. **List two advantages of inhalation anesthesia.**
   a. ______________________________
   b. ______________________________

4. **List at least five disadvantages of inhalation anesthesia.**
   a. ______________________________
   b. ______________________________
   c. ______________________________
   d. ______________________________
   e. ______________________________

5. **The drug most commonly used for intravenous anesthesia is: ______________________________.**

6. **List two complications of intravenous anesthesia.**
   a. ______________________________
   b. ______________________________

Answers

1. Maternal regurgitation and aspiration of gastric contents can be prevented by: (a) limiting oral intake and administering drugs to increase gastric emptying, (b) decreasing the acidity of gastric contents, and (c) applying cricoid pressure during intubation to prevent regurgitation during induction of general anesthesia.

2. When administering inhalation anesthesia for delivery, the most important consideration is the *amount of time between the onset of administration and the birth of the baby*.

3. Advantages of inhalation anesthesia are: (a) greater overall body muscle relaxation, (b) decreased possibility of convulsions due to central nervous system depression, and (c) rapid induction.

4. Disadvantages of inhalation anesthesia are: (a) additive CNS depressant effect when combined with agonists or sedatives, (b) rapid placental diffusion of anesthesia, causing fetal anesthesia with respiratory depression and anoxia of the newborn, (c) increased possibility of maternal aspiration of gastric contents, causing pneumonia or even death, (d) no participation in the delivery by the mother, (e) makes father's presence at the delivery undesirable, (f) need a trained anesthetist present to administer the agent, (g) recovery period for the mother longer, with postpartum nausea and vomiting often present, and (h) uterine relaxation likely causing postpartum hemorrhage.

5. *Sodium pentothal* is most commonly used for intravenous anesthesia.

6. Complications of intravenous anesthesia are: (a) depression of maternal vital

centers with bronchospasms, laryngospasms, and hypotension, (b) rapid placental transfer causing fetal depression, and (c) fetal hypoxia due to maternal hypotension.

• •

CONCLUSION

The process of labor and delivery is considered a stressful event to which women respond in a variety of ways. If the woman is unprepared for the experience, she may interpret the contractions of labor as being excessively painful. Excessive pain can be detrimental. Therefore, it must be interrupted through supportive nursing interventions and the careful and proper use of analgesics and anesthetics. Drugs given to a woman in labor affect not only her but may also have undesirable effects upon the fetus or newborn. What to give and when to give it can sometimes be a very difficult decision to make. Ideally, the woman who is able to progress normally through the process of labor and delivery should be given as little medication as possible. *Perhaps, none at all may be best.*

REFERENCES

1. Simkin, P: Stress, pain, and catecholamines in labor: Part 1. A review. Birth 13(4):227, 1986.
2. Lagercrantz, H and Slotkin, TA: The stress of being born. Sci Am 12:100, 1985.
3. Lederman, E, et al: Maternal psychological and physiologic correlates of fetal-newborn health status. Am J Obstet Gynecol 139:956, 1981.
4. Oxorn, DC: Obstetric analgesia and anesthesia. In Oxorn, H: Oxorn-Foote Human Labor and Birth, ed 5. Appleton-Century-Crofts, New York, 1986, p 466, 437, 453.
5. Fox, HA: The effects of catecholamines and drug treatment on the fetus and newborn. Birth Fam J 6:157, 1979.
6. McCaffery, M: Nursing Management of the Patient with Pain, ed. 2. JB Lippincott, Philadelphia, 1979, p 63.
7. Adamatsu, TJ and Bonica, JJ: Pain pathway during labor. In Clark, AL and Affonso, DD: Childbearing: A Nursing Perspective, ed 2. FA Davis, Philadelphia, 1979, p 421.
8. Swonger, AK and Matejski, MP: Nursing Pharmacology, An Integrated Approch to Drug Therapy and Nursing Practice, Scott Foresman & Co., Boston, 1988, p 377, 992, 974, 233, 235.
9. Shnider, SM and Moya, F: Effects of meperidine on the newborn infant. Am J Obstet Gynecol 89:1009, 1964.
10. DeVoe, SJ, et al: Effects of meperidine on uterine contractility. Am J Obstet Gynecol 105:1004, 1969.
11. Riffel, HD, et al: Effects of meperidine and promethazine during labor. Obstet Gynecol 42:738, 1973.
12. Kuhnert, BR, et al: Meperidine and normeperidine levels following meperidine administration during labor. II. Fetus and neonate. Am J Obstet Gynecol 133(8):909, 1979.

13. Belfrage, P, et al: Neonatal depression after obstetrical analgesia with pethidine. The role of the injection-delivery time interval and of the plasma concentrations of pethidine and norpethidine. Acta Obstet Gynecol Scand 60(1):43, 1981.
14. Belsey, EM, et al: The influence of maternal analgesia on neonatal behavior: I. Pethidine. Br J Obstet Gynecol 88(4):398, 1981.
15. Hodgkinson, R and Husain, FJ: The duration of effect of maternally administered meperidine on neonatal neurobehavior. Anesthesiology 56:51, 1982.
16. Kuhnert, BR, et al: Effects of low doses of meperidine on neonatal behavior. Anesth Analg 64(3):335, 1985.
17. Olds, SB, London, ML and Ladewig, PA: Maternal-Newborn Nursing, A Family-Centered Approach, ed 3. Addison-Wesley, Menlo Park, 1988, p 694, 695, 1007.
18. Baer, CL and Williams, BR: Clinical Pharmacology and Nursing, Springhouse Publishing, Pennsylvania, 1988, p 427, 426, 489, 450.
19. Hodgkinson, R, et al: Neonatal neurobehavior in the first 48 hours of life: Effect of the administration of meperidine with and without Naloxone in the mother. Pediatrics 62(3):294, 1978.
20. Kron, RE, Stein, M and Goddard, DE: Newborn sucking behavior affected by obstetric sedation. Pediatrics 37:1012, 1966.
21. Scanlon, JW, et al: Neurobehavioral responses of newborn infants after maternal epidural anesthesia. Anesthesiology 40:121, 1974.
22. Scanlon, JW, et al: Neurobehavioral responses and drug concentrations in newborns after maternal epidural anesthesia with bupivacaine. Anesthesiology 45:400, 1976.
23. Murray, AD, et al: Effects of epidural anesthesia on newborns and their mothers. Child Dev 52:71, 1981.
24. Rosenblatt, DB, et al: The influence of maternal analgesia on neonatal behavior. II. Epidural bupivacaine. Br J Obstet Gynecol 88:407, 1981.
25. Abboud, TK, et al: Maternal, fetal and neonatal responses after epidural anesthesia with bupivacaine, 2-chloroprocaine, or lidocaine. Anesth Analg 61:638, 1982.
26. Abboud, TK, et al: Lack of adverse neonatal neurobehavioral effects of lidocaine. Anesth Analg 62:473, 1983.
27. Abboud, TK, et al: Epidural bupivacaine, chloroprocaine, or lidocaine for cesarean section—maternal and neonatal effects. Anesth Analg 62(10):914, 1983.
28. Abboud, TK, et al: Continuous infusion epidural analgesia in parturients receiving bupivacaine, chloroprocaine, or lidocaine—maternal, fetal, and neonatal effects. Anesth Analg 63(4):421, 1984.
29. Lester, BM, Als, H and Brazelton, TB: Regional obstetric anesthesia and newborn behavior: A reanalysis toward synergistic effects. Child Dev 53:687, 1982.
30. Hoult, IJ, Maclennan, AH and Carrie, LES: Lumbar epidural analgesia in labour. Relation to foetal malposition and instrumental delivery. Br Med J 3:114, 1977.
31. Fulbert, MN and Marx, GF: Extradural pressures in the parturient patient. Anesthesiology 40:499, 1974.
32. Haight, K: What you should know about epidural analgesia. Nurs 87 17(9):58, 1987.
33. Pritchard, JA, McDonald, PC and Gant, NF: Williams Obstetrics, ed 17. Appleton-Century-Crofts, Norwalk, Connecticut, 1985, p 359.

BIBLIOGRAPHY

Avard, DM and Nimrod, CM: Risks and benefits of obstetric epidural analgesia: A review. Birth 12(4):215, 1985.

Baer, CL and Williams, BR: Clinical Pharmacology and Nursing, Springhouse Publishing, Springhouse, PA, 1988.

Bloom, KC: Assisting the unprepared woman during labor. J Obstet Gynecol Neonatol Nurs 13(5):303, 1984.

Brucker, MC: Nonpharmaceutical methods for relieving pain and discomfort during pregnancy. Matern Child Nurs J 9(5):390, 1984.

Clark, RB: Conduction anesthesia. Clin Obstet Gynecol 24(2):603, 1981.

Dick-Reed, G: Childbirth Without Fear, ed 4. Harper and Row, New York, 1972.

Fishburne, JI: Systemic analgesia during labor. Clin Perinatol 9(1):29, 1982.

Holmes, J and Magiera, L: Maternity Nursing, Macmillan, New York, 1987.

Howe, CL: Physiologic and psychologic assessment in labor. Nurs Clin N Amer 17(1):49, 1982.

Kuhnert, BR, et al: Obstetric medication and neonatal behavior. Current controversies. Clin Perinatol 12(2):423, 1985.

Mathewson, MK: Pharmacotherapeutics: A Nursing Approach, FA Davis, Philadelphia, 1986.

Melzack, R, et al: Severity of labour pain: Influence of physical as well as psychologic variables. Can Med Assoc J 130:579, 1984.

Moir, DD: Local anesthetic techniques in obstetrics. Br J Anaesth 58(7):747, 1986.

Neesom, JD and May, KA: Comprehensive Maternity Nursing: Nursing Process and the Childbearing Family, JB Lippincott, Philadelphia, 1986.

Olsson, G and Parker, G: A model approach to pain assessment. Nurs 87 17(5):52, 1987.

Oxorn, H: Oxorn-Foote Human Labor and Birth, ed 5. Appleton-Century-Crofts, Norwalk, Connecticut, 1986.

Pritchard, JA, McDonald, PC and Gant, NF: Williams Obstetrics, ed 17. Appleton-Century-Crofts, Norwalk, Connecticut, 1985.

Roberts, JE: Factors influencing distress from pain during labor. Matern Child Nurs J 8(1):62, 1983.

Shnider, SM: Choice of anesthesia for labor and delivery. Obstet Gynecol 58:24S, 1981.

Simkin, P: Stress, pain, and catecholamines in labor: Part 1. A review. Birth 13(4):227, 1986.

Smith, CM: Epidural anesthesia in labor. Various agents employed. J Obstet Neonatol Nurs 13(1):17, 1984.

Swonger, AK and Matejski, MP: Nursing Pharmacology: An Integrated Approach to Drug Therapy and Nursing Practice, Scott Foresman & Co., Boston, 1988.

POST-TEST 6

1. Pain is a subjective phenomenon that exists when an individual:
   a. experiences ______
   b. interprets ______
   c. exhibits ______

2. Describe the positive and negative roles of catecholamines in labor.
   Positive ______
   ______
   ______
   ______

   Negative ______
   ______
   ______
   ______

3. Differentiate among the following factors that may accompany an individual's reaction to pain: P. physiologic, V. verbal, or N. nonverbal. Place the appropriate letter (P, V, or N) in front of each descriptive term.

____ a. depression	____ h. cries for help
____ b. increased BP	____ i. increased muscle tension
____ c. moaning	____ j. hostility
____ d. rigidity	____ k. groaning
____ e. grimacing	____ l. increased respiration
____ f. fear	____ m. pacing
____ g. dilated pupils	____ n. withdrawal

4. List at least four reasons why pain may occur during labor.
   a. ______
   b. ______
   c. ______
   d. ______

5. What nonpharmacologic interventions might the nurse use to help decrease a laboring woman's perception of pain?
   a. ______
   b. ______

c. ______
d. ______
e. ______

6. What three factors must be carefully considered when deciding on a program of drug intervention for the woman in labor?
a. ______
b. ______
c. ______

7. Name the direct maternal effects of drug intervention that can indirectly affect the fetus or newborn.
a. ______
b. ______
c. ______

8. What is analgesia? What is the most common narcotic agonist used during labor to provide analgesia? ______

9. What desirable effects should narcotic agonists have on the mother? What is the major undesirable effect? ______

10. How might narcotic agonists administered to the mother affect the fetus? What nursing interventions are appropriate? How might it affect the newborn? ______

11. What subtle behavioral changes have been observed in the newborn during the first 24 hours of life following the administration of meperidine to the mother in labor? ______

How might the new mother feel about these behavioral changes in the newborn? ______

What are the appropriate nursing interventions? ______

12. Key: A. Narcotic Agonists
B. Narcotic Antagonists
C. Mixed Agonists/Antagonists
D. Sedatives

The following statements need to be completed. Insert the appropriate letter(s) (using the above key) to make the statements correct.

a. _____ may be given alone in false labor or early prodromal labor to decrease fear, apprehension, anxiety, and promote sedation.
b. _____ Respiratory depression is a major side effect of _______.
c. _____ When __________________ is administered to the mother during labor, subtle behavioral changes may be observed in the newborn during the first 24 hours of life.
d. _____ During the first 4 days of life, the newborn may exhibit poor sucking reflex, fewer sucks per minute, lower sucking pressure and decreased formula intake when __________________ have been administered to the mother during labor.
e. _____ Respiratory depression of the newborn caused by sedatives may be increased when _______ are administered.
f. _____ Maternal hypotension is a major side effect of ________ drugs.
g. _____ _____ administered at the appropriate time in labor may promote cervical dilatation, thereby enhancing labor progress.

13. Key: A. Epidural
B. Caudal
C. Saddle
D. Spinal
E. Paracervical
F. Pudendal
G. Local Infiltration

The following statements need to be completed. Insert the appropriate letter(s) (using the above key) to make the statements correct. There may be more than one correct answer.

a. _____ The episiotomy site is desensitized just prior to delivery with ____.
b. _____ A puncture through the dura into the subarachnoid space is necessary for administration of _____ and ________.
c. _____ Dural puncture is the major complication of ___________.
d. _____ Transient fetal bradycardia is the major side effect of ____.
e. _____ Although the urge to push is slightly diminished, the mother is able to push effectively following _______________.
f. _____ The space that is level with the last sacral vertebra is the site of injection for ______________________________.

g. ____ A continuous anesthetic effect during labor and delivery can be obtained with ____________ and ____________.

h. ____ ______ is used to block nerves at the ischial spine level to provide anesthesia to the perineal area, vulva and vagina.

i. ____ A headache may occur as a side effect of ____________ and ____________.

j. ____ The major side effect of maternal hypotension is associated with ______, ______, ______, and ______ anesthesia.

k. ____ The __________ is effective only during Stage I of labor.

l. ____ The ______ provides anesthesia to the perineum, lower pelvis, and upper thighs only.

m. ____ ______ anesthesia is administered into the space surrounding the dura between L2–L3 and L3–L4.

14. Discuss the use of epidural morphine for labor and delivery. What is the major side effect? Describe the appropriate nursing interventions. ____________

15. Since anesthetic agents might cause maternal hypotension or fetal bradycardia, what five nursing interventions would be appropriate if one or both did occur?
   a. ____________
   b. ____________
   c. ____________
   d. ____________
   e. ____________

Answers

1. Pain is a subjective phenomenon that exists when an individual: (a) experiences a sensation, (b) interprets the sensation as painful, and (c) exhibits a psychologic and physiologic reaction to the sensation.

2. *Positive effects of catecholamines*: catecholamines are produced in response to the stress of labor. They prepare the mother's body for action and assist the fetus to adapt to decreased oxygen during contractions.
   Negative effects of catecholamines: excess catecholamines may be produced in response to distress (excess pain) which leads to shunting of maternal blood to the vital organs with prolonged fetal hypoxia.

3. a. V and N;
   b. P
   c. V
   d. N
   e. N
   f. V and N
   g. P
   h. V
   i. N
   j. V and N
   k. V
   l. P
   m. N
   n. V and N

Physiologic reactions to pain include: increased blood pressure, heart rate, respirations, pupil diameter, muscle tension, and muscle activity. Verbal reactions to pain include: cries for help, moaning, and groaning. Nonverbal reactions to pain include: depression, hostility, fear, and withdrawal.

4. The following are theories of the causes of pain in labor:
   a. hypoxia of compressed muscle cells of the uterus brought about with each contraction
   b. compression of the nerve ganglia in the cervix and lower uterine segments during contractions
   c. stretching of the cervix during dilatation and effacement
   d. stretching and displacing of the perineum as the fetus descends the birth canal
   e. pressure on the urethra, bladder, and rectum as the fetus descends
   f. fear resulting in tension causing pain and more fear as a spontaneous occurrence

5. Nonpharmacologic interventions that the nurse can use to help decrease the perception of pain are:
   a. alleviate fear
   b. praise positive efforts
   c. promote rest between contractions
   d. assist with distraction, cutaneous stimulation, relaxation and guided imagery
   e. accurately assess reactions to pain
   f. accurately assess need for drugs
   g. assess the effectiveness of drugs

6. Three important considerations regarding drug intervention are:
   a. potency of the drug
   b. side effects on the mother and fetus/newborn
   c. stage in labor and progress made

7. Direct maternal effects of drug intervention may cause the following indirect effects on the fetus or newborn:
   a. Impaired maternal ventilation or arterial hypotension can cause decreased fetal heart rate.
   b. Maternal hypertension can cause abruption of the placenta with fetal anoxia and possible death.
   c. Alteration in the forces of labor can cause fetal trauma due to prolonged labor.

8. Analgesia is the absence or decreased awareness of a normal sensation of pain. The narcotic agonist, *meperidine (Demerol)* is the most common analgesic used in labor.

9. The desirable effects of narcotic agonists upon the mother are relief of pain, antispasmodic action, decreased anxiety, euphoria, and sedation. The major undesirable effect is that it may cause respiratory depression.

10. Narcotic agonists administered to the mother in labor may cause respiratory depression of the fetus. No specific nursing intervention is required as long as placental sufficiency is maintained for adequate oxygenation of the fetus.

However, at birth, if the newborn exhibits signs of narcotic depression, resuscitative measures will be necessary.

11. Meperidine administered to the mother during labor may produce subtle behavioral changes in the newborn during the first 24 hours of life. These newborns tend to be less alert and generally demonstrate sluggish behavior. They exhibit a decreased response to maternal stimuli such as startling, cuddling, and consoling. The nurse should try to help the new mother understand that the newborn will become more alert and responsive with time. She needs much assurance that the unresponsiveness of her baby is not a reflection of her mothering ability.

12. The following statements are correct.

a. D
b. A, C, D
c. A
d. D
e. A, C
f. A, D
g. A

a. *Sedatives* may be given alone in false labor or early prodromal labor to decrease apprehension, fear, anxiety, and promote sedation.
b. Respiratory depression is the major side effect of *Narcotic Agonists*, *Mixed Agonists/Antagonists*, and *Sedatives*.
c. When *Narcotic Agonists* are administered to the mother during labor subtle behavioral changes may be observed in the newborn during the first 24 hours of life.
d. During the first 4 days of life, the newborn may exhibit poor sucking reflex, fewer sucks per minute, lower sucking pressure, and decreased formula intake when *Sedatives/Barbiturates* have been administered to the mother during labor.
e. Depression from sedatives may be increased when *Narcotic Agonists*, *Mixed Agonists/Antagonists* are administered.
f. Maternal hypotension is the major side effect of *Narcotic Agonists*, and *Sedatives*.
g. *Narcotic Agonists* administered at the appropriate time in labor may promote cervical dilatation, thereby enhancing labor progression.

13. The following statements are correct.

a. G
b. D, C
c. A
d. E
e. F
f. B
g. B, A
h. F
i. D, C
j. A, B, C, D
k. E
l. C
m. A

a. The episiotomy site is desensitized just prior to delivery with *Local*.
b. A puncture through the dura into the subarachnoid space is necessary for administration of *Spinal* and *Saddle*.
c. Dural puncture is the major complication of *Epidural*.
d. Transient fetal bradycardia is the major side effect of *Paracervical*.
e. Although the urge to push is slightly diminished, the mother is able to push effectively following *Pudendal*.
f. The space that is level with the last sacral vertebra is the site of injection for *Caudal*.

g. A continuous anesthetic effect during labor and delivery can be obtained with *Caudal* and *Epidural*.
h. *Pudendal* is used to block nerves at the ischial spine level to provide anesthesia to the perineal area, vulva, and vagina.
i. A headache is a side effect of *Spinal* and *Saddle*.
j. The major side effect of maternal hypotension is associated with *Epidural*, *Caudal*, *Saddle*, *Spinal*.
k. The *Paracervical* is effective only during stage I of labor.
l. The *Saddle* provides anesthesia to the perineum, lower pelvis and upper thighs.
m. *Epidural* anesthesia is administered into the space surrounding the dura between L2–L3 or L3–L4.

14. Epidural morphine may be given during the first stage of labor to relieve pain. Although a smaller dose is needed, the onset of action is slow. The major side effect is respiratory depression. Nursing interventions include: assess respiratory function for at least 24 hours (apnea monitor recommended), provide alternative methods of pain relief while waiting for drug to take effect, and have resuscitative equipment available.

15. If maternal hypotension or fetal bradycardia occurs following anesthetic administration, the appropriate nursing interventions are:
    a. Turn the mother on her left side to relieve uterine pressure on the iliac veins and inferior vena cava, and promote venous return, thereby increasing oxygen supply to the fetus.
    b. Administer oxygen at 5 or 7 to 10 liters per minute via face mask.
    c. Discontinue oxytocic drug.
    d. Increase intravenous flow rate to expand circulatory volume.
    e. Elevate the woman's legs to increase blood volume in the central circulation.
    f. Assess fetal heart rate pattern.
    g. Notify the physician.
    h. DO NOT LEAVE THE WOMAN ALONE.

7 CONTEMPORARY APPROACHES TO THE LABOR PROCESS

Celeste R. Phillips

OBJECTIVES

Upon completing this chapter, you will be able to:

- ▶ Identify major trends occurring in today's dynamic maternity care system.
- ▶ Explain the philosophy of care which is the driving force for contemporary maternity programs.
- ▶ Describe the "pillars" that support contemporary maternity care.
- ▶ Discuss vaginal birth after cesarean (VBAC) as an acceptable method for childbirth after cesarean birth.
- ▶ Differentiate LDR, LDRP, and SRMC.
- ▶ Compare and contrast three methods of preparation for birth currently taught in the United States.
- ▶ Describe the three specific breathing patterns widely used in Lamaze birth classes.
- ▶ Explain exhalation breathing for pushing in second stage.
- ▶ Describe five nonpharmaceutical methods for relieving pain during labor.
- ▶ Explain how labor and birth can affect all family members.
- ▶ Discuss out-of-hospital options for the place of birth that are available in today's practice.

A restructuring of the health care delivery system is mandating alterations in traditional approaches to care. In this dynamic setting, labor and birth present unique challenges to today's nurses. Childbirth preparation, women's conscious involvement in birth, and family participation are fast becoming the norm. As the average length of hospital stay shortens dramatically, consideration of the woman's requested, as well as bio-socio-physical, needs becomes essential. This chapter provides an overview of (1) health care trends in general, (2) preparation for birth, and (3) nonpharmaceutical pain relief methods. This chapter also promotes awareness of nursing responsibilities in contemporary approaches to labor and birth.

DYNAMIC MATERNITY CARE SYSTEM

Health Care Trends in General

Never before has so much occurred so fast, affecting the very survival of facilities and personnel in the health care industry. The traditional practice of health care is being altered dramatically. Rising costs of medical care, an oversupply of qualified doctors, the medical malpractice crisis, and the changing demands of the health care consumer are just a few of the causes of this radical transformation.

When increased yearly costs of 15 percent or more for hospital care became routine in the late 1960s, efforts began to deal with shrinking resources for payment of these costs. After Medicare's implementation of diagnostic related groupings (DRGs) for reimbursement of hospital and physician costs, many third-party payers also adopted similar prospective payment systems (PPS).[1]

These first moves into cost-conscious health care were followed by numerous new delivery systems offering lower priced services. Examples of the new systems include ambulatory care centers, health maintenance organizations (HMOs), individual practice associations (IPAs), preferred provider organizations (PPOs), and other innovative practice arrangements now being designed.

The shift from the traditional fee for service medical care to prepaid, preventive-oriented, group health management affected maternity care directly. Maternity departments in hospitals have reduced the average length of stay (ALOS) to win HMO and PPO contracts. By 1995, hospital stays for normal vaginal births may average 24 hours with accompanying home care nursing services and support for the family. As a result, the way maternity care is perceived, delivered, and directed will be dramatically different in the near future.[2]

• •

Review Questions

1. Four causes of the radical transformation occurring in health care today are:
   a. ______________________________

b. ________________________________
c. ________________________________
d. ________________________________

2. The major move to cost-conscious health care involves a shift from traditional fee for service medical care to ________________________________

____

Answers

1. Four causes of the radical transformation in health care today are:
   a. *Rising costs of medical care.*
   b. *An oversupply of qualified doctors.*
   c. *The medical malpractice crisis.*
   d. *The changing health care consumer.*

2. The major move to cost-conscious health care involves a shift from traditional fee for service medical care to *prospective payment systems.*

• •

FAMILY-CENTERED MATERNITY AND NEWBORN CARE

Historical Perspectives

To understand today's conventional maternity care, a brief look at the past is necessary. Since the beginning of time, childbirth has reflected society's most fundamental attitudes. Two main attributes of childbirth have been traditionally common to all cultures. The first is the birthing woman's need for a support system to help with both the woman's emotional and physical needs. In only rare cases have societies sent their women off to bear children in isolation. Women of almost all cultures prepare for childbirth by establishing a network of support that involves the participation of other women or family members. In this context, birth is a cultural and social event.

The second childbirth characteristic common to all cultures is the upright position for birth. Up until about 250 years ago, women gave birth in some kind of upright position: squatting, sitting, kneeling, or standing. The use of a birth stool, which was fairly common, dates back to 2500 B.C. This was a horseshoe-shaped chair with a cutout seat through which the baby was delivered into the waiting hands of the midwife, who knelt or sat in front. Egyptian hieroglyphics show women seated during childbirth, and the Bible refers repeatedly to the Hebrew custom of giving birth upright. Upright positions for birth were common until 1738 when François Mauriceau, celebrated obstetrician to the Queen of France, proposed the recumbent position in bed as an alternative to the birth stool. This change was made because it was easier for the birth attendant (or accoucheur) to do vaginal examinations, to perform obstetrical maneuvers, and to use forceps, not because it might be beneficial to the mother or fetus. At the same time, obstetric practitioners were becoming more interventionistic, as demonstrated by the use of forceps and introduction of anesthesia.

Although for thousands of years women attended other women during labor and birth in their homes, at the beginning of the twentieth century hospital birth instead of home birth gradually became the norm, adding medical control to the process of delivery. With hospitalization and use of analgesia and anesthesia, the childbearing woman became a patient rather than a woman giving birth. With this shift in attitude, the childbearing process became an illness. Maternity unit designs were patterned after a multi-transfer surgical system. All but maternity team personnel were barred from delivery rooms and measures were taken to separate infants from their families within moments of their birth.

Birth became a procedure that women endured alone. Women were delivered . . . instead of giving birth. Although one advantage of in-hospital birth in the United States has been a dramatic reduction in maternal and newborn morbidity and mortality, the dehumanization of hospital routines was felt by many women.[3]

Consumer Influence

In the 1960s, women began to talk openly about their dissatisfaction with the dehumanizing routines of hospital maternity wards. With the publication of *Thank you, Dr. Lamaze,* natural or prepared childbirth gained popularity. Consumer groups demanded husbands enter the delivery rooms. Midwives became more prevalent, and although often not permitted to be independent practitioners, their concept of personal, continual care was again valued.

Consumer pressure resulted in birthing rooms and sibling visitation in some hospitals, in the establishment of free-standing birth centers, and in a small but tenacious home birth movement. Birthing rooms or alternative birth centers (ABCs) were hospitals' answer to people choosing home birth over hospital birth. They were often small, converted, windowless labor rooms. Restrictive screening criteria for ABC use excluded most women from using them. The few who were admitted to ABCs often needed to be transferred to a labor or delivery room after developing a "risk factor" during labor. Examples of such risk factors would often include meconium-stained amniotic fluid, fetal distress, or even need for pitocin stimulation or intravenous fluids.

However, in spite of limited usage in many institutions, it is estimated that over 70 percent of U.S. hospitals have ABCs today. These "birthing rooms" became essential marketing tools for hospitals because more and more women began to request them in the 1980s. Women appreciated the ambience their ancestors had known for centuries. In ABCs, women had family and friends to support them and usually had the freedom to choose positions of comfort for labor and upright positions for birth. Those initial responses to consumer requests were the beginning of a new way to practice maternity care which will hereafter be described as "contemporary."

Contemporary Maternity Care

In visualizing contemporary maternity care as the house in which maternity care can be conducted, the roof has support pillars: philosophy, clinical care, design, and education and marketing (Fig. 7–1).

The philosophy of care, which consists of the statements of values and beliefs held by the staff and the institution collectively, determine the clinical care practiced. For example, if it is a commonly held belief that pregnancy is an experience of well-being, a time of social, emotional, and physical change and stress rather than an illness, then all pregnant women will not routinely have IVs, continuous fetal monitoring, and anesthesia for birth. Because form follows function, the design of the maternity unit will depend on what kind of clinical care is practiced. For example, tertiary care centers will have differing space needs from facilities where the acuity rates are much lower. And finally, the type of patient and/or nursing education and marketing done will incorporate all of the above.

Philosophic Foundation

The philosophy of care which is *the* driving force for contemporary maternity programs is that of Family-Centered Maternity Care. The definition of family-centered care (ACOG, 1978) is as follows:

> Family-centered maternity/newborn care can be defined as the delivery of safe, quality health care while recognizing, focusing on, and adapting to both the physical and psychological needs of the client-patient, the family, and the newly born. The emphasis is on the provision of maternity/newborn care which fosters family unity while maintaining physical safety.

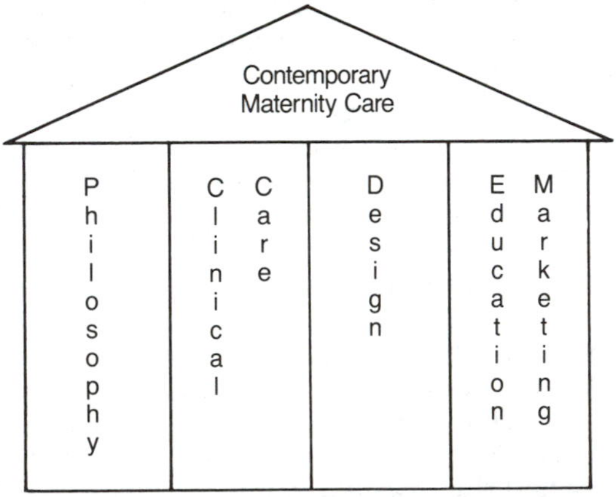

Figure 7–1. The Pillars of Contemporary Maternity Care.

The attitude of the health care providers is the most important aspect of family-centered care. Family-centered care recognizes birth as a vital life event and not a surgical procedure. The philosophic approach to family-centered care and alternative childbirth programs is aimed at combating paternalism in the health care system by giving the pregnant family the right to make informed choices regarding their childbirth experiences.

Clinical Practice

There is a movement towards providing comprehensive, individualized, and non-fragmented care. The family is educated about childbearing and childrearing and is provided flexible, individualized, and supportive medical and nursing care. To accomplish this, nursing staff are cross-trained to care for the mother-infant unit during the entire hospital stay. The most prevalent practice is when the postpartum and nursery staffs are cross-educated and combined into one staff, and one nurse provides comprehensive couplet (mother-baby) care for both the mother and her infant. In some instances, labor and delivery nurses are cross-trained to couplet (mother-baby) nursing and mother-baby nurses to labor and delivery care. When this comprehensive approach to cross-training has been accomplished, each member of the maternity nursing staff will be capable of providing "primary care" for any phase of the childbearing process. This allows for optimal use of staff with resultant increases in nursing productivity.

Obstetric practice also is changing in contemporary programs so that a physiologic approach to care is promoted. Women are encouraged to ambulate in early labor and to assume positions of comfort for labor and birth. See Table 7–1 for comparison of conventional and family-centered care.

A good example of how clinical practice has been changed is the option of VBAC (vaginal birth after previous cesarean) being offered.

VBAC (Vaginal Birth After Previous Cesarean)

Since 1916, obstetricians in the United States have routinely practiced a policy of "once a cesarean, always a cesarean," a dictum attributed to Edward Cragin of the Eastern Medical Society of New York. However, because of the rising cesarean birth rate, high costs, and greater maternal morbidity and mortality associated with cesareans, renewed interest in vaginal delivery after prior cesarean birth has again been evident. It is obvious that if the elective repeat cesarean birth rates can be lowered, the overall cesarean rate can be lowered.[5]

The concern generated by this trend of rising cesarean rates has been the subject of numerous publications, a National Institutes of Health (NIH) task force review, and a 1984 revision and relaxation of the American College of Obstetricians and Gynecologists (ACOG) Guidelines regarding cesareans. Both NIH and ACOG concluded that

Table 7–1. COMPARISONS OF CONVENTIONAL AND FAMILY-CENTERED MODELS OF OBSTETRIC CARE

CONVENTIONAL MEDICAL MODEL	FAMILY-CENTERED MODEL
No childbirth education required.	Prepared childbirth education required.
Pregnancy, labor, and delivery considered an illness.	Pregnancy, labor, and delivery considered a time of emotional, social, and physical change/stress.
Care is task oriented, routinized.	Care is individualized.
Staff, in position of authority, make treatment decisions. Family is dependent.	Staff uses expertise to inform family of options; family makes decision; family and staff create team for treatment.
Staff is rigid.	Staff is flexible.
Mother and infant considered separate patients.	Mother and infant served as a unit.
Labor, delivery, recovery, postpartum, and neonatal care take place in different locations.	Labor, delivery, recovery, postpartum, and neonatal care occur in one location.
Infant care primarily in nursery.	Infant remains with mother.
Visiting hours prescribed.	Family and friends encouraged to be present at any time mother wishes.
Father or supportive person informed of labor progress and birth.	Father or supportive person present and actively involved in labor, delivery, postpartum, and neonatal care.

vaginal birth after cesarean is an appropriate and important option. Highlights of these criteria, combined with those selected from the literature, can be found in Figure 7–2.[6]

However, in spite of these reports and favorable clinical experience with thousands of VBACs, there are still many communities in the United States where trial of labor after a prior cesarean is not allowed.

Risks. The primary concerns about VBACs voiced by health professionals and clients is that the old uterine scar may rupture and have catastrophic results. In reality, statistics show that risk is minimal, ranging from as little as 0.5 percent to 3.2 percent in studies of trials of labor.[6]

Options. Increasing numbers of parents do not wish to elect repeat cesarean birth, unless they are convinced it is absolutely necessary. Although theoretically, the ultimate decision-making responsibility rests with the parents, obstetrician acceptance and enthusiasm for a trial of labor are directly related to successful outcomes.[7]

Special Needs. A woman seeking a VBAC has distinct special needs. She and her family are likely to have **anxiety** [specify] **and knowledge deficit (of the implications of VBAC) related to lack of exposure.** Since the woman may not have resolved her previous cesarean, questions to explore with her include the following:

- Why do you wish to attempt vaginal birth?
- What are your fantasies of birthing?
- What are your fears?
- Is your family supportive/fearful of your plans?
- What did you find most helpful in your previous delivery/labor experiences?
- What procedures/treatments/supportive measures did you find least helpful/tolerable?

In preparing for this trial of labor she needs help to become sensitive to her body signals concerning sensations of labor and birth. Tools are needed to work with in labor in order to create a supportive environment. Relaxation and breathing techniques are useful.

Who is a Candidate for VBAC?

A woman who:

- wants a normal labor and delivery
- has had a previous low transverse uterine incision
- has no recurring problem (fetal distress, placenta previa)
- is in good health
- has had a normal pregnancy—vertex position, fetal weight less than 4000 g
- understands the risks and the possibility of repeat cesarean delivery
- understands that analgesics may be limited during labor
- will be admitted to a hospital when labor begins where:
  - fully privileged obstetrician must attend the birth
  - large-bore IV catheter must be in place throughout active labor and birth
  - two units of blood must be available
  - delivery room staff, anesthesiologist, and nursery staff must be advised of VBAC (and the potential of a cesarean delivery)
  - physician and hospital personnel must be prepared for emergency cesarean section within 15 minutes
  - continuous monitoring must be done
  - woman must be adequately informed of the trial of labor process and give her consent
  - uterine scar must be evaluated after delivery

Figure 7–2. Who is a candidate for VBAC?

Prenatal instruction for VBAC should also include:

- participating in choice of anesthetic
- father (significant other) being present during procedures/birth
- father present in recovery
- audio recording/photos of birth
- delayed eye treatment of infant to promote eye contact between parent and infant
- physical contact or holding newborn immediately post birth
- breast-feeding on delivery table/recovery room
- preparation for repeat cesarean, if needed

With careful screening, many women can choose trial labor, regardless of their previous cesareans. Through education, advocacy, and cost containment measures, the option of vaginal birth after cesarean will one day be a standard of practice.

Obstetrical Design Trends

The physical setting in which birth takes place is important, both in itself and for its potential effect in modifying professional attitudes. A pleasant, warm, non-clinical environment is less strange and less frightening to women in labor than is the conventional labor or delivery room. Aesthetically pleasing surroundings are not expensive and no less sterile than traditional hospital furnishings.

Currently, there are two major trends in obstetrical hospital design in the United States: the LDR (labor/delivery/recovery) room and the LDR/P (labor/delivery/recovery/postpartum) room.

Designed in the early 1980s, the LDR is an enlarged birthing room equipped to accommodate all but cesarean births. Women labor, deliver, and recover in these LDR rooms, and then are transferred to a postpartum room for the remainder of their hospital stay. Since the word "birthing" had negative connotations at the time for most obstetricians, the room was called an LDR (for the traditional terms labor/delivery/recovery) room. The LDR room, designed for both high-risk and low-risk vaginal deliveries, is equipped well enough to give physicians the confidence that everything they need will be available. It is large enough to prevent crowding, and its interior design creates a pleasant, home-like atmosphere.

The LDR/P room is an extended version of the LDR room concept. The laboring woman is admitted to one room and she and her newborn essentially remain in that room until they are discharged together.

When only LDR/Ps are in use in a facility, a single-room maternity care (SRMC) system is in place. The SRMC system typically includes an optional system of care for the infant in which the infant remains in the mother's room with mother-baby nursing. Rather than designing a traditional nursery complex, baby holding areas adjacent to the nurse control station are available. Holding areas are intended for infants needing more than routine observation or for an infant whose mother, along with the nursing staff, cannot partake in the care of the infant, usually due to the mother's fatigue or medical complications.

Marketing and Education

Childbirth education is an important product line for hospitals in competitive times. Because such programs attract private pay patients, childbirth education is often used to make the public aware of the services of the hospital and to establish hospital name recognition. Childbirth education also provides feedback for understanding what the consumers want from the maternity service.

A comprehensive education program can serve the community in many ways. It serves the practitioners and patients by teaching people how to care for themselves during the many months of pregnancy. Good nutrition and exercise have been shown to reduce the incidence of many complications, including pregnancy-induced hypertension and low-birth-weight babies. The casual, friendly atmosphere of the classroom often encourages women to speak more candidly about themselves and their body changes. Students often ask advice of their teachers concerning seemingly minor aches and pains. A well-trained teacher serves as a frontline screener in this regard, identifying symptoms of abnormality early and directing women to contact their practitioners in time to prevent more serious complications.

• •

Review Questions

1. The "pillars" that support the roof of a contemporary maternity care program are:
   a. ______________ c. ______________
   b. ______________ d. ______________
2. The philosophy of care which is the driving force for contemporary maternity programs is that of Family-Centered Maternity Care. Explain this philosophy of care.
   ____
   ____
   ____
   ____
3. Three reasons for renewed interest in vaginal delivery after prior cesarean birth are:
   a. ______________
   b. ______________
   c. ______________
4. What is the primary risk perceived to be associated with VBACs?
   ____
   ____

5. Who is a candidate for VBAC?

____

____

____

____

____

____

Answers

1. The "pillars" that support contemporary maternity care are: (a) *philosophy*, (b) *clinical care*, (c) *design*, and (d) *education and marketing*.
2. Family-Centered Maternity Care can be defined as the delivery of safe, quality health care while recognizing, focusing on, and adapting to both the physical and psychological needs of the client-patient, the family, and the newly born. The emphasis is on the provision of maternity/newborn care while maintaining physical safety.
3. Three reasons for renewed interest in vaginal delivery after previous cesarean birth are:
   a. *rising cesarean birth rate*
   b. high costs
   c. greater maternal morbidity and mortality associated with cesareans
4. What is the primary risk perceived to be associated with VBACs? *Rupture of the uterine scar.*
5. Who is a candidate for VBAC?
   See Figure 7–2 for a list of who is a candidate for VBAC.

• •

PREPARATION FOR BIRTH

Self-Care Concepts

When birth is perceived as a dimension of, not deviation from, wellness, and as a transition to parenthood, the nursing emphasis is on self-care. Instead of the maternalistic approach of "I am here to take care of you," the nurse uses the helping relationship of "I am here to assist you in taking care of yourself." In this self-care approach, families are active, rather than passive, participants in health care. Such an approach promotes self-worth and dignity for the laboring family.

The foundation of family-centered care is based on a strong, open, trusting relationship between the pregnant woman and her family and the health care provider. The provider must have the capacity to remain open and responsive to the needs and desires of the woman and her family, and the woman and family must have confidence in the clinical judgment, technical expertise, and motivations of the provider.

PREPARED CHILDBIRTH METHODS

Childbirth Education

In order to function as partners with the care provider, the family must be knowledgeable. Most partners have a **knowledge deficit (of prepared childbirth methods) related to a lack of experience**. Important benefits of childbirth education include understanding of the processes of pregnancy, labor, and childbirth, as well as the roles of sound nutrition, physical conditioning, and the avoidance of drugs, alcohol, caffeine, and tobacco. Inclusion of techniques for adapting to labor, emphasizing active participation of the partner, are known to have a positive effect on the birth process.[8] A major focus of childbirth education is on ways to deal with **comfort, alterations in: pain, acute related to lack of information about the labor process**.

Family-centered maternity care implies a personalized environment for the childbirth process. The partners benefit from learning about the environment in which childbirth will occur prior to the onset of labor. Such an approach allows for the resolution of most potential problems between the family and provider, and provides for attention to the family's needs during the birth process.

Childbirth preparation is a vehicle to accomplish this. Currently, there are numerous methods of preparation for birth being taught throughout the world. These methods became popular because they gave control back to the woman and stressed the "wellness" approach to childbirth. Included here are the *Dick-Read method*, the *Bradley method*, and the *Lamaze method*. Although these methods differ, they all have three similarities:

1. psychophysical components
2. psychological components
3. intellectual components

Read Method: Childbirth without Fear

An English physician, Dr. Grantly Dick-Read, published works in which he theorized that pain in childbirth is socially conditioned. In his books *Natural Childbirth* (1933) and *Childbirth Without Fear* (1944), Dr. Read described his theory. He explained that when a woman approaches labor with fear and anxiety, her natural protective tensions are aroused, thus creating tension in the muscles that open the cervix. Dr. Read termed this negative process the fear—tension—pain cycle (Fig. 7–3).[9]

In order to discuss Dr. Read's theory, *a review of uterine musculature* is appropriate. Refer to Chapter 3 and Figure 3-2 for an explanation of uterine activity.

Psychophysical Component. Dr. Dick-Read's response to this fear—tension—pain cycle was to teach women to use passive relaxation of the muscle groups in their entire bodies. He basically recom-

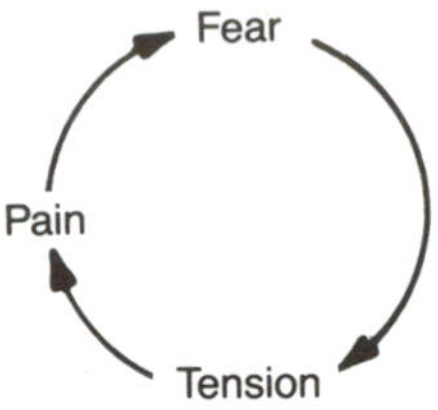

Figure 7–3. Fear—tension—pain cycle

mended increasing the depth and rapidity of abdominal breathing as the intensity of the contractions of first stage increased, with panting and breath-holding during the second stage of labor. Strenuous physical exercise was also incorporated to prepare the body for labor.

Psychological Component. As the women relaxed, the circular muscles of the cervix relaxed and uterine contractions became effective in dilating and effacing the cervix. Thus, as their anxiety returned to normal levels, sympathetic nervous system responses and the resultant contracting effects on uterine muscle did not occur. As a result, labor progress was positively affected.[10]

Intellectual Component. Dr. Read's teachings attempted to reverse the negative influence of cultural conditioning by educating women about the labor and birth process. If they are prepared for what is likely to occur, they experience less fear, tension, and pain.

Dr. Grantly Dick-Read's work became the basis for the first organized series of programs in preparation for birth by pregnant couples and for teacher certification. The first group to organize was the consumer-oriented International Childbirth Education Association (ICEA) founded in 1960. It continues today as a leading organization for education of childbearing families dedicated to freedom of choice based on knowledge of alternatives.

•   •

Review Questions

1. What are three methods of preparation for birth currently taught?
   a. ______________________________
   b. ______________________________
   c. ______________________________

2. Diagram Dr. Read's basic three-part cycle that he theorized caused the pain of labor.

3. Match column I with column II:

COLUMN I	COLUMN II
a. **Psychophysical component of the Read method.**	______**Reversal of negative influence of cultural conditioning through education.**
b. **Intellectual component of the Read method.**	______**Passive total body relaxation, abdominal breathing, panting, and breath-holding.**
c. **Psychological component of the Read method.**	______**Relaxation facilitating effective cervical dilatation and effacement.**

Answers

1. What are three methods of preparation for birth currently taught in the U.S.?
   a. *the Read method*
   b. *the Bradley method*
   c. *the Lamaze method*
2. Figure 7–3 presents the diagram of Dr. Read's basic cycle that he theorized caused the pain of labor.
3. Match column I with column II:

COLUMN I	COLUMN II
a. Psychophysical component of the Read method.	b Reversal of negative influence of cultural conditioning through education.
b. Intellectual component of the Read method.	a Passive total body relaxation, abdominal breathing, panting, and breath-holding.
c. Psychological component of the Read method.	c Relaxation facilitating effective cervical dilatation and effacement.

• •

Bradley Method

An American physician, Dr. Robert Bradley, developed a method that he claims emphasizes "true natural childbirth," which is unmedicated, using a "husband-coach." The first edition of Dr. Bradley's book, *Husband-Coached Childbirth*, was published in 1965. The American Academy of Husband-Coached Childbirth (AAHCC) was founded to make the Bradley method widely available and to certify teachers of the method.

Dr. Bradley observed the manner in which other mammals instinctively conduct labor. Using these observations and extensive experience with women's births, he developed a technique that works in harmony with the woman's body. Use of medication of any kind during labor and birth is strongly discouraged.

Psychophysical Component. As a result of Bradley's studies, breath control is utilized for labor using abdominal breathing while in a position imitating the sleep position, which may differ for each individual woman. Rigorous prenatal exercise prepares the woman for the athletic qualities of labor. Although pushing techniques are used, the major breathing taught for all of labor is abdominal breathing.

Psychological Component. Deep mental relaxation is used. The role of the husband is central to this method, thus it is called "husband-coached." Some critics find the role of the husband in this method to be almost domineering.

Intellectual Component. Preparation for birth through classes teaches nonintervention of obstetrical technologies and avoidance of analgesics and anesthetics.[11]

• •

Review Questions

1. Explain Dr. Bradley's "natural childbirth."

____

____

____

2. Briefly describe the psychophysical, psychological, and intellectual components of the Bradley method.

____

____

____

Answers

1. Dr. Bradley's natural childbirth uses a technique that works in harmony with the woman's body. Use of medication of any kind during labor and birth is discouraged.

2. *Psychophysical*: Breath control is utilized for labor using abdominal breathing while in a position imitating the sleep position, which may differ for each individual woman.
   Psychological: Deep mental relaxation is utilized.
   Intellectual: Preparation for birth provides education about labor and birth and focuses on nonintervention of obstetrical technologies and avoidance of analgesics and anesthetics.

• •

Lamaze Method (PPM)

Marjorie Karmel introduced the Lamaze method to the United States in her book, *Thank You, Dr. Lamaze*, which was published in the United States in 1959. The Lamaze method, also known as psychoprophylactic method (PPM), emphasizes mental control of pain in labor. In 1960, the American Society for Psychoprophylaxis in Obstetrics (ASPO) began in New York to promote the Lamaze method and certify teachers.

In his work on the higher nervous activity of humans, the Russian scientist, Pavlov, proposed that every vital activity of an organism is a complex reflex process capable of conditioning. The classic Lamaze method is based on Pavlovian conditioning. This conditioning raises the woman's pain threshold by creating a zone of inhibition in her cerebral cortex.

Dr. Fernand Lamaze of France was in Russia for a medical convention in 1951 when he first saw women using Pavlovian conditioning for childbirth. Upon his return to France, he began to teach women how to give birth using basic concepts of reflexology:

1. The nervous system functions as a reception (stimulus) → response mechanism.
2. Reception → response is reflex activity.
3. There are inborn reflexes. An example is that eyes blink when an object approaches them quickly.
4. There are conditioned reflexes by which stimuli move up nerves to the spinal cord and to the brain. When the stimulus reaches the brain, it fires off a focus of activity which directly stimulates functions in the absolute reflexes. A famous example is the following: Ring a bell → dog turns his head. Now place meat in front of dog → dog salivates. For one focus of activity, the reflex of orientation was stimulated; while for the other, the reflex of salivation. Now if both foci of activity are activated at once and with repetition, a connection is established between the two foci. As a result, one focus of activity can activate the other so that when you ring the bell, the dog will salivate. This is an example of a conditioned reflex.[12]

As a result of Lamaze preparation as it is taught today in the United States, behavioral conditioning of the woman produces reliable and constructive responses to the pain associated with uterine contractions. Lamaze-trained women respond to the pain of uterine contractions by using learned breathing techniques.

Psychophysical Component. There are four parts to the Lamaze method: (1) controlled muscular relaxation and release, (2) rhythmic breathing, (3) concentration on a focal point, and (4) active relaxation. The woman may be taught neuromuscular dissociation exercises in which she relaxes uninvolved muscle groups while contracting a specific muscle group. By using this technique, the woman is able to relax her body muscles while her uterine muscles contract (Fig. 7–4).

The diaphragmatic breathing patterns are rhythmic—slow to shallow—and vary according to the intensity of the contractions and progress of labor. More is said about breathing patterns in the

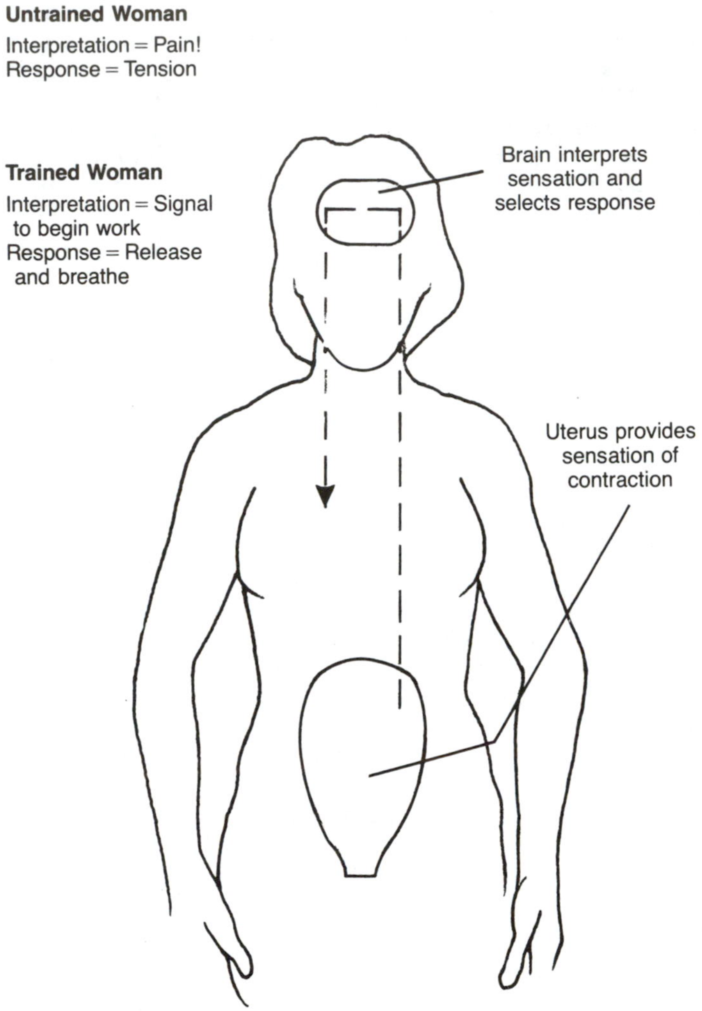

Figure 7–4. Psychophysical pathway as explained by Lamaze.

next few pages. A nonstrenuous program of physical fitness is also advocated to prepare the woman's body for labor.

Psychological Component. In the Lamaze method, the woman uses concentration and active relaxation as appropriate responses to pain stimulus.

Intellectual Component. Lamaze preparation is comprehensive, offering a structured program to remove fear by education, thus eliminating distressing associations.

• •

Review Questions

1. **Give the classic example of a conditioned reflex.**

2. **Briefly describe the psychophysical, psychological, and intellectual components of the Lamaze method.**

Answers

1. The famous example of a conditioned reflex is:
Ring a bell → dog turns his head. Meat is placed in front of the dog → dog salivates.

2. The components of the Lamaze method are described as follows:
Psychophysical: Controlled muscular relaxation and release, rhythmic breathing, concentration on a focal point, and refined active relaxation are parts of the Lamaze system.
Psychological: In the Lamaze method, the woman uses concentration and active relaxation as appropriate responses to pain stimulus.
Intellectual: Lamaze preparation is comprehensive, offering a structured program to remove fear by education, thus eliminating distressing associations.

• •

BASIC BREATHING FOR LABOR AND BIRTH

Few women are taught a pure (single) method of breathing techniques. Most often an eclectic approach is used—that is, the best of many. Lamaze techniques are often the basis upon which variations are made. Therefore, the following is a description of Lamaze breathing patterns that can be used to help laboring women. Awareness of these patterns is to help laboring women. Awareness of these patterns is useful when caring for women who use these patterns or those who need additional teaching. Below is a description of basic Lamaze breathing rhythms that are beneficial in reducing stress and managing pain, as well as supplying a good oxygen level. The reader is encouraged to practice the breathing progressions in order to support Lamaze-prepared women in labor.

BASIC BREATHING AWARENESS

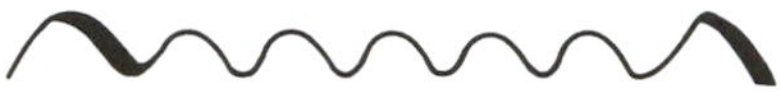

Find a comfortable position. With eyes relaxed, breathe in comfortably, blow or sigh the air out slowly, letting your body go limp.

Allow the breathing to continue on its own, quietly, easily, and rhythmically.

Concentrate on letting yourself go completely loose with each outward breath.

Soon your body will begin to feel very heavy and any exertion will be difficult.

When ready to rouse yourself, breathe in deeply, stretching arms and legs, then relax as you sigh or blow the air out.

Having learned a conscious breathing pattern based on normal respiratory physiology, women can adapt both simple "breath awareness" and three basic types of *paced* breathing to individual needs according to demands of contractions and other possible stressful labor procedures.

I. For mild to strong contractions, use:

SLOW PACED BREATHING

Approximately half (6 to 9 breaths per minute) of a normal resting rate

A "cleansing/greeting" breath is taken at beginning of contraction

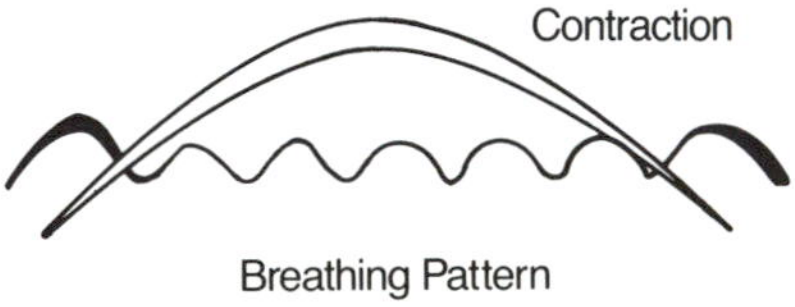

Continue to breathe in and out, slowly, easily, and evenly; movement is relaxed motion in chest and abdomen.

One or more of these Breathing Focusing Techniques may be used:
- inhale/exhale through nose
- inhale/exhale through mouth
- inhale through nose/exhale through mouth

- timing, counting, imagery (mental strategies), or
- relaxation, massage, movement (physical strategies)

As contraction ends, take a "cleansing/resting" breath, breathing out slowly.

Approximately half of an individual's resting respiratory rate is encouraged for use throughout as much of labor as possible for mild to even strong contractions if tolerated, and during the increment/ decrement of contractions (see Chapter 3) requiring modification of the pace for comfort and relaxation. Research shows that slow breathing induces and reinforces both physiological and psychological relaxation.

II. For strong contractions, use:

MODIFIED PACED BREATHING

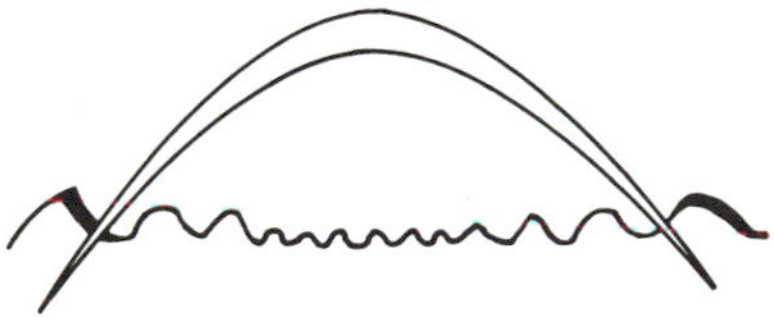

Take a deep relaxing breath.

Use breathing frequency up to twice a normal resting rate.

Relax chest and abdomen.

Focus may be on: Same strategies as Slow Paced Breathing.

May be used as needed for challenging contractions.

Can be combined with Slow Paced Breathing in same contraction, using Modified Paced at the peak.

End with deep relaxing breath.

Modified Paced Breathing may be done for over the peak of strong contractions, gradually increasing the pace of breathing, *not to exceed twice the normal resting rate.*

III. For very strong contractions, use:

PATTERNED PACED BREATHING

Take a deep relaxing breath.

Frequency is increased up to maximum rate of twice the normal rate.

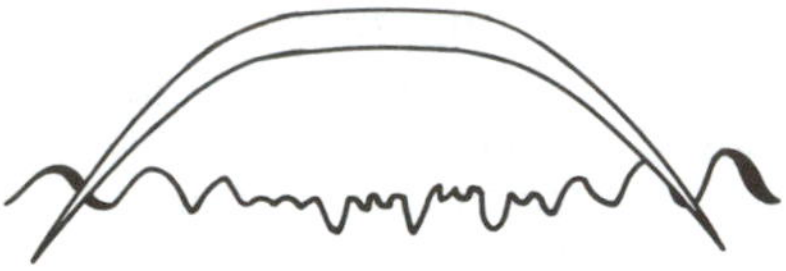

Movement is relaxed—face, chest, abdomen relaxed.

Focus may be same as in Slow or Modified Paced Breathing.

Strategy is rhythmic breathing patterned with gentle blows, no rate change—variations may be: 1 breath/1 blow . . . 2 breaths/1 blow . . . 3, 4, 5, 6 breaths/1 blow.

Again, the pace is not to exceed twice the resting rate; this is a "counted" breathing pattern in which modified paced breathing is interrupted at rhythmic intervals with soft blows (puffs) that do not change the rate or volume of air exchange. A repetitive, defined rhythm has a psychologically and physiologically calming influence.

The cleansing/organizing breaths used to "greet" and "bid farewell" to contractions are similar to those used in traditional Lamaze breathing. To avoid inducing tension at the onset of contractions, the woman should take only a moderate breath before exhaling (or simply breathe out) in response to the contraction's onset. A deeper complete breath is appropriate at the end of contractions.

Choosing whether to breathe in/out through nose or mouth, or in through nose, out through mouth, is an individual choice. As in normal breathing, gentle movement of both abdominal and chest wall will be observed. To discourage tension and fatigue, and particular placement of tongue or lips generally is to be avoided, except for the rhythmic puffs in patterned paced breathing.

• •

Review Questions

1. What are the three specific breathing patterns widely used in Lamaze birth classes?
   a. ______
   b. ______
   c. ______
2. Identify the appropriate breathing rate for each of these three breathing patterns.
   ______
   ______
   ______

Answers

1. The three breathing patterns widely used in Lamaze birth classes are:
   a. slow paced breathing.
   b. modified paced breathing.
   c. patterned paced breathing.

2. For *slow paced breathing*, the appropriate rate is approximately one-half the normal resting rate.
For *modified paced breathing*, the frequency is twice the normal resting rate.
For *patterned paced breathing*, frequency is increased up to a maximum rate of twice the normal rate.

• •

Pushing

The common practice of prolonged breath-holding while bearing down with maximum force has until recently been taught in preparation for birth classes and supported by hospital staff. Women were encouraged to "push, push, keep it going as long as you can, now grab another breath, and push again." Fixing her thorax, the woman holds her breath and pushes against a closed glottis.[14]

Fortunately, most women of childbearing age are in good health and suffer only minor effects, such as facial petechiae or ruptured blood vessels in the sclera of the eye from closed-glottis pushing. However, more serious complications can result if the woman has cardiac problems or an unknown aneurysm.

When a woman holds her breath and pushes with a closed glottis (Valsalva Maneuver) the intrathoracic and arterial pressures increase. These increases cause a decrease in venous return from outside the abdomen and thorax that results in decreased cardiac output, blood pressure, inflation of the eustachian tubes, and engorgement of the neck veins. Reflex vasoconstriction follows as the woman holds her breath and bears down for a sustained period. This sustained bearing down can result in fetal head compression and resultant fetal hypoxic effects. When the woman quickly gasps one or more breaths, the abdominal muscles retract vigorously and the pushing effect is lost. In addition, a sudden surge of blood is delivered to the heart. If the heart is not functioning properly, tachycardia and possible cardiac arrest can result.[15] During a normal second stage, a woman may employ the prolonged breath holding valsalva-type push over a period of hours with potentially serious maternal and fetal consequences.

Exhalation Breathing

Immediately following complete dilatation of the cervix there is a resting phase and contractions are less frequent and intense. Bearing down efforts are minimal. With descent of the fetus the Ferguson reflex is activated as the presenting part presses stress receptors in the pelvic musculature. There is a surge of endogenous oxytocin, and as contractions increase in strength, the urge to push increases.

Studies have shown the best amplitude of push is obtained when the push is no more than 4 to 5 seconds and there is no closure of the glottis. Holding the breath more than 6 to 7 seconds seems to endanger the fetus by reducing placental perfusion which can result in fetal hypoxia and acidosis.[16]

Other studies have also suggested that supporting the involuntary bearing-down efforts of women is compatible with good maternal and fetal outcomes.[17] Many studies suggest using some form of exhalation breathing, which is described in the next paragraph. With this type of breathing, rapid fluctuations in blood pressure and cardiovascular dynamics are minimized and a near normal O_2-CO_2 exchange is maintained.

The directions for exhalation breathing are as follows:

1. Assume a physiologic position suitable for second stage (i.e., squatting or sitting in a C-shaped position).
2. Take a few deep breaths as the urge to push builds.
3. When ready, hold your breath for about 5 seconds to "fix" your thorax and abdominal muscles.
4. Begin slow light exhalation through slightly pursed lips.
5. As you inhale spontaneously for 5 to 6 seconds, the thorax and abdominal muscles will continue to stay fixed, preventing upward retraction or movement of the fetus. Inhale slowly, straightening the neck. Take as many inhalations and exhalations as needed during a contraction.
6. Only as you feel the urge to push, use the abdominal muscles to push with contractions.
7. Concentrate on keeping the pelvic floor muscles relaxed.
8. When the contraction is over, take a deep breath and relax.

This type of pushing works best when there is a strong urge to push.

• •

Review Question

Give directions for exhalation breathing for pushing in second stage.

____
____
____
____
____
____
____
____
____
____

Answer

The directions for exhalation breathing are as follows:

a. Assume a physiologic position suitable for second stage (i.e., squatting or sitting in a C-shaped position).

b. Take a few deep breaths as the urge to push builds.
c. When ready, hold your breath for about 5 seconds to "fix" your thorax and abdominal muscles.
d. Begin slow light exhalation through slightly pursed lips.
e. As you inhale spontaneously for 5 to 6 seconds, the thorax and abdominal muscles will continue to stay fixed, preventing upward retraction or movement of the fetus. Inhale slowly, straightening the neck. Take as many inhalations and exhalations as needed during a contraction.
f. Only as you feel the urge to push, use the abdominal muscles to push with contractions.
g. Concentrate on keeping the pelvic floor muscles relaxed.
h. When the contraction is over, take a deep breath and relax.

• •

OTHER NONPHARMACEUTICAL METHODS

The pain of labor can be altered, blocked, or modulated through both childbirth preparation and other nonpharmaceutical methods.

According to Melzack and Wall's *Gate Control Theory* (1965), in the periphery of the nervous system are specialized large- and small-diameter nerve fibers. The small-diameter fibers carry impulses to the area of spinal cord called the substantia gelatinosa where they intersect with large-diameter cutaneous fibers. Large-diameter cutaneous nerves on the surface of the skin can be stimulated by vibration (electronic nerve stimulation), acupuncture, scratching, or rubbing, to act as negative charges to the incoming positive charges of the small-diameter excitatory fibers. This inhibitive or negative action closes the "gate" to pain signals at their level of entry into the spinal cord. In addition to the gate's control by these afferent signals, there are theorized to be descending control systems or signals from the brain that can close the spinal gate and block pain signals from the affected part.

Another popular explanation of the pain of labor is the *Endogenous Pain Control Theory*. According to this theory, there are internally produced morphine-like substances from the pituitary gland, called *Endorphins* (Fig. 7–5). Endorphins are produced during the stress of labor. They, in turn, stimulate prolactin which causes pleasurable feelings that reinforce the behavior which began the cycle.

This theory suggests natural pain control reward systems occur when stressful activities stimulate endorphin release. In a laboring woman, an increase in prolactin secretion causes feelings of warmth and pleasure which facilitate mothering. Endorphin production is increased by laboring women and believed to be beneficial in decreasing the perception of pain. Pain medications interfere with endorphin production. Therefore, other options for pain relief are desirable.

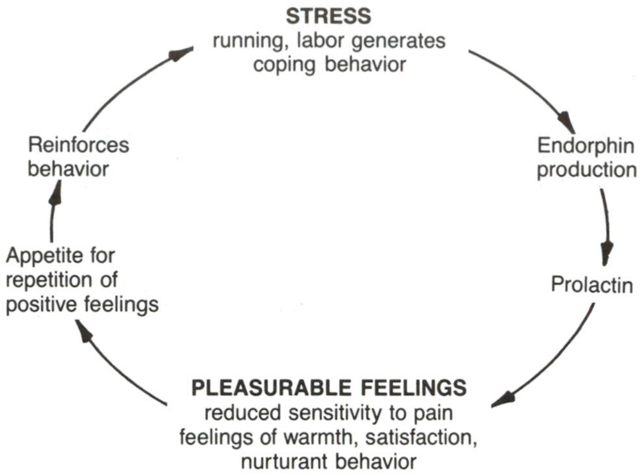

Figure 7–5. Endogenous pain control cycle.

OTHER OPTIONS

Physical Means

All of the following nonpharmaceutical methods for relieving pain use relaxation or an altered state of consciousness called the *alpha state*. In the alpha state, which falls between full consciousness and unconsciousness, thought processes become less logical and more associative and creative. Sense of time and body may be distorted, and there is a heightened ability to focus on an idea or image.[18] The intent is to relieve **comfort, alteration in: pain, acute related to generalized muscle tension during labor**. By overcoming the **knowledge deficit** (of cutaneous stimulation and other relaxation techniques) **related to lack of exposure; unfamiliarity with information resources**, the pain of labor can be decreased considerably.

Hydrotherapy

Bathing or showering has hydrokinetic and hydrothermal effects causing local vasodilatation, increasing the velocity of nerve conduction and relaxing muscles. A warm bath during labor helps decrease pressure of abdominal muscles on the uterus.

Therapeutic Touch

Therapeutic touch is a natural healing method developed by Dolores Krieger, R.N., Ph.D., at New York University. This pain relief method operates on the principle that the human body has an electromagnetic energy field that is responsive to healing. By directing or channeling energy from a healthy person to someone who is ill, that person's own recuperative powers are stimulated. In the technique there are three main stages:

1. Centering: healer (nurse or other) calms self
2. Assessing the field (electromagnetic): healer runs hands over patient's body (2 to 4 inches away from it); healer experiences heat, cold, prickliness, sticky, or congested feeling.
3. Applying treatment: "unruffle" field with gentle sweeping hand motions by healer on patient; as this occurs, the healer visualizes healing energy to area; the process takes 15 to 20 minutes.

The use of therapeutic touch is not well understood for pregnancy because the mother and fetus are two energy fields. However, some studies have shown decreased stress in laboring women following therapeutic touch.

Acupressure

Acupressure has been widely used in the Orient for years. It is based on the belief that an illness or pain is an imbalance of energy within the body. In labor, to mediate the imbalance, pressure from the fingertips is put on three major points (adapted to individuals according to their body size):

Point Co 4	Between 1st and 2nd metacarpal bones (thumb and index fingers) on dorsum of hand
Point St 36	Below the tibial tuberosity on the side of the tibalis anterior muscle
Point St 6	Behind the tibia, above the medial malleolus

Acupuncture

Acupuncture is based on the same belief and uses the same three major points but needles are inserted at these points. The use of acupuncture is limited to those licensed to do it, and is not normally used by nurses. Both acupressure and acupuncture are thought to stimulate the release of endorphins which can provide total anesthesia.

Massage

Massage can combine touching therapeutically and pressure. Massage can be in the form of gentle stroking or firm pressure to the body of a laboring woman.

Psychological Support

Restful music can relax. Rhythms can be soothing to both mother and fetus in utero. Most people have their own favorite relaxation music. In some cases, women are encouraged to bring their own to the labor room.

Imager/Visualization: With this technique the person pictures desired effects. A laboring woman would picture muscles spreading out and becoming soft, cervix opening, baby coming down and out, thus facilitating the labor process. Numerous publications describe this process, including one by Samuels.[19]

Biofeedback

This relaxation method of pain relief is founded on the concept that individuals can be trained to recognize signals of internal physiologic events and then manipulate those events. A machine known as an electromyograph can be used to measure neuromuscular tension and a thermometer to measure skin temperature at extremeties. If biofeedback is to be used during labor, training must begin long before labor begins.

Transcutaneous Electrical Nerve Stimulation (TENS)

The Gate Control Theory provides a theoretical foundation for TENS. Electrical stimulation by pulsed alternating current of large, afferent, high-velocity pain-carrying fibers prevents smaller, slow-velocity pain-carrying fibers from transmitting pain signals to higher brain centers. TENS electrodes can be placed on back and lower sacrum of a mother in labor. The effectiveness of TENS for pain control in labor is equivocal. Controlled clinical trials using non-functioning and functioning TENS units suggests that TENS therapy may have a placebo effect. TENS is not ordinarily available in labor units. Special arrangements must be made.

Autogenic Training

Such training occurs through mental suggestions about various bodily functions; for example, "my right arm is heavy" or "my left arm is warm." As a result, mental control modifies muscular and autonomic systems responses.

Hypnosuggestion

Hypnosuggestion was used in childbirth for the first time in 1823. It became popular in the late nineteenth century and then fell into disuse. Hypnosuggestion is defined as a temporarily altered state of consciousness in which the individual has increased suggestibility. There are a variety of techniques. Most involve the rhythmic, monotonous voice of a hypnotist. The voice continues in a monotone and the subject becomes increasingly open to suggestions. This approach is often used when giving verbal cues to use various breathing techniques (take a relaxing breath; breathe in through the nose).

Physical dissociation – eye techniques include *eye fixation* (most often used): the woman is told to fix her eyes on a subject in a way that will produce fatigue of the ocular muscles. Coins, pendulums, and hands with fingers spread can be used as the object on which the woman fixes her eyes.

Success depends on the hypnotist, the environment, the time, the subject's motivation, and the circumstances.

With hypnosuggestion an advantage is that the mother can be pain-free, and baby not affected by anesthesia. However, a disadvantage is the time it takes. For hypnosuggestion to be effective, sessions of one and one-half hours are needed once a week for 4 or 5 months.[13] Also, the father or significant other is left out of the labor support role.[20]

• •

Review Question

Match column I with column II:

COLUMN I		COLUMN II
1. therapeutic touch	____	principle that the body's electromagnetic energy field is responsive to healing.
2. acupressure/acupuncture	____	based on belief that a pain is an imbalance of energy within the body.
3. imagery	____	once trained to recognize signals of internal physiologic events, individuals can manipulate those events
4. biofeedback	____	pictures desired effects.
5. autogenic training	____	mental control modifies muscular and autonomic systems responses.

Answer

COLUMN I		COLUMN II
1. therapeutic touch	1	principle that the body's electromagnetic energy field is responsive to healing.
2. acupressure/acupuncture	2	based on belief that a pain is an imbalance of energy within the body.
3. imagery	4	once trained to recognize signals of internal physiologic events, individuals can manipulate those events.
4. biobeedback	3	pictures desired effects.
5. autogenic training	5	mental control modifies muscular and autonomic systems responses.

• •

LABOR AND BIRTH SUPPORT

Passage to Parenthood

Birth is a transition to parenthood. With birth, two people become a family. Wives become mothers. Husbands become fathers. Along generation lines, previous children become siblings, and parents become grandparents. Childbearing is a developmental opportunity and/or a situational crisis, during which all family members can benefit from the supporting solidarity of the family unit. When provided with education, support, guidance, and sensitive care, families are able to achieve a sense of mastery over the childbearing experience. Thus, there is increased self-esteem for each family member.[21]

Bonding is the affectional connection that takes place between infants and parents in the hours and days after birth, and forms a basis for a lifelong deeper emotional attachment. Attachment is an affectional tie between infants and parents that begins during pregnancy and continues through birth and flourishes over a lifetime. Attachment often begins during pregnancy when the parents first feel their baby move or hear their baby's heart beat. Attachment is reciprocal and is influenced by many variables.[22]

Supportive Roles

Having prepared for birth with her, a woman's primary support person has worked with her during the preparatory period and is ready to give both emotional support and practical coaching in specific techniques they have learned. Enhancement of the support of the pregnant woman is very important. Without it there is potential **coping, ineffective individual related to inadequate support during labor**.

When siblings will be present during the labor and birth, it is important to prepare them for the birth experience. A support person, other than the father, should be designated specifically for the sibling(s). Although theories of sibling relationships are still quite primitive, the goal of sibling participation in the childbearing experience is to minimize separation anxiety (from parents) and jealousy toward the new baby. For older siblings, attachment and bonding may be facilitated by early involvement and contact with the newborn. Otherwise there is likely to be a **family process, alteration in related to the birth of the new baby**.

Many grandparents don't understand new trends in prepared childbirth and feel left out. Yet because biological links and generational ties are profound, most grandparents want to see and hold the new baby. Efforts can be made to include grandparents in the childbirth experience. They often welcome the opportunity to be responsible for the siblings who are present at, or nearby, the birth. Grandparents, too, can experience **family process, alteration in related to lack of involvement in birth process**.

Nursing Implications for Labor Support

In addition to the many approaches already mentioned as ways to relieve pain, the nurse needs to recognize that many traditional labor approaches may not be the best.

A woman in labor should be encouraged to choose the position that is most comfortable. Vertical positions (standing, walking, and sitting) are helpful if no contraindications exist, such as bleeding, fetal distress, premature labor, or ruptured membranes with an unengaged presenting part or breech presentation. In some hospitals there are routine orders for a woman to remain in bed, recumbent, after membranes rupture. The reason for this order is concern that the umbilical cord may prolapse if the woman stands. The cord has been known to prolapse in women who are supine when the membranes rupture and the fetus is in a breech presentation or when the head is not yet engaged. If the presenting part of the fetus is engaged, it is very unlikely that the cord will drop below the fetus. Some investigators state that they have not seen prolapse happen when the woman is ambulating but still they monitor the woman with a telemetry unit to detect any undesirable change in the fetal heart rate. During the later phases of labor or when a woman is more comfortable in bed, she should be at a 45° angle or on her left side.

During the second stage of labor, a woman's back should be supported until she is almost in a sitting position or a squatting position. The woman's freedom to select her own positions for labor and birth is conducive to a comfortable experience which has the orientation of wellness . . . of giving birth instead of being delivered.

Because of widespread use, social custom, or convenience, many obstetrical practices have become deeply entrenched. Although these "routine" practices persist in some communities, they are being replaced by contemporary maternity care. Evidence is mounting that clearly indicates lack of any benefits to preps and enemas. The value of episiotomies as "routine" is also being questioned. Consumer pressure for a "better birth experience" is responsible for much of this change.[23]

Out-of-Hospital Options

Out-of-hospital births have remained almost constant at one percent of total births occurring in the United States since 1975. However, since many states include with these totals those births that take place in freestanding birth centers, it would appear that the number of births occurring in the home is decreasing.

Freestanding Birthing Centers

Despite the surge of popularity of birth centers in the early 1980s, their numbers are decreasing. It is theorized that this decline is due to more options and choices being offered in contemporary local childbirth programs in hospitals. A major problem for freestanding birth centers is acquiring adequate liability insurance. Although freestanding centers offer services at one-half to two-thirds the cost of hospitals in their communities, another problem is lack of reimbursement by some health care coverage plans. While the American Public Health Association endorses freestanding birth centers, other professional organizations indicate that more research is needed concerning their safety.[24]

Home Birth

Families choose home birth for many reasons, but mainly because they want to keep their child's birth as personal as possible. Although in some instances physicians do attend home births, attendants are often certified nurse midwives (CNMs), professional or lay/empirical midwives. According to the *American College of Nurse Midwives* (ACMN), "Certified nurse midwifery practice is the independent management of care of essentially normal newborns and women, antepartally, intrapartally, postpartally, and/or gynecologically, occurring within a health care system which provides for medical consultation, collaborative management, or referrals and is in accord with the qualifications, standards, and functions for practice of nurse midwives." A lay or empirical midwife is someone who is trained outside of the medical system or is self-trained, who is neither under the control of, nor subscribes to the approach of the American College of Obstetricians and Gynecologists (ACOG). This type of midwife is licensed in some states but licensing for empirical midwives is opposed by ACOG and the ACNM.[24]

CONCLUSION

Pregnancy, labor, and birth comprise a life experience that can be described as a "passage to parenthood." In the actual labor and birth, averaging 12 to 24 hours, women and their partners cross a bridge to new roles that will last the rest of their lives. Even if the pressures of life may divide them and their love relationship ends, they will remain parents forever.

Supporting couples through this significant life experience can be both exhausting and exhilarating for the nurse. To support a woman and her partner in labor means to strengthen their ability to give birth. In supporting, instead of controlling, the nurse helps to build each family member's ego and concept of self. All people, no matter how well prepared, enter labor with some level of anxiety. Even if the laboring woman and her partner are well prepared, the nurse is an important member of the childbirth team.

When involved with couples in the childbearing process, it helps for nurses to consider their own feelings and attitudes related to childbirth. Self-analysis of personal and professional values is important. Providing support demands active involvement and continued assessment of two or more persons and their relationship, rather than of one isolated laboring woman. It is exhausting but rewarding work.

A Vision of the Future

Facilities and functional programs in the 21st century will be very different from what they were in the 1950s. The following are some of the factors which may exert a major effect on future maternity care:

Maternity marketing will increase. To maintain overall occupancy, hospitals will target new parents, hoping that they will bring their families back for future care. Maternity departments will be very attractive, resembling hotels more than hospitals. Some will be showplaces of innovative design. Restrictive signs, bare corridors, and windowless labor and delivery rooms will be relics of the past. In assessing quality of care, hospitals will include community satisfaction with care along with standard measurements such as morbidity and mortality rates.

Maternity units will drastically reduce length of stay and cut costs to win HMO and PPO contracts. The average length of stay for maternity care will decrease until normal childbirth is an outpatient procedure by the turn of the century. Hospital stays for cesarean births will be less than four days.

Consumers and third-party payers will avoid hospitals whose clinical practices increase length of stay for mother or baby. Clinical care will emphasize physiologic management to encourage spontaneous childbirth and reduce recovery times. Physiologic labor and birth management, along with individualized care, will replace routine active management (for example, confinement to bed in labor and lithotomy positioning for delivery) as the standard.

Single-room maternity systems (SRMC) will be standard facility design. By 1995, almost all new maternity care facility construction will use the SRMC system.

As women have more physiologic births and shorter stays, hospitals will no longer staff normal newborn nurseries for custodial care of well babies. Babies will be cared for, not in newborn nurseries, but with their mothers, and by mother/baby couplet nursing. Nurseries will eventually be phased out because of changing community education and expectations. Only babies in need of constant medical attention will continue to be cared for in intensive-care nurseries.

A well-organized and supportive education program will be the cornerstone to any successful maternity service. The very philosophy of contemporary care is based on informed consent so that women make choices that are pertinent to the needs of their individual families. Prenatal classes will be the key to these choices.

As explained at the beginning of this chapter, this is a time of great concern and a time of great challenge in the health care delivery system. Clearly the deciding factor between who will survive and who will flounder rests in the hands of the marketplace. Nurses have been in a position of consumer advocacy for many years. The financial constraints of the 1980s are requiring a new consideration of the needs and desires of birthing women. The time is ripe for nurses to offer their expertise in this area and assume a significant role in shaping the maternity care of the future.

REFERENCES

1. Powills, S: Hospital industry price wars heat up. Hospitals 59(19) 69, 1985.
2. Bajo, K and Phillips, C: Changing times and changing opportunities: Innovative maternity facility designs and the childbirth educator. NAACOG Update Series, Vol. 5, Lesson 18, CPEC, Princeton, New Jersey, 1986.
3. Leavitt, JW: Brought to bed. Oxford University Press, New York, 1986.
4. Interprofessional Task Force on Health Care of Women and Children. Joint position statement of the development of family-centered maternity/newborn care in hospitals. Interprofessional task force on Health Care of Women and Children, Chicago, 1978.
5. Meier, P and Porreco, R: Trial of labor following cesarean section: A two-year experience. AM J Obstet Gynecol 6:671, 1982.
6. Brengman, S, and Burns, M: Vaginal delivery after C-section. Am J Nurs 83:1545, 1983.
7. Farley, AA: Vaginal birth after cesarean section. NAACOG Update Series 5:23, 1987.
8. Buxton, CL: A Study of Psychological Methods for Relief of Pain in Childbirth. WB Saunders, Philadelphia, 1962.
9. Dick-Read, G: Natural Childbirth. Harpers & Bros., New York, 1933.
10. Dick-Read, G: Childbirth Without Fear, ed. 2. Harper & Row, New York, 1959.
11. Bradley, R: Husband-Coached Childbirth. Harper & Row, New York, 1965.
12. Karmel, M: Thank you, Dr. Lamaze. JB Lippincott, Philadelphia, 1959.
13. Hassid, P: Textbook for Childbirth Educators. Harper & Row, 1986.
14. McKay, S: Second stage labor—has tradition replaced safety?. Am J Nurs 81(5):1016, 1981.
15. Caldeyro-Barcia, R: The influence of maternal bearing-down effects during second stage on fetal well-being. Birth Fam J, 6(2)17, 1979.
16. Caldeyro-Barcia, R, et al: The bearing down efforts and their effects on fetal heart rate, oxygenation, and acid base balance. J Perinat Med 9:63, 1981.
17. Roberts, J, et al: A descriptive analysis of involuntary bearing-down effects during the expulsive phase of labor. J Obstet Gynecol Neonatal Nurs 16(1):48, 1987.
18. Brucker, M: Nonpharmaceutical methods for relieving pain and discomfort during pregnancy. Matern Child Nurs J 9(6):390, 1984.
19. Samuels, M and Samuels, N: Seeing with the mind's eye: The history, techniques, and uses of visualization. Random House, New York, 1975.
20. Vadurro, F and Butts, P: Reducing the anxiety and pain of childbirth through hypnosis. Am J Nurs 82(4):620, 1982.
21. McKay, S and Phillips, CR: Family-centered maternity care: Implementation strategies. Aspen Systems, Rockville, MD, 1984.

22. Klaus, MH and Kennell, JH: Parent-infant bonding, ed. 2. CV Mosby, St. Louis, 1982.
23. Young, D: Changing childbirth: Family Birth in the Hospital. Childbirth Graphics, Ltd., Rochester, NY, 1982.
24. White, WG: Debate, Part II: Out of hospital. Childbirth Educator 33, 1983.
25. Fisher, L: A crying shame. Medicenter Management, 16, 1987.

BIBLIOGRAPHY

Alternatives for Obstetric Design. Ross Laboratories, Columbus, OH, 1980.

Bajo, K and Shidaker, T: Innovations in obstetric design that meet professional and consumer demands. Hospital Administration Currents 28:7, April-June 1984.

Carlson, JM, et al: Maternal position during parturition in normal labor. Obstetrics and Gynecology 68:443, October 1986.

Fenwick, LF and Dearing, RH: The Cybele Cluster: A Single-Room Maternity Care System for High- and Low-Risk Families. The Cybele Society, Spokane, WA, 1981.

McKay, S and Phillips, CR: Family Centered Maternity Care: Implementation Strategies. Aspen Systems, Rockville, MD, 1984.

Nathanson, M: Single-room maternity care seen as a way to attract patients, cut costs. Modern Healthcare March, 1985.

Notelovitz, M: The single-unit delivery system: A safe alternative to home deliveries. Am J Obstet Gynecol 132(8):889, 1978.

Phillips, C: Single room maternity care for maximum cost efficiency. Perinatology and Neonatology March/April 1988.

7 POST-TEST

1. Four causes of the radical transformation occurring in health care today are:
   a. ______
   b. ______
   c. ______
   d. ______

2. The major move to cost-conscious health care involves a shift from traditional fee for service medical care to ______
______

3. The "pillars" which support the roof of a contemporary maternity care program are:
   a. ______
   b. ______
   c. ______
   d. ______

4. The philosophy of care which is the driving force for contemporary maternity programs is that of Family-Centered Maternity Care. Explain this philosophy of care.
______
______
______
______
______
______

5. Three reasons for renewed interest in vaginal delivery after prior cesarean birth are:
   a. ______
   b. ______
   c. ______

6. What is the primary risk perceived to be associated with VBACs?
______
______
______

7. Who is a candidate for VBAC?

____
____
____
____
____
____
____
____

8. What are three methods of preparation for birth currently taught?
   a. ________________________________
   b. ________________________________
   c. ________________________________

9. Diagram Dr. Read's basic three-part cycle that he theorized caused the pain of labor.

10. Match column I with column II:

COLUMN I		COLUMN II
a. Psychophysical component of the Read method.	____	Reversal of negative influence of cultural conditioning through education.
b. Intellectual component of the Read method.	____	Passive total body relaxation, abdominal breathing, panting, and breath-holding.
c. Psychological component of the Read method.	____	Relaxation facilitating effective cervical dilatation and effacement.

11. Explain Dr. Bradley's "natural childbirth."

____
____
____

12. Briefly describe the psychophysical, psychological, and intellectual components of the Bradley method.

____
____
____

13. Give the classic example of a conditioned reflex.

____
____
____

14. Briefly describe the psychophysical, psychological, and intellectual components of the Lamaze method.

____

____

____

15. What are the three specific breathing patterns widely used in Lamaze birth classes?
(1) ____
(2) ____
(3) ____

16. Identify the appropriate breathing rate for each of these three breathing patterns.

____

____

____

____

____

____

17. Give directions for exhalation breathing for pushing in second stage.

____

____

____

____

____

____

____

____

18. Match column I with column II:

COLUMN I	COLUMN II
a. therapeutic touch	_____ principle that the body's electromagnetic energy field is responsive to healing.
b. acupressure/acupuncture	_____ based on belief that a pain is an imbalance of energy within the body.
c. imagery	_____ once trained to recognize signals of internal physiologic events, individuals can manipulate those events.
d. biofeedback	_____ pictures desired effects.
e. autogenic training	_____ mental control modifies muscular and autonomic systems responses.

Answers to Post-Test

1. Four causes of the radical transformation in health care today are:
   a. *rising costs of medical care*
   b. *an oversupply of qualified doctors*
   c. *the medical malpractice crisis*
   d. *the changing health care consumer*

2. The major move to cost-conscious health care involves a shift from traditional fee for service medical care to *prospective payment systems.*

3. The "pillars" which support contemporary maternity care are: (a) *philosophy,* (b) *clinical care,* (c) *design,* and (d) *education and marketing.*

4. Family-Centered Maternity Care can be defined as the delivery of safe, quality health care while recognizing, focusing on, and adapting to both the physical and psychological needs of the client-patient, the family, and the newly born. The emphasis is on the provision of maternity/newborn care while maintaining physical safety.

5. Three reasons for renewed interest in vaginal delivery after previous cesarean birth are:
   a. *rising cesarean birth rate*
   b. *high costs*
   c. *greater maternal morbidity and mortality associated with cesareans*

6. What is the primary risk perceived to be associated with VBACs? *Rupture of the uterine scar.*

7. Who is a candidate for VBAC?
   See Figure 7–2 for a list of who is a candidate for VBAC.

8. What are three methods of preparation for birth currently taught in the U.S.?
   a. *the Read method*
   b. *the Bradley method*
   c. *the Lamaze method*

9. Figure 7–3 presents the diagram of Dr. Read's basic cycle that he theorized caused the pain of labor.

10. Match column I with column II:

COLUMN I	COLUMN II
a. Psychophysical component of the Read method.	_b_ Reversal of negative influence of cultural conditioning through education.
b. Intellectual component of the Read method.	_a_ Passive total body relaxation, abdominal breathing, panting, and breath-holding.
c. Psychological component of the Read method.	_c_ Relaxation facilitating effective cervical dilatation and effacement.

11. Dr. Bradley's natural childbirth utilizes a technique that works in harmony with the woman's body. Use of medication of any kind during labor and birth is discouraged.

12. *Psychophysical:* Breath control is utilized for labor, using abdominal breathing while in a position imitating the sleep position, which may differ for each individual woman.
Psychological: Deep mental relaxation is utilized.
Intellectual: Preparation for birth provides education about labor and birth and focuses on nonintervention of obstetrical technologies and avoidance of analgesics and anesthetics.

13. The famous example of a conditioned reflex is: Ring a bell ⟶ dog turns his head. Meat is placed in front of the dog ⟶ dog salivates.

14. The components of the Lamaze method are described as follows:
Psychophysical: Controlled muscular relaxation and release, rhythmic breathing, concentration on a focal point, and refined active relaxation are parts of the Lamaze system.
Psychological: In the Lamaze method, the woman uses concentration and active relaxation as appropriate responses to pain stimulus.
Intellectual: Lamaze preparation is comprehensive, offering a structured program to remove fear by education, thus eliminating distressing associations.

15. The three breathing patterns widely used in Lamaze birth classes are:
(1) slow paced breathing
(2) modified paced breathing
(3) patterned paced breathing

16. For *slow paced breathing*, the appropriate rate is approximately one-half the normal resting rate.
For *modified paced breathing*, the frequency is twice the normal resting rate.
For *patterned paced breathing*, frequency is increased up to a maximum rate of twice the normal rate.

17. The directions for exhalation breathing are as follows:
    a. Assume a physiologic position suitable for second stage (i.e., squatting or sitting in a C-shaped position).
    b. Take a few deep breaths as the urge to push builds.
    c. When ready, hold your breath for about 5 seconds to "fix" your thorax and abdominal muscles.
    d. Begin slow light exhalation through slightly pursed lips.
    e. As you inhale spontaneously in 5-6 seconds, the thorax and abdominal muscles will continue to stay fixed, preventing upward retraction or movement of the fetus. Inhale slowly, straightening the neck. Take as many inhalations and exhalations as needed during a contraction.
    f. Only as you feel the urge to push, use the abdominal muscles to push with contractions.
    g. Concentrate on keeping the pelvic floor muscles relaxed.
    h. When the contraction is over, take a deep breath and relax.

18. Match column I with column II:

COLUMN I		COLUMN II
a. therapeutic touch	a	principle that the body's electromagnetic energy field is responsive to healing.
b. acupressure/acupuncture	b	based on belief that a pain is an imbalance of energy within the body.
c. imagery	d	once trained to recognize signals of internal physiologic events, individuals can manipulate those events.
d. biofeedback	e	pictures desired effects.
e. autogenic training	c	mental control modifies muscular and autonomic systems responses.

8 SELECTED MATERNAL COMPLICATIONS

Janet S. Malinowski

OBJECTIVES

Upon completing this chapter, you will be able to:

- Explore how nursing care during labor is altered when caring for:
  a. a young adolescent
  b. an older woman
  c. a substance abuser
- Identify the special aspects of care necessary for a laboring woman experiencing:
  a. abnormal bleeding
  b. pregnancy induced hypertension
- Discuss the physical and emotional care of the pregnant woman experiencing a cesarean delivery.
- Apply the assessment, nursing diagnosis, and intervention steps of the nursing process for selected complications.

Throughout this book, several complications of labor are discussed as they appropriately fit into the content of various chapters. For example, general problems related to pelvic dimension and fetal position are found in Chapter 2, uterine dysfunction in Chapter 3, prolonged labor in Chapter 4, and preterm and post-term labor in Chapter 9. Other complications are briefly addressed elsewhere. For example, diabetes is in Chapters 1, 3, and 8, multiple gestation is in Chapters 1 and 8, hydramnios is in Chapters 1 and 8, breech presentation is in Chapters 1 and 2, use of forceps is in Chapters 2 and 8, and vaginal birth after cesarean delivery is in Chapters 1 and 7.

This chapter deals with selected maternal complications that are not addressed in other parts of the book. Included here are maternal age (the very young and the older mother), substance abuse, maternal health status alterations (bleeding and hypertension), and cesarean delivery. The emphasis is on how these complications alter the nursing care during labor and immediately following delivery. Another source should be consulted for the in-depth pathophysiology involved.

THE ADOLESCENT IN LABOR

The young adolescent is considered to be a complicating factor for labor for several reasons. Some of the major ones are that she is usually poorly informed about birth, not prepared to cope with the stresses of labor, and may lack a strong support system. The nurse, therefore, often finds it challenging to meet the young woman at her individual intellectual and psychological level.

Adolescents frequently do not choose (subconsciously or consciously), or lack the opportunity, to gain accurate and comprehensive information about childbirth. Without knowing what to expect of labor and without being prepared with specific coping methods to deal with the stresses of labor, the adolescent is likely to experience a great deal of emotional and physical distress.

The implications of being a pregnant adolescent are a result of her maturational stage and her individual situation, rather than her chronological age. The pregnancy, labor, and birth change her previous roles of child and daughter to adult and mother. Not only is there an expected change in role performance and personal identity, but there is a disturbance in self-concept. Her body image and her self-image are altered. Her cultural background will also influence the stresses imposed by her family and her home community.

Many pregnant adolescents lack a strong support system as a result of financial impoverishment, single parent (her mother) head of household, and absence of a husband.[1] Some adolescents come from an environment where the family relationships were faulty in the first place, and the pregnancy is a form of rebellion.[2] Usually the pregnancy results in social isolation from her usual peer group—those at school.[3] During pregnancy, she is likely to associate with other pregnant teens, her boyfriend (two thirds of the pregnant adolescents are unwed[4]), and relatives who will accept her. Often the adolescent is resistant to help and prefers only her mother and/or boyfriend, if he remains supportive.[5] The adolescent's response to labor frequently indicates a low pain threshold. She may view labor as a punishment rather than the means to the outcome of birth. Anxiety is heightened by the use of technology, such as monitors, and the complications that may occur. There is an increased incidence of prolonged labor and cesarean delivery, especially in the 12- to 14-year-old, due to cephalopelvic disproportion resulting from her physiologic immaturity. Intrauterine growth retardation (IUGR) and anemia (both due to poor nutrition), pregnancy-induced hypertension (PIH), sexually transmitted diseases (STD), and substance abuse also may complicate the pregnancy and labor. Many of these conditions are influenced by insufficient prenatal care, race, and poverty.

The following nursing strategies are useful when caring for adolescents in labor. By involving the adolescent in decision making and keeping her informed about her status, her self-esteem and personal development can be fostered. The nurse should assist the adolescent to feel that she is in control. It is important to be direct but not to talk down to her as if she is a young child. A relaxed approach provides support and reassurance. Repetition should be done as necessary. In tense situations, most people do not hear correctly and comprehend the first time something new is said. Her modesty must be respected by providing privacy and explaining why certain procedures, including repeated vaginal exams, are necessary. Her support persons should be involved if they are willing and able. If conflict exists between the baby's father and the adolescent's mother, the nurse may need to assist the laboring woman to decide which one she wants at the bedside. If a cesarean is necessary, the nurse should recognize that it is likely to be perceived as disfiguring to the adolescent, even more so than to the mature adult. An understanding explanation of the purpose and what is involved is important.

• •

Review Questions

1. In nursing diagnosis format, state five problems the nurse often finds in the adolescent in labor:
   a. ______________________________
   ____
   b. ______________________________
   ____
   c. ______________________________
   ____
   d. ______________________________
   ____
   e. ______________________________
   ____

2. Identify five complications of labor that adolescents are at risk for:
   a. ______________________________
   b. ______________________________
   c. ______________________________
   d. ______________________________
   e. ______________________________

3. List five nursing strategies that foster self-esteem and personal development in the laboring adolescent:
   a. ______________________________
   b. ______________________________
   c. ______________________________

d. ____
e. ____

Answers

1. Nursing diagnoses appropriate for a laboring adolescent include:
   a. **Knowledge deficit [about the birth process] related to lack of exposure, unfamiliarity with sources of information, cognitive limitation, and/or lack of interest in learning in the adolescent.**
   b. **Coping, ineffective individual related to the situational and maturational crisis of labor.**
   c. **Self-concept, disturbance in: role performance related to the biophysical, psychosocial, intellectual, and cultural factors of adolescent pregnancy.**
   d. **Family process, alteration in related to situational and developmental transition/crisis involved in adolescent giving birth.**
   e. **Social isolation related to adolescent pregnancy.**
   f. **Comfort, alteration in: pain, acute related to low pain threshold during labor.**
   g. **Anxiety [specify] related to situational and maturational crises, threat to self-concept, threat of death, and unmet needs.**
   h. **Injury, potential for; (fetal) trauma related to maternal malnutrition, physiologic immaturity, and inadequate health care.**

2. Labor complications that adolescents are at risk for include:
   a. prolonged labor
   b. cesarean delivery
   c. cephalopelvic disproportion
   d. intrauterine growth retardation
   e. anemia
   f. pregnancy-induced hypertension
   g. sexually transmitted diseases
   h. substance abuse

3. Nursing strategies that are effective in fostering self-esteem and personal development with laboring adolescents include:
   a. Assist her to feel she is in control.
   b. Be direct but do not talk down to her.
   c. Use a relaxed, supportive approach.
   d. Repeat explanations as necessary.
   e. Respect her modesty.
   f. Involve the support person(s) of her choice.
   g. Recognize her perception of disfigurement from cesarean delivery.

• •

THE OLDER WOMAN IN LABOR

In contrast to the adolescent pregnant woman is the "older" one, the woman over 35 years of age. These women, up until the age of 47, make up a growing segment of the North American childbearing population. Pregnancy after age 47 is uncommon.[6]

The fetus of the older woman is at risk for chromosomal abnormalities (especially Down syndrome), postmaturity, and twinning.

The frequency of Down syndrome is 1 in 885 at age 30, 1 in 465 at age 34, 1 in 365 at age 35, and significantly greater, 1 in 85 or less, in women over 40.[7] As a result, in addition to routine antepartal assessment, ultrasound, amniocentesis, or chorionic villi sampling, and genetic screening should be offered. Although younger mothers tend to have more post-term pregnancies, the woman past 35 more often has a neonate with more severe effects of postmaturity.[8] (See Chapter 9.) This in part is due to her cardiovascular status. There are also effects of increased maternal age (up to about 40) and parity (up to 7) on the incidence of twinning.[9] The maximum twinning rate is between ages 35 and 39.[10]

Recent studies suggest that pre-existing medical problems (such as hypertension and diabetes) are more influential than the mother's age on the mother's well-being and the pregnancy's outcome.[11,12] In a 1977 study of pregnant women ages 40 to 54, hypertensive disorders were common. Abruptio placenta occurred in almost 5% of them.[6] "The increasing frequency of hypertension with advancing years and the greater tendency to uterine hemorrhage contribute significantly to the elevation of the mortality rate. Advanced age and high parity act independently to increase the risk of childbearing, but their effects are usually additive."[13]

Nurses who care for the older pregnant woman need to recognize that she has special needs. For example, there may be other family members at home about whom the woman is concerned. Often she has a career outside of her home which must be altered. In addition, she may have to deal with others' negative attitudes about her late pregnancy. On the positive side, the older woman has a variety of life experiences and, thereby, possesses ability to cope with many changes, including most of those occurring due to pregnancy. She may plan her life and have high expectations of herself and her health caretakers. She also may have a great desire to learn. In a study done by Winslow,[14] the older primigravidas were extremely knowledgeable about pregnancy. This was a result of their own individual research rather than through childbirth education classes in which they felt out of place. These women sought genetic testing and the best maternity care possible. Similar to the adolescent, the older pregnant woman considered labor and delivery to be a time when she would lack control.

The above statements have several implications for labor nurses. Age probably increases the independence and assertiveness of the pregnant woman. This may pose a problem for the very young nurse when attempting to establish rapport. Since certain medical problems are more prevalent in this age group, specific assessment should be done for them. This woman, like all others in labor, needs to be treated as an individual who, regardless of how well prepared and confident she appears, is going through a stressful situation during which time she needs understanding care.

• •

Review Question

List two problems for the fetus and two for the mother that may be experienced as a result of her being over 35 years of age:
a. Fetus: ______________________
b. Mother: ______________________

Answer

Problems that may occur because the mother is over 35 include:
a. Fetal: Down syndrome, post-mature problems, and twinning.
b. Maternal: hypertension, abruptio placenta, uterine hemorrhage.

• •

THE SUBSTANCE ABUSER

Substance abuse is a prevalent problem in today's pregnant population. The addictive substances of particular importance to the labor nurse are heroin, methadone, cocaine (including crack), amphetamines, barbiturates, hallucinogens (LSD and PCP), and alcohol. When substance abuse is present, it is common for the person to take multiple substances (including alcohol, caffeine, and nicotine) so the outcome is a combined effect.

The effect of these substances on the newborn is dramatic and, in some states under child abuse protection laws, reportable by professionals before discharge. Substance withdrawal in the newborn includes a variety of symptoms such as central nervous system irritability, shrill cry, tremors, hypertonia, nasal stuffiness, fever, feeding problems, yawning, tachypnea, vomiting, and diarrhea. Therapy involves a controlled thermal environment, fluid and electrolyte monitoring, and drugs (diazepam, chlorpromazine, phenobarbital, or paregoric) given to the newborn for several days to weeks depending on the presence of symptoms. Heroin-addicted babies show neurologic disturbances within the first 24 hours of life. Methadone-addicted babies may not show symptoms of withdrawal for a week or so following birth. Fetal alcohol syndrome (FAS) is apparent in congenital anomalies distinctively seen in the face, as well as elsewhere.

A high percentage of pregnant substance abusers do not seek prenatal care until the onset of labor, thus they are "walk-ins." They come to the labor unit with numerous complications associated with their substance abuse (Table 8–1). They may also possess behavioral characteristics which make them more difficult to care for. For example, they may show irritability, uncoordinated movements, disorientation, and marked mood changes.

It is no easy task to meet the needs of the complex problems of the substance abuser. Usually the substance abuser is distrustful of professionals and fearful of legal action. The nurse should use a

Table 8–1. COMPLICATIONS ASSOCIATED WITH SUBSTANCE ABUSE

Preterm labor	Hypertension/Pregnancy-induced hypertension
Bleeding (placenta previa or abruptio placenta)	Malpresentation
Infections (hepatitis, pneumonia, endocarditis, cystitis, urethritis, pyelonephritis, abcess at injection sites, septic thrombophlebitis, sexually transmitted diseases, acquired immunodeficiency syndrome)	Stillbirth
	Puerperal morbidity
	Nutritional deficits
	Intrauterine growth retardation
	Poor dental hygiene
	Anemia
	Liver disease (jaundice)
	Signs of abuse

tactful, nonjudgmental approach. Attempts should be made to accurately assess the prenatal history and to determine the current risk factors. These women are notorious for being manipulative and giving unreliable information. They may give misleading information because of the way a question is asked. For example, when asked if they take drugs they may say "No" because they do not ingest or inject them. A more accurate answer may come if they are also asked what substances they snort or smoke. An alternate approach to the question about substance abuse that receives immediate denial is a natural appearing pause. During the silent moment the woman may reconsider her answer. Substance abusers also typically have inadequate financial and social support systems, and lack knowledge about the labor/delivery process.

Subtle or overt signs of substance abuse may be evident in the woman's mood, personal grooming, and affect. The presence of scars ("tracks") from venipuncture is a definite clue to substance abuse. These, coupled with any complications identified in Table 8–1, indicate that the nurse needs to attempt to determine the pattern of drug use: the type(s), frequency, amount, mode of administration, use of detoxification programs, and (very important) time of last usage. Abruptio placenta usually occurs within an hour of cocaine administration, and "a sudden onset of uterine contractions, fetal tachycardia, and excessive fetal activity within hours or even minutes of [cocaine] ingestion."[15]

The baby will have more severe substance withdrawal symptoms the closer the drug ingestion is to the delivery. However, the onset and symptoms will depend on the substance. The nurse should also take precautions against AIDS (see Appendix D). At the same time, the nurse must assess for unstable emotional behaviors in order to assess the safety of this mother and her infant.

Assessment of fetal status is equally important. Because these women often have irregular menstrual cycles and/or amenorrhea, their EDC cannot be determined solely on their LMP. Ultrasound may be performed to assess fetal status and gestational age. To assess fetal well-being, continuous electronic fetal monitoring is also needed. The combination of uterine contractions and maternal withdrawal may increase the stress on the fetal oxygen requirements. The nurse must recognize that intrauterine hypoxia is likely to result. In order to promote optimum oxygen exchange, the mother should be placed in a left lateral position and be well hydrated. Since her veins may be thrombosed, an intravenous line is usually established early in labor and kept open for 24 hours following delivery. Oxygen by mask may be needed. A fetal scalp pH (see Chapter 9) may be warranted as labor progresses.

Since the pain threshold is low in substance abusive women, analgesia is needed, as well as possibly epidural anesthesia. Medications can be administered on the order of the obstetrician. Usually consultation is sought with the anesthesiologist since respiratory depression, hypotension, and fetal narcotism are plausible.[16] The nurse should expect that the effect of narcotics will be shortened due to the abuser's tolerance. The usual doses of Demerol, Dilaudid, or morphine can be given.[16] If the woman is on a methadone maintenance program, that, too, may be given during labor[16,17] to decrease fetal compromise resulting from maternal and fetal withdrawal. Talwin, a narcotic antagonist analgesic, is contraindicated since it can precipitate a withdrawal reaction.[16]

The nurse should provide support and reassurance to this woman who is likely to have minimal knowledge of the labor process and procedures. Comfort measures and verbal encouragement may decrease her need for pain relief medication. The support person should be involved as appropriate.

A high-risk birth should be anticipated. Therefore, the delivery should occur in a regional perinatal center whenever possible. Often there is intrauterine distress, a low birth weight infant (LBW is less than 2500 g), and neonatal distress.[18] The delivery team should be prepared to suction, and to provide warmth, respiratory and fluid support, medications, and ventilation to the newborn. A pediatrician, neonatologist, or perinatologist should be present at the time of delivery. Approximately 50 percent of the heroin-addicted babies develop withdrawal symptoms and without treatment most of them die.[19]

Several nursing problems are identified for the substance abuser in labor in the above paragraphs. A sample of the appropriate nursing diagnoses include:

Knowledge deficit [of labor process] related to lack of prenatal care of substance abuser.

Infection, potential for (in numerous sites) related to substance abuse.

Nutrition, alteration in: less than body requirements related to substance abuse.

Injury, potential for; trauma related to drug abuse and impaired mental processes.

Coping, ineffective individual related to dependence and/or denial of substance abuse.

Family process, alteration in related to substance abuse.

Communication, impaired: verbal related to withdrawal symptoms of substance abuse.

• •

Review Question

List six ways that nursing care is altered when the laboring woman is a substance abuser:

a. ______________________________

b. ______________________________

c. ______________________________

d. ______________________________

e. ______________________________

f. ______________________________

Answer

Nursing care is altered in the following ways when the laboring woman is a substance abuser:

a. In some states, report addicted baby (based on child abuse law).
b. Observe for symptoms of drug withdrawal in the newborn and treat as necessary.
c. Assess "walk-ins" and others with bizarre behavior for substance abuse and associated complications.
d. Use tact and nonjudgmental approach to woman who probably is distrustful and fearful of legal action.
e. Try to determine drug use pattern, especially time of last usage.
f. Be concerned about the woman's safety, especially in the presence of unstable emotional behaviors.
g. Recognize the need to determine accurate gestational age and fetal well-being status.
h. Use continuous electronic fetal monitoring.
i. Keep woman in left lateral position and well hydrated.
j. Anticipate need for intravenous line early, oxygen and scalp pH.
k. Provide ordered analgesia (except Talwin) more frequently than for non-addicted woman.
l. Give methadone if on maintenance program.
m. Anticipate high-risk newborn and involve medical caretaker for newborn at time of delivery.

• •

BLEEDING

Some women are at risk for excessive bleeding during labor—bleeding other than the normal bloody show of labor. Among those most commonly at risk are women with chronic hypertension, pregnancy-induced hypertension, parity of five or more, multiple gestation, large fetus, or history of previous hemorrhage.

As a woman and her family experience excessive bleeding, emotional support is very important. She rightfully has **anxiety [specify] related to the well being of herself and her baby**. She understandably has a **knowledge deficit [of the cause of the bleeding and the therapy involved] related to lack of exposure, lack of recall.** She should be mentally prepared for a possible cesarean delivery, and informed of the anticipated care that will be involved. She also needs to know that although the nurse will be assessing her frequently, she can help by letting the nurse know if there is increased bleeding or uterine changes such as in pain sensation.

Management of the bleeding pregnant woman varies dependent on the extent of the bleeding and the cause. The extent is not always visible since the bleeding may be concealed behind the attached portions of the placenta or by the fetal presenting part as it blocks the cervical opening. Therefore, the nurse must not rely solely on the apparent bleeding, but also on other signs of pending shock—for example, decreased blood pressure, weak rapid pulse, rapid shallow respirations, pallor, restlessness, and results of serial (every 4 to 6 hours) hemoglobin or hematocrit and coagulation profiles.

There are several possible causes of bleeding, including:

- abnormal placenta—previa (low implantation), abruption (premature separation),
- coagulation problems (disseminated intravascular coagulation, DIC, which is common in severe abruption),
- uterine rupture,
- lacerations in the cervix or vagina.

Trauma from a car accident or physical abuse can be the precipitating factor for all of the above. In cases of minimal painless bleeding, assessment by ultrasound may be performed in the physician's office. When there is more than minimal bleeding, the pregnant woman should be hospitalized even though she may not be in labor. In the hospital she is put on bed rest and placed on a continuous electronic monitor to assess both the fetal heart rate and contraction patterns. A side lying position increases uterine blood perfusion and elevation of the head 20 to 30 degrees may help the fetus to press against a low-lying placenta. Vital signs must be frequently (at least hourly) assessed, as well as the amount of external bleeding found on perineal pads or Chuxs. The attending physician needs to be immediately informed of the woman's initial status, as well as the occurrence of non-reassuring fetal heart rates (see Chapter 3), signs of pending shock, a hypertonic uterus, or abnormal labor progress (see Chapter 4). If the bleeding is life threatening, the admission history taking is kept to a minimum and preparation for delivery (usually cesarean) is done. The first priority is correction of coagulopathies and hypovolemia.[20] If the gestation is less than 37 weeks, the woman should be stabilized and transferred to, if not already at, a regional perinatal center.

Several characteristics of vaginal bleeding are noteworthy. The amount may be described by the pregnant woman in lay terms (cupful vs. tablespoon) or in terms of saturated perineal pads. A saturated pad contains 30 ml of blood, and if weighed, 1 g equals 1 ml of blood. The color of blood is usually dark red for abruption and bright red for previa. The consistency may or may not include clots. Fetal vs. maternal blood can be differentiated relatively simply by the Apt test. This involves mixing a dilute solution of bloody fluid with *N*-sodium hyroxide. Within 30 seconds maternal blood turns the solution greenish-brown and in 1 to 2 minutes the solution turns pink for fetal or cord blood.

• •

Review Questions

1. Since the amount of blood loss is not always externally evident, what other five signs of pending shock should the nurse look for?
   a. ______ d. ______
   b. ______ e. ______
   c. ______
2. When a laboring woman experiences excessive bleeding, what six actions should the nurse initially take?
   a. ______ d. ______
   b. ______ e. ______
   c. ______ f. ______
3. Identify three characteristics of blood loss that the nurse should note:
   a. ______, b. ______
   and c. ______.

Answers

1. Other than external blood loss, pending shock can be noted in: (a) decreased blood pressure, (b) weak rapid pulse, (c) rapid shallow respirations, (d) pallor, (e) restlessness, and (f) abnormal hemoglobin, hematocrit and/or coagulation lab results.
2. If excessive bleeding exists: (a) anticipate an order to keep the woman in the hospital, (b) enforce bedrest, in a lateral position, with the head of the bed slightly elevated, (c) monitor fetal heart rate and contractions continuously, (d) assess vital signs at least hourly, (e) assess external blood loss, and (f) notify her physician immediately.
3. The characteristics of blood loss that a nurse should note are: (a) amount, (b) color, (c) consistency, and (d) if possible whether it is fetal or maternal blood.

• •

Abruptio Placenta and Placenta Previa

Abruptio placenta is partial or complete separation of the normally implanted placenta from the uterine wall prior to the delivery of the fetus. The bleeding is termed *concealed* or *apparent* depending on whether it is visible as it flows from the vagina. Due to the accumulation of blood behind the placenta or in the uterus in abruptio placenta, the woman ordinarily experiences pain. Concealed hemorrhage produces an area of extreme uterine sensitivity and rigidity that increases the uterine size. Retroplacental bleeding causes a rise in the fundal height and is detectable if the fundal height is initially marked on the abdomen with a felt-tipped pen. The pain is constant and the relaxing phase of contractions is usually non-existent. When there are signs of abruption, most authorities say oxytocin should not be infused because the drug hastens further separation.

Placenta previa is a placenta that is abnormally implanted in the lower uterine segment. It is labeled according to its proximity to the internal cervical os. *Total* or *complete* placenta previa completely covers the os, *partial* or *incomplete* covers part of the os, and *marginal* or *low-lying* encroaches on the margin, but does not cover any of the internal cervical os.

In contrast to abruptio placenta, with placenta previa there is no pain except that which normally occurs with contractions. In placenta previa the initial amount of bleeding is usually small, but it increases with recurrent bleeding. The presence of the placenta in the lower uterus causes the fetal presenting part to assume a higher than normal station, often accompanied by malpresentation.

Several factors will determine the medical management in abruptio placenta and placenta previa. The first factor is the extent of the actual bleeding. Besides maternal vital signs, the fetal heart rate pattern must be considered. As long as the condition is stabilized and there is no immediate threat to the mother's or baby's life, immediate delivery is not needed. The preference then is to allow the pregnancy to get as close to term as possible. Ultrasound is done to verify the exact diagnosis—abruption vs. (degree of) placenta previa. Whether vaginal or cesarean delivery is to be done is in part dependent upon the cervical opening. If it is not completely dilated or is blocked by 30 or more percent of the placenta, vaginal delivery is not possible. When only moderate bleeding exists in a term gestation, a trial of labor is usually attempted as long as there are not other contraindications.

If there is a suspicion of placenta previa, vaginal (internal digital) examinations are ordinarily not done since they may precipitate massive hemorrhage. Initially the physician may do a gentle speculum exam of the birth canal to rule out a friable cervix or polyps that might be the source of bleeding. For a woman who is a candidate for a vaginal exam, a double set-up vaginal examination may be done. This is performed in the delivery room with preparations made so that a cesarean delivery could be immediately done, if necessary. Occasionally the physician chooses to rupture the membranes to promote fetal descent and compression of the placenta by the presenting part, thus decreasing the active bleeding in placenta previa. When the source of bleeding is determined, infrequent vaginal exams may be permitted if the diagnosis is placental abruption or with extreme caution in marginal previa. Whenever vaginal exams are done, they must be done with strict sterile technique, since there is **infection, potential for related to the open sinuses at the placental site and/or nearness of the placenta to the cervix**. Temperatures should be taken hourly to detect a threatening infection.

When delivery is imminent, the woman should be kept NPO, have a #16 or #18 intracatheter with IV fluid infusing, and be typed and cross-matched for 2 to 4 units of blood. She has **fluid volume deficit, potential related to altered blood flow at the placental site**. She should have a Foley catheter inserted, and be maintained on intake and output. There is potential **tissue perfusion, alteration in: cardiopulmonary related to hypovolemia**. Some institutions use central venous pressure lines which are more accurate in determining fluid needs and preventing fluid overload. The left lateral position is desirable, and oxygen at 7 to 12 liters may be needed to stabilize the woman's vital signs. Coagulation studies may be done for either abruptio placenta or placenta previa since disseminated intravascular coagulation (DIC) can occur with either condition.

Some women with a confirmed diagnosis of placenta previa are sent home after the bleeding ceases. These women usually are not at term and do not have a complete previa. Involvement of a supportive partner (or other) is preferred. Discharge instructions should include weekly visits to the physician, no insertion of anything into the birth canal, no tub baths, and information about occurrences which warrant immediate medical attention.

Uterine rupture is a rare cause of bleeding in labor. It is often associated with injudicious use of oxytocin (see Chapter 5). Less than one percent[21] of the time does it occur in vaginal births after cesarean (VBAC). Signs of rupture include severe pain, boardlike abdomen, cessation of contractions and possibly fetal heart rates, and shock. Immediate assistance from the medical team is needed. Vital signs must be assessed frequently, Trendelenburg position assumed with legs elevated (and use of Mast Trousers, if available), oxygen administered, and an intravenous infused. The woman must be prepared for immediate surgery, in most cases a hysterectomy.

Lacerations are the final cause of bleeding in labor that will be mentioned. Due to the increased incidence of spousal abuse and auto accidents, consideration should be given to the possibility of vaginal bleeding occurring as a result of lacerations to the labia, perineum, vagina, or cervix, as well as from the vaginal birth process. Initial examination with a speculum usually is diagnostic and repair is done with sutures by the physician or midwife, depending on the severity of the laceration. Blood replacement and antibiotic administration may be appropriate. Heat or cold applications and analgesic are used to promote healing and comfort.

• •

Review Questions

1. State at least three distinguishing symptoms for abruptio placenta and placenta previa.
   a. Abruptio placenta: (a) ________, (b) ________, (c) ________.
   b. Placenta previa: (a) ________, (b) ________, (c) ________.

2. Fill in the blanks for the following statements dealing with the medical management of abruptio placenta and placenta previa:
   a. If there is no immediate threat to the mother's or baby's life, delivery does not have to be done ________.
   b. It is desirable to have a ________ gestation.
   c. Cesarean will be necessary if the cervix is ________ dilated or ________ percent or more of the cervical os is covered by placenta.
   d. If there is no severe bleeding, term gestation, and no other contraindications, a ________ of labor is probable.
   e. Initially a vaginal exam is ________ done since this might precipitate massive hemorrhage.
   f. Double set-up is performed in the ________ room.

3. What preparation for delivery is routine for a bleeding woman?
   a. ________ e. ________
   b. ________ f. ________
   c. ________ g. ________
   d. ________

4. What is uterine rupture closely associated with? ________

5. What are signs of uterine rupture?
   a. ________ c. ________
   b. ________ d. ________

6. Having already notified the physician, what should the nurse do next when suspecting a uterine rupture?
   a. ________ d. ________
   b. ________ e. ________
   c. ________

7. What kind of examination is likely if vaginal lacerations are suspected? ________

Answers

1. (a) Abruptio placenta involves (constant) pain, extreme uterine sensitivity, uterine rigidity, no relaxation between contractions, and dark red bleeding.
   (b) Placenta previa is painless (except during contractions which cause the uterus to tense and then relax), the initial (bright red) bleeding episode is slight and

succeeding ones increasingly more, fetal station is unusually high, and frequently there is malpresentation.

2. The completed statements dealing with the medical management of abruptio placenta and placenta previa should read as follows:
   a. If there is no threat to the mother's or baby's life, delivery does not have to be done *immediately*.
   b. It is desirable to have a *term* gestation.
   c. Cesarean will be necessary if the cervix is *not completely* dilated or 30 percent or more of the cervical os is covered by placenta.
   d. If there is no severe bleeding, term gestation, and no other contraindications, *trial* of labor is probable.
   e. Initially a vaginal exam is *not* done since this might precipitate massive hemorrhage.
   f. Double set-up is performed in the *delivery or operating* room.
3. In preparation for delivery of a bleeding woman, the following is routine: (a) keep NPO, (b) infuse IV with blood administration tubing, (c) insert Foley catheter, (d) maintain intake and output, (e) place woman in left lateral position, (f) administer oxygen as necessary, and (g) anticipate an order for coagulation studies.
4. Uterine rupture is closely associated with poor judgment when oxytocin is given.
5. Signs of uterine rupture include: (a) severe uterine pain, (b) boardlike abdomen, (c) no more uterine contractions and possibly fetal heart rate, and (d) shock.
6. Having already notified the physician, the nurse should do the following when suspecting uterine rupture: (a) take vital signs, (b) place woman in Trendelenburg position, (c) administer oxygen, (d) anticipate an order for an IV, and (e) anticipate an order for preparation for surgery (hysterectomy).
7. A *speculum* examination is adequate for diagnosis of vaginal lacerations.

• •

Postpartum Hemorrhage

A number of conditions during early stage IV are likely to result in postpartum hemorrhage. The most common ones are listed in Table 8–2. Uterine atony is the most frequent cause. If the uterus

Table 8–2. CONDITIONS THAT PREDISPOSE POSTPARTAL HEMORRHAGE

Dysfunctional labor	History of previous PP hemorrhage
Grand multiparity	Hydramnios
Multiple gestation	Large fetus
Induction with oxytocin	Abruptio placenta, placenta previa
Precipitous or difficult delivery: lacerations	Fibroids

did not contract effectively during labor, it often does not contract well following delivery either. A less frequent, yet significant, cause of hemorrhage is lacerations from a traumatic delivery, for example, following the use of forceps. Hematomas and retained placental fragments also can result in hemorrhage.

Uterine atony is evident in a soft, boggy uterus and heavy vaginal bleeding with clots. According to a standard for assessing lochial volume developed by Jacobson, a heavy amount saturates one peripad within one hour.[22] Nursing management of uterine atony usually involves uterine massage and administration of (ordered) oxytocin.

Massage should be done with the uterus cupped between both hands — one just above the mother's symphysis and the other on the uterine fundus. This method provides support to the uterus. The uterus must be massaged until firm and followed by expression of the collected blood, clots, and placental fragments from the uterus. Massage decreases blood loss by stimulating contraction of the uterine muscles. Caution must be taken to avoid overzealous massage that contributes to muscle fatigue and relaxation. Because massage may be painful to the delivered woman, she may need to use the relaxation techniques used in labor. Analgesia may also be necessary.

Most often, administration of 20 units of oxytocin mixed in 1000 ml intravenous solution is effective for uterine atony. Methergine, or less frequently ergotrate, may be used in place of, or in addition to, oxytocin. Methergine should be given cautiously in the hypertensive woman. Ergotrate should not be used if she is hypertensive. Breast feeding the baby may also be successful in stimulating uterine contractions.

If the above methods do not sufficiently firm the uterus, the physician or midwife may perform bimanual massage with one hand compressing the uterus from the top and the other fist placed up the vagina anterior to the uterus. By exerting pressure from both hands at the same time, the uterine arteries are compressed. If this technique does not work, surgery will be necessary to stop the excessive bleeding. Surgery can involve ligation of uterine or internal iliac arteries, or a hysterectomy. If retained fragments of the placenta are assumed to be the cause of the hemorrhage, and massage is unsuccessful in expelling the tissue as evident by ultrasound, the physician or midwife needs to remove the placental fragments manually or by curettage under anesthesia.

Lacerations require inspection by the physician or midwife, and probable suturing. They should be suspected when blood spurts upon palpation of a firm fundus. Hematomas may be reduced by the application of cold, which ordinarily is a nursing function permissible by hospital protocol. If the hematoma still progresses in size, excision by the physician is indicated. Pain from a hematoma is usually severe enough to require analgesia.

Similar nursing problems exist in postpartal hemorrhage to those identified during bleeding in labor: anxiety, knowledge deficit, fluid volume deficit, alteration in tissue perfusion, and infection. In addition there is the **parenting, alteration in: potential related to the physical status of the hemorrhaging mother**. This is a stressful time for the woman, who now has the additional role of mother. The astute, caring nurse can help her to make the numerous adjustments necessary at this time.

• •

Review Question

State the nursing actions that need to be taken in the presence of:

a. Uterine atony: ______________________________

____

b. Lacerations: ______________________________

c. Hematoma: ______________________________

____

d. Retained placental fragments: ______________________________

____

Answer

Nursing actions for the following causes of postpartal hemorrhage should be: (a) Uterine atony: massage uterus using "cupping" method, administer oxytocin and/or methergine or ergotrate, have mother breast feed (if appropriate); if unsuccessful in firming uterus, notify physician (midwife). (b) Lacerations: notify physician (midwife). (c) Hematoma: apply cold compresses and provide analgesia; if unsuccessful in decreasing size of hematoma, notify physician (midwife). (d) Retained placental fragments: massage uterus to firm uterus and to promote expulsion of contents; if uterus does not remain firm, notify physician (midwife). An order for an oxytocic agent should be anticipated.

• •

PREGNANCY-INDUCED HYPERTENSION

Pregnancy-induced hypertension (PIH) is the onset of hypertension, proteinuria, and edema after 20 weeks' gestation. The condition is considered to be mild when the hypertension is in the range of 140/90 or an increase of +30/+15, and the proteinuria is 1+ to 2+. A severe condition exists when the blood pressure is greater than 160/110 and the proteinuria 3+ to 4+.

Most women with controlled PIH continue to be closely monitored and medically managed until labor begins spontaneously, or, when near term, labor is induced by amniotomy and/or oxytocin. Because of the irritability of the uterus in PIH, even an unfavorable cervix tends to respond to oxytocin.

When there is severe PIH and the gestational age is less than 38 weeks, fetal maturity and growth studies such as ultrasound are done and lung immaturity therapy may be administered (see Chapter 9). If symptoms of uncontrolled PIH fail to decrease within 24 to 48 hours despite medical management, termination of the pregnancy is warranted since the severity of the PIH will be intensified by continuing the pregnancy. If at any time fetal deterioration is evident (for example, based on NST, OCT or BPP—see Chapter 9), delivery is preferred. Cesarean delivery is usually reserved for obstetrical indications, even in the presence of severe PIH.[23] A variety of anesthetics can be used. Continuous lumbar epidural anesthesia may be used because of its hypotensive effect.[24,25]

Nursing care of the woman with PIH during labor and delivery should be carried out with a calm, matter-of-fact attitude, providing brief explanations of the therapy involved. The environment should be as quiet, softly lit and unstimulating as possible. The labor room should not be occupied by another patient. Visitors should be kept to a minimum, but a non-anxious support person is desirable. Absolute bedrest, with the side rails up and a left side lying position are necessary. If the woman insists on the supine position, the head of the bed should be slightly raised and a wedge placed under her right hip. Only essential procedures (not even baths) should be done. The blood pressure must be taken at least every hour. Preferably the blood pressure is taken more frequently with the cuff left in place and continuous electronic monitoring done. Intravenous fluids should be run at a keep open rate and an indwelling catheter inserted with output and proteinuria levels recorded every one to two hours. The woman should be NPO if seizure activity is suspected. Only small doses of analgesia should be given. The nurse should be aware of laboratory values, such as medication levels, fibrinogen and platelets, and urine specific gravity. In preparation for an emergency, blood should be typed, cross-matched, and kept available, and emergency equipment kept in the room, including an airway, padded tongue blade, oxygen and suction equipment, and medications. The "preeclamptic tray" of medications should contain magnesium sulfate, calcium gluconate, cardiac stimulants, and anti-hypertensives (hydralazine or nipride), as well as syringes, needles, and alcohol sponges. A delivery pack should be readily available.

Symptoms indicating progression of PIH require prompt reporting to the physician. These symptoms include those listed in Table 8–3. Further progression of PIH is evident in the onset of convulsions. It is at this time that the woman is said to be *eclamptic*.

If a convulsion should occur, the nurse should:

- Turn the woman to her left side to prevent aspiration of vomitus, discourage supine hypotension syndrome, and increase renal perfusion. Initially Trendelenburg position may be used.
- Protect her from injury during the convulsion.
- Insert an object other than a finger into the side of the woman's mouth, if the jaws are not clamped down yet, to prevent her from biting her lips or tongue and to maintain the airway.

Table 8–3. SYMPTOMS INDICATING PROGRESSION OF PREGNANCY-INDUCED HYPERTENSION

Rapid rise in blood pressure	Severe headache
Quantitative increase in proteinuria	Epigastric pain
Increased edema	Visual disturbances
Less than 30 ml/hr urine output	Drowsiness
Marked hyperflexia (especially transient or sustained ankle clonus)	Listlessness
	Extreme irritability

- Suction food and fluids from her glottis and trachea.
- Administer medications as ordered (e.g., magnesium sulfate and hydralazine).
- Document occurrences on the chart including a description of the convulsion, and all nursing and medical actions taken.
- Be alert for signs of abruptio placenta, hemorrhage, and shock to which the eclamptic woman is prone.
- Keep her NPO.

The nurse should anticipate that following the convulsion, there may be a rapid onset of labor and/or an increase in the labor progress due to uterine hyperactivity. Delivery can usually be postponed until the woman's status is stable.[26]

• •

Review Questions

Fill in the blanks or circle the correct response in the following statements which deal with the special aspects of nursing care needed for a laboring woman with pregnancy induced hypertension:

1. Anticipate that despite an unfavorable cervix, oxytocin may stimulate labor because of the ______________________ uterus.
2. Delivery is usually ______________________ (type).
3. The labor room should be ______________ and ______________.
4. The woman is kept (confined to bed *or* up to bathroom only), on her ______________________ side, and with the side rails ________.
5. Frequent monitoring is done of ______________________, ______________________ and ______________________.
6. Emergency items that are kept in her room include ______________, ______________ and ______________________.
7. The following subjective symptoms, which the woman relates, are immediately reportable to the physician: ______________________, ______________________, and ______________________.

8. In general terms, the following nursing actions are implemented when a convulsion occurs:

a. ______________	d. ______________
b. ______________	e. ______________
c. ______________	f. ______________

Answers

Aspects of nursing care for a PIH laboring woman include:

1. Anticipate that despite an unfavorable cervix, oxytocin may stimulate labor because of the *irritable* uterus.
2. Delivery is usually *vaginal.*
3. The labor room should be *nonstimulating* and *private.*
4. The woman is kept *confined to bed,* on her *left* side, and with the side rails *up.*
5. Frequent monitoring is done of *blood pressure, intake and output,* and *proteinuria.*
6. Emergency items that are kept in her room include *special equipment (such as airway, padded tongue blade, oxygen, suction apparatus), medications,* and *delivery pack.*
7. Subjective symptoms related by the woman that are immediately reportable to the physician are: *headache, epigastric pain,* and *visual disturbances* and others listed in Table 8–3.
8. The following nursing actions are taken at the time of a convulsion: (a) *position woman,* (b) *protect her,* (c) *maintain airway,* (d) *administer CNS depressant and antihypertensive medications,* (e) *document occurrences and actions taken,* and (f) *watch for additional complications.*

• •

Pregnancy-Induced Hypertension Treatment

Magnesium sulfate is the central nervous system depressant used to decrease the possibility of convulsions. A secondary action, although not always effective by itself, is to decrease the blood pressure in the patient with PIH. Before each administration, the nurse should assess for the presence of deep tendon reflexes, respirations of at least 12 per minute, and urine output of at least 30 ml per hour. (Some hospital protocol also call for a urine specific gravity of at least 1.018.) Absence of any of these criteria indicates a need to decrease the magnesium sulfate dosage.

An initial dose of magnesium sulfate is given intravenously, usually 4 g in 250 ml of 5% D/W injected slowly at a rate of 10 ml per minute. The IV effect is immediate and lasts for about 30 minutes. The woman should be told in advance to expect hot flashes, and possible nausea and vomiting with the initial dose. There is some experiential support for using 20% D/W instead of 5% to decrease the vomiting potential. The initial dose is followed by a maintenance dose of 1 to 2 g per hour via infusion pump, or an intramuscular dose that can be given at 4-hour intervals. When given IM a 3 inch 20-gauge needle is used to inject 4 or 5 g of medication deep in each buttock. The Z-track technique is used since magnesium sulfate is extremely irritating to the tissue. One percent procaine may be added to the solution to decrease the pain of the injection. The IM onset of action is approximately 1 hour and the effect lasts 3 to 4 hours. Hourly intake and output, and blood pressure and respirations need to be documented every 15 to 30 minutes when this medication is given.

Magnesium sulfate toxicity is first observable in the loss, absence, or sharp decrease of the deep tendon reflexes (DTR). This appears when the magnesium sulfate blood level is 7 to 10 mEq per liter. DTR are elicited by tapping the involved tendon briskly which causes a brief jerk of the body part affected by the contracting muscle. The *knee-jerk or patellar reflex,* which is the easiest to determine, involves knee extension and leg jerk. The normal jerk is given a 2+ on a scale of 0 to 4+ (Table 8–4). The normal finding is neither sluggish nor brisk. 3+ indicates possible, but not absolute, central nervous system (CNS) disorder. No reflex and very brisk reflex response require physician notification.

The knee-jerk reflex is elicited by positioning the woman's knee somewhat flexed and relaxed. If in a lying position, the nurse supports the knee by placing a hand under the knee. It is not necessary to have the woman's foot off the bed. If she is sitting, her lower leg should be dangling freely. After palpating the patella and the tendon below it, the nurse taps the patellar tendon with the pointed end of the reflex hammer. In the presence of dependent edema, the *brachioradialis reflex* is more reliable. This involves resting the forearm in the lap or on the abdomen and striking the radial bone 1 to 2 inches above the wrist with the pointed or broad end of the reflex hammer.[27]

In the presence of a 3+ or 4+ DTR response, *clonus,* which indicates the presence of CNS disease such as uncontrolled PIH, should be checked. In obstetrics, clonus is elicited most commonly in the ankle and feels like jerks called "beats." With the knee partially flexed and a hand providing support under the knee, the foot is maintained sharply dorsiflexed. If there is clonus, beats can

Table 8–4. DEEP TENDON REFLEX EVALUATION SCALE

0	= no response
1+	= sluggish, diminished
2+	= normal, average
3+	= brisk, hyperactive without clonus
4+	= very brisk, usually associated with clonus

be felt and seen, and range from 1 to 2 to sustained beating.[27] The presence of more than 3 beats is classified as clonus.[28]

With no DTR, clonus present, and a 10 mEq blood level, respiratory distress is likely. If such occurs, 10 to 20 ml of the antidote, 20% calcium gluconate, must be given immediately via a slow intravenous route. At this time it is desirable to use a cardiac monitor, such as that available on the crash cart to observe the cardiac patterns for dysrhythmias.

The ideal magnesium sulfate level is 4 to 7.5 mEq per liter. This dose is therapeutic in preventing convulsions.[29–31] Since body weight and compromised renal function will alter the drug level of magnesium sulfate in the blood stream, it is not surprising that seizures have occurred in the presence of therapeutic levels of magnesium sulfate. For this reason, Seconal or Valium may be given in conjunction with magnesium sulfate.[32]

Oxytocin frequently is given to stimulate labor at the same time that magnesium sulfate is given. They are always administered in separate intravenous lines due to oxytocin's effects on contractions. Only a small amount of oxytocin may be needed since labor progress can be rapid.

Hydralazine (Apresoline) is the choice antihypertensive medication. When the diastolic is hovering around 110, the nurse is justified in seeking an order for the antihypertensive medication. Usually, a 5 mg dose of hydralazine is given slowly IV push. Up to 20 mg may be given gradually to decrease the diastolic blood pressure to the 90 to 100 mm Hg range. Careful monitoring should assure that it does not lower the diastolic below 80 mm Hg. During such administration, the blood pressure should be taken every 5 minutes, if not constantly by an electronic monitor.

Although the way to cure PIH is to terminate the pregnancy by delivery, PIH can persist into, or occur for the first time in, the postpartal period. For 24 to 48 hours following delivery of a woman medically treated for PIH, magnesium sulfate and anti-hypertensive therapy are generally continued since eclamptic convulsions are still possible. An early sign of improvement is increased urinary output. Phenobarbital is likely to be continued throughout the hospitalization. Nursing care should involve frequent monitoring of vital signs, reflexes, and urinary proteins. If the platelet count is low, the nurse should watch for excessive bleeding. (The complex condition of HELLP is PIH in combination with low platelets or DIC.) The woman needs to be assessed for weakness and dizziness due to a fall in hemoglobin and hematocrit. This fall is due to excessive diuresis occurring shortly following delivery, at which time the extravascular fluid shifts to the intravascular compartment.

PIH does present risks for the fetus. As much as 30 to 50 percent of the placental blood flow is decreased regardless of the severity of the PIH.[33] Intrauterine growth retardation is associated with significant increase in proteinuria,[34] as well as placental dysfunction. This is a good reason to use continuous electronic fetal monitoring during a PIH woman's labor. Furthermore, with the use of magnesium sulfate therapy, decreased beat-to-beat variability often occurs. If magnesium sulfate was given shortly before delivery, hypocalcemia and hypermagnesemia are likely in the neonate. For these reasons, at the time of delivery, a pediatrician and NICU nurse (if appropriate) should be present.

Based on the above information about PIH, the following nursing diagnoses may be appropriate:

Urinary elimination, alteration in patterns related to PIH as evidenced by diuresis and excess fluid retention.

Anxiety [specify] related to fear of unknown and lack of predictable outcomes in the presence of PIH.

Coping, ineffective individual/family: compromised related to stress of PIH.

Fluid volume, alteration in: excess related to decreased urine production.

Self-care deficit: bathing/hygiene, dressing/grooming, toileting related to absolute bedrest status.

Comfort, alteration in: pain, acute related to uterine contractions in the presence of anxiety, possible abruptio placenta, and oxytocin infusion.

Injury, potential for; trauma related to sedation (from medications administered), eclamptic episode(s), aspiration of gastric or oral secretions.

Knowledge deficit [of intrapartal hypertension] related to lack of exposure, cognitive limitation.

(Fetal) Gas exchange, impaired related to inadequate uteroplacental perfusion as evidenced by vasospasms, and/or decreased uterine relaxation.

(Fetal) Gas exchange, impaired related to placental abruption or oxytocin infusion as evidenced by decreased or inadequate uterine relaxation between contractions.

• •

Review Questions

Fill in the blanks in the following statements that deal with the special aspects of nursing care needed for a laboring woman with pregnancy-induced hypertension:

1. Contraindications to giving magnesium sulfate include:
   a. ______________________
   b. ______________________
   c. ______________________
2. The toxic blood level of magnesium sulfate is __________ mEq/L.
3. Oxytocin and magnesium sulfate are always administered on ______________________ intravenous lines.
4. Antihypertensive drugs should maintain a diastolic blood pressure of no lower than __________ and no higher than __________.

5. **The cure for PIH is ______________________________.**

6. **The onset of PIH can be as late as ______________________.**

7. **Continuous electronic fetal monitoring is used in labor because of potential ______________________ and ______________________.**

Answers

Aspects of nursing care for a PIH laboring woman includes:

1. Contraindications to giving magnesium sulfate are: (a) *lack of deep tendon reflexes,* (b) *respirations less than 12 per minute,* and (c) *urine output less than 30 ml per hour.*

2. The toxic blood level of magnesium sulfate is *7 to 10* mEq per liter.

3. Oxytocin and magnesium sulfate are always administered on *separate* intravenous lines.

4. Antihypertensive drugs should maintain a diastolic blood pressure of *80* to *110.*

5. The cure for PIH is *delivery.*

6. The onset of PIH can be as late as *48 hours after delivery.*

7. Continuous electronic fetal monitoring is used in labor because of potential *uteroplacental insufficiency (late decelerations) from the PIH* and *decreased beat-to-beat variability from the magnesium sulfate.*

• •

CESAREAN DELIVERY

Cesarean is an alternative to vaginal delivery and is the method of childbirth for nearly 20 percent of all deliveries in the United States. It is abdominal surgery requiring an incision through the uterine wall. The first cesarean a woman has is a *primary cesarean.* Those that follow are *repeats,* or *elective repeats.* The delivery may occur before any uterine contractions occur, or as late as after many hours of labor. Several variations of vertical and transverse uterine incisions can be made but the low segment transverse is the incision of choice due to increased healing ability, less bleeding, low infection rate, and feasibility of having a vaginal delivery with subsequent pregnancies.[35]

The operative procedure may be preplanned (elective) for a variety of reasons including obvious feto-pelvic disproportion, a uterus with an upper segment vertical scar, the presence of active herpes genitalia, or a chronic state of maternal distress such as severe cardiac disease. In these cases, the mode of delivery may be determined long before the surgery is performed. The cesarean delivery may also be an unanticipated emergency as in the case of severe maternal bleeding, or failure to progress despite quality contractions that become increasingly stressful to the fetus. Women who are eligible for a "trial of labor" but do not progress normally also become candidates for cesarean births. Examples include when a fetus is suspected of being slightly large for the pelvis, when the woman's hypertensive state is initially stable but becomes out of control and contributes to fetal distress, or when the induction following spontaneous rupture of membranes fails to cause labor progress. (A more extensive list is presented in Table 8–5.)

Emotional Aspects Prior to Cesarean Delivery

Emotional sequelae are inherent in all major surgeries. Cesarean delivery is no exception. There is **injury, potential for; trauma (to the mother and baby) related to the reasons for and the procedure involved in the cesarean.** Although the surgery is relatively safe, there are physical sequelae such as increased incidence of maternal infection and hemorrhage, and increased neonatal morbidity, especially transient tachypnea. Mothers experience a sense of guilt or failure, uncertainty, and disappointment. There is **self-concept, disturbance: self-esteem related to cesarean birth implying failure in the ability to give birth "normally."** There may also be a sense of **fear (of the unknown) related to the condition of self/fetus, pain, procedures, and outcomes.** Support is a vital ingredient that needs to be provided by the hospital staff, as well as family members. One form of support is to alleviate fear that occurs from **knowledge**

Table 8–5. REASONS FOR CESAREAN DELIVERIES

PREPLANNED, ELECTIVE	UNANTICIPATED, EMERGENCY
Fetal (or cephalo) pelvic disproportion	Severe maternal bleeding (abruptio placenta, placenta previa)
Uterine scar tissue, previous cesarean	Fetal distress when vaginal delivery impossible (at times)
Active herpes genitalia	Prolapsed cord
Severe cardiac disease	Failed forceps delivery
Severe preeclampsia/eclampsia	
>30% placenta previa	
Malpresentation (transverse lie, breech in nullip/possibly others)	
Pending fetal distress, evident in biophysical profiles, non-stress or stress tests	
Chronic fetal distress (severe Rh disease, etc.)	
Locked twins	
DETERMINED FOLLOWING TRIAL OF LABOR	
Failure to progress (FTP), prolonged labor	
Unstable maternal blood pressure causing fetal distress	
Failed induction	

deficit [about the reasons for the cesarean, the procedures, methods of relaxation and pain relief] related to lack of exposure, lack of recall. The nurse should anticipate decreased **coping, ineffective individual related to being tired from labor or lacking sleep.**

Confirming Diagnostic Procedures

For several reasons, including legal, physicians must be certain that a cesarean is the best medical management for a particular woman. When in doubt, additional tests or advice must be sought. Ultrasound is often used to verify the location of the placenta or extent of uterine bleeding, the presentation of the fetus, and so forth. Amniocentesis may be necessary to confirm mature fetal age. Continuous fetal monitoring provides data about the contractions and fetal heart rate. Fetal pH may confirm the suspicions about fetal well-being. (Ultrasound, amniocentesis and fetal pH are discussed in Chapter 9; monitoring is in Chapter 3.) At times, another physician will be consulted to verify the attending physician's conclusions. The decision to perform the cesarean must be discussed by the physician with the woman, and she must sign a consent form. These activities, as well as the physical preparation for the cesarean, are stressful to the pregnant woman who becomes increasingly concerned about both her well-being and that of her baby.

• •

Review Questions

1. Under what three general circumstances is a cesarean delivery performed?
   a. ______
   b. ______
   c. ______
2. What are four emotional problems the nurse is likely to find in a woman experiencing a cesarean delivery?
   a. ______
   b. ______
   c. ______
   d. ______
3. What are five procedures often done to confirm the need for a cesarean delivery?
   a. ______ d. ______
   b. ______ e. ______
   c. ______

Answers

1. A cesarean delivery can be done under the following general circumstances: (a)

preplanned, elective; (b) emergency (unanticipated); (c) following an unsuccessful trial of labor.

2. Emotional problems the nurse is likely to find in a woman experiencing a cesarean delivery include: (a) fear of potential injury to self and baby; (b) self-esteem deficit; (c) fear of pain, procedures, and outcome; (d) fear due to knowledge deficit about cesarean delivery; and (e) decreased coping ability.

3. Procedures that are often done to confirm the need for a cesarean delivery include: (a) ultrasound, (b) amniocentesis, (c) continuous electronic fetal monitoring, (d) fetal pH, and (e) consultation with another physician.

• •

Preparation Prior to Cesarean Delivery

A nursing assessment is done in order to plan nursing care. In addition, a history and physical is usually done by the physician on all women just prior to or upon admission to the labor unit. In women who are given a trial of labor, a blood type and screen may be part of the admission workup. "If unusual antibodies are present, then cross-matched blood is necessary."[36] Two units of blood need to be made available in case of excessive blood loss. There is **cardiac output, alteration in: decreased related to excessive blood loss, positional changes, anesthetic/analgesic reactions**. When a cesarean is decided on, if a CBC and serology have not already been drawn, they are done now. A hematocrit of 33 or higher is preferred in order to have a good post-operative period.[37]

The physician is responsible for discussing the contents of the Informed Consent Form—the need for the operation, the anesthesia to be used, and consequences of alternate approaches—with the woman and preferably her support person. The nurse should be present to repeat and clarify the information as necessary. Preferably the couple senses that they are involved in the decision to do the cesarean. Such couples are likely to view the birth more positively. In an emergency, there is little time for lengthy discussion but clear explanations and emotional support are needed. Either the physician or nurse can obtain the woman's signature (or that of the support person's in some places, if she is unable to sign) on the consent form that grants permission for the operation and anesthesia. The woman's preference for the type of anesthesia to be used may be expressed and considered but often her physical condition or the preference of the physician and anesthesiologist is the determinant. (See Chapter 6.) If time permits, the nurse should explain what to expect during and following the cesarean, and provide an opportunity for expression of any concerns.

If an IV is not already running, the nurse is then involved in starting one to provide an open route for administration of medications, fluids, and blood. Commonly, blood administration tubing is used and Ringers lactate or 5% dextrose in water is hung. One to two liters is infused during and immediately following the operation. The nurse should anticipate that 20 units of oxytocin will be added following the birth of the infant's shoulders or the placenta. In order to prevent bladder distention, a retention (Foley) catheter is inserted and attached to dependent drainage. The nurse must be certain that there is proper drainage. Hospital routine and the situation (preplanned versus emergency) may determine whether the Foley is inserted before or after anesthesia is administered. A specimen for urinalysis is usually collected immediately after insertion.

The nurse also must remove all valuables, providing for their safe keeping, and take routine preop precautions (remove fingernail polish or artificial nails, dentures, glasses, contact lenses, etc.). An abdominal scrub is done with antiseptic soap/solution followed by a shave from the xiphoid cartilage just below the breasts, to and including the upper pubic area, and out to the far sides. Care must be taken to avoid **skin integrity, impairment of: potential related to knicks in the skin from the shaving process.**

In some hospitals, preop medications are given. Except for these medications, the woman should be kept NPO for at least 8 hours pre-op. Some medications decrease the **anxiety [specify] related to the cesarean procedure.** Secobarbital may be given at bedtime in the hospital or at home the night before if the cesarean was preplanned. Atropine and a narcotic may be ordered "on call." A nonparticulate antacid (such as sodium citrate, 30 ml) is often given approximately 15 minutes before the anesthesia to decrease the risk of lung irritation from gastric hydrochloride if aspiration occurs. Aspiration could result in aspiration pneumonitis. Antibiotics may be indicated as in the presence of prolonged rupture of membranes and/or labor, or numerous vaginal examinations.

In addition to the above, the woman having an elective cesarean (not in labor) should be observed for prodromal signs of labor since they may alter the timing of the operation. For all women anticipating a cesarean, fetal heart rate, maternal vital signs, and labor status must be assessed periodically until transfer to the delivery/operating suite, with the frequency depending on the status of the labor, mother and fetus. At some hospitals a baseline fetal monitor strip is done prior to the cesarean.

The nurse is also responsible for notifying, or designating another responsible person to notify, other members of the delivery team (such as the anesthesia team, pediatrician, and nursery). She also inspects the delivery/operating room for adequacy of all equipment (including infant warmer, suction and cautery machine), and sets up as necessary. The support person is also dependent on the nurse since he/she needs to be readied for the delivery room and kept informed of the occurrences.

As time permits, it is helpful if the nurse explains to the woman and her support person (since he/she is often included in the delivery room and seated at the woman's head) the anticipated sequence of events and what sensations the mother is likely to experience.

Realistically, under regional anesthesia, the mother may feel a pulling sensation during the surgery. She will be awake, may not be able to move her legs, may smell and hear equipment used to ligate blood vessels and suction fluids, and may see the sponge count initially and at the end. She can also see and touch the baby if appropriate. Upon leaving the delivery room, she will go to the post-anesthesia recovery unit (PARU) or return to her LDR (see Chapter 7) where she will receive frequent nursing care and be given analgesia for her discomfort. For the woman experiencing an elective cesarean, preferably she received this information individually or in group classes prior to hospital admission.

At the time of transfer to the delivery suite, the nurse must ensure the presence of the correct patient and provide assistance in placing her securely on the delivery table. A left lateral tilt position (achieved with a blanket roll or other means) may be the routine position, or used only in the presence of hypotension. By shifting the uterus to the left side, it moves off the vena cava and prevents supine hypotension. The nurse assists the physicians with gowning and gloving, times and documents all events, and provides the necessary support to the mother and her support person. (Roles specific for the scrub and circulating nurses have been omitted here.)

Postoperative Care

Postoperatively, both post-delivery and post-operative needs must be immediately met. The uterine fundus must remain firmly contracted. While under the influence of anesthesia and/or analgesia, gentle palpation for assessment should be tolerable. Minimal to moderate vaginal bleeding (lochia) will normally occur. Assessment of the fundus, lochia, pulse, and blood pressure should be done every 15 minutes for at least the first hour, as in the vaginally delivered mother. The temperature is taken only once the first postoperative hour. The volume and consistency of urine output must be noted, as well as any drainage on the abdominal dressing. The rate of the intravenous fluid is dependent on the vital signs and uterine firmness, since ordinarily 20 units of Pitocin is added to the initial one or two IVs. Analgesia, especially for incisional pain, is likely to be given initially intramuscularly (ordinarily a total of 75 mg Demerol or 10 mg Morphine every 3 to 4 hours) or as a morphine epidural. Alternative forms of pain relief involve the use of patient-controlled analgesia (PCA) pump[38] and transcutaneous electrical nerve stimulation (TENS) (see Chapter 7). Consideration must be given to any previous medications given because a cumulative effect could cause respiratory depression and/or hypotension. Assessment is also done for the level of consciousness and, for the woman who received spinal anesthesia, the return of sensation to the lower extremities. Coughing and deep breathing (C&DB) and leg movements should be done. It is desirable that C&DB be practiced before the surgery but that is not always feasible. The effects of various anesthesias were discussed in Chapter 6. Except when the mother received general anesthesia or a large dose of narcotic, she is usually alert enough and eager to see, touch, and even hold her baby. Some wish to breast feed while in the delivery room or recovery room. The individual situation will determine the feasibility of maternal/infant interaction. It is the nurse's role to facilitate breast feeding and maternal-infant bonding in the early postpartal period. It is desirable to include family members whenever the situation permits.

• •

Review Questions

1. Put a check mark (✓) in front of those items which are routine preparation for a cesarean delivery:
 ____type and cross match for 2 units of blood ____CBC, serology ____x-ray ____enema ____signed informed consent form ____IV infusing ____retention (Foley) catheter inserted ____valuables, nail polish, contacts, etc. removed ____NPO ____abdominal scrub and shave ____preop medications, if ordered ____assess fetal heart rate, VS, labor progress until transferred to delivery suite ____notify delivery team (anesthesia, pediatrician, nursery, etc.) ____ready support person as necessary ____explain anticipated occurrences to woman and support person.

2. List 10 things the nurse assesses (monitors) during the immediate postoperative period:

a. ____	e. ____	h. ____
b. ____	f. ____	i. ____
c. ____	g. ____	j. ____
d. ____		

Answers

1. All of the above stated items except x-ray and enema are routine preparation for a cesarean delivery.
2. Immediately postoperatively, the nurse assesses/monitors: (a) fundus, (b) lochia, (c) pulse, and (d) blood pressure every 15 minutes; (e) temperature first hour; (f) urine volume and consistency; (g) IV rate; (h) need for analgesia; (i) level of consciousness and sensation; (j) coughing and deep breathing; and (k) desire/ability to handle baby.

• •

CONCLUSION

The selected maternal complications presented in this chapter, as well as those dispersed throughout this book, have implications for nursing care during the labor process. A critical nursing role is assessment—distinguishing normal from abnormal data, recognizing potential and actual complications. The nurse is responsible for making accurate assessments, for formulating nursing diagnoses, and for responding in an appropriate manner. Interventions must be consistent with established protocols (standards), and carried out in a timely fashion. Legally, the nurse is responsible for documenting the assessment data, actions taken, and results based on the nurse's evaluation. When complications occur, the nurse must think clearly and respond appropriately as the situation could be life threatening.

REFERENCES

1. U.S. Bureau of the Census: Statistical Abstracts of the United States, ed. 103. Government Printing Office, Washington, DC, 1982.
2. Bobak, IM and Jensen, MD: Essentials of Maternity Nursing: The Nurse and the Childbearing Family. CV Mosby, St. Louis, 1987, p 950.
3. Auvenshire, MA and Enriquez, MG: Maternity Nursing: Dimensions of Change. Wadsworth Health Sciences Division, Monterey, Calif., 1985, p 634.
4. National Center for Health Statistics: Monthly Vital Statistics Report 1980, No. 8. DHHS Publication No. (PHS) 83-1120, Nov. 1982.
5. Doenges, ME, Kenty, JR and Moorhouse, MF: Maternal/Newborn Care Plans: Guidelines for Client Care. FA Davis, Philadelphia, 1988, pp 92–97.
6. Pritchard, JA, MacDonald, PC and Gant, NF: Williams Obstetrics, ed. 17. Appleton-Century-Crofts, Norwalk, Connecticut, 1985, p 205.
7. Simpson, J and Verp, M: The prenatal diagnosis of genetic disorders. Cl Obstet Gynecol 25(4):640, 1982.
8. Gilbert, ES and Harmon, JS: High-Risk Pregnancy and Delivery: Nursing Perspectives. CV Mosby, St. Louis, 1986, p 423.
9. Pritchard, JA, MacDonald, PC and Gant, NF: Williams Obstetrics, ed. 17. Appleton-Century-Crofts, Norwalk, Connecticut, 1985, pp 504–505.
10. Knuppel, RA and Drukker, JE: High-Risk Pregnancy: A Team Approach. WB Saunders, Philadelphia, 1986, p 335.
11. Kirz, DS, et al: Advanced maternal age. The mature gravida. Am J Obstet Gynecol 152:7, 1985.
12. Stein, Z: Pregnancy in gravidas over age 35. J Nurse-Midwife 28:17, 1983.
13. Pritchard, JA, MacDonald, PC and Gant, NF: Williams Obstetrics, ed. 17. Appleton-Century-Crofts, Norwalk, Connecticut, 1985, p 3.
14. Winslow, W: First pregnancy after 35: What is the experience? Matern Child Nurs J 12(2):92, 1987.
15. Smith, J: The dangers of prenatal cocaine use. Matern Child Nurs J 13(1):174, 1988.
16. Jensen, MD and Bobak, IM: Maternity and Gynecologic Care: The Nurse and the Family, ed. 3. CV Mosby, St. Louis, 1985, p 1008.
17. Ouimette, J: Perinatal Nursing: Care of the High-Risk Mother and Infant. Jones and Bartlett, Boston, 1986, p 269.
18. Pritchard, JA, MacDonald, PC and Gant, NF: Williams Obstetrics, ed. 17. Appleton-Century-Crofts, Norwalk, Connecticut, 1985, p 259.
19. Pritchard, JA, MacDonald, PC and Gant, NF: Williams Obstetrics, ed. 17. Appleton-Century-Crofts, Norwalk, Connecticut, 1985, p 788.
20. Angelini, DJ, Knapp, CMW and Gibes, RM (eds): Perinatal/Neonatal Nursing: A Clinical Handbook. Blackwell Scientific Publications, Boston, 1986, p 210.

21. Lanvin, J, et al: Vaginal delivery in patients with a prior cesarean section: A review of the literature from 1950–1980. Obstet and Gynecol 59:135–150, 1982.
22. Jacobson, H: A standard for assessing lochia volume. Matern Child Nurs J 10(3):174, 1985.
23. Pritchard, JA and Pritchard, S: Standardized treatment of 154 consecutive cases of eclampsia. Am J Obstet Gynecol 123(5):543, 1975.
24. Ouimette, J: Perinatal Nursing: Care of the High-Risk Mother and Infant. Jones and Bartlett, Boston, 1986, p 130.
25. Oxorn, H: Oxorn-Foote Human Labor & Birth, ed. 5. Appleton-Century-Crofts, Norwalk, Connecticut, 1986, p 849.
26. Angelini, DJ, Knapp, CMW and Gibes, RM (eds): Perinatal/Neonatal Nursing: A Clinical Handbook. Blackwell Scientific Publications, Boston, 1986, p 199.
27. Varney, H: Nurse-Midwifery, ed. 2. Blackwell Scientific Publications, Boston, 1987, pp 638–688.
28. Ouimette, J: Perinatal Nursing: Care of the High-Risk Mother and Infant. Jones and Bartlett, Boston, 1986, p 118.
29. Paul, RH, Koh, KS and Bernstein, SG: Changes in fetal heart rate-uterine contraction patterns associated with eclampsia. Am J OB Gynecol 130(2):165–169, 1978.
30. Pritchard, JA: The use of magnesium sulfate in preeclampsia-eclampsia. J Reprod Med 23(107):107–114, 1979.
31. Zuspan, FP: Hypertension in pregnancy. In Quillan, EJ and Kretchmer, N (eds): Fetal and Maternal Medicine. John Wiley & Sons, New York, 1982.
32. Angelini, DJ, Knapp, CMW and Gibes, RM (eds): Perinatal/Neonatal Nursing: A Clinical Handbook. Blackwell Scientific Publications, Boston, 1986, pp 196–197.
33. Gant, N and Worley, R: Hypertension in pregnancy: Concepts and management. Appleton-Century-Crofts, New York, 1980.
34. Ouimette, J: Perinatal Nursing: Care of the High-Risk Mother and Infant. Jones and Bartlett, Boston, 1986, p 129.
35. Oxorn, H: Oxorn-Foote Human Labor & Birth, ed. 5. Appleton-Century-Crofts, Norwalk, Connecticut, 1986, p 804.
36. Knuppel, RA and Drukker, JE: High-Risk Pregnancy: A Team Approach. WB Saunders, Philadelphia, 1986, p 260.
37. Pritchard, JA, MacDonald, PC, and Gant, NF: Williams Obstetrics, ed. 17. Appleton-Century-Crofts, Norwalk, Connecticut, 1985, p 881.
38. White, PF: Patient-controlled analgesia: a new approach to the management of postoperative pain. Seminars in Anesthesia 4(3):155, 1985.

BIBLIOGRAPHY

Angelini, DJ, Knapp DMW and Gibes, RM (eds): Perinatal/Neonatal Nursing: A Clinical Handbook. Blackwell Scientific Publications, Boston, 1986.

Auvenshire, MA and Enriquez, MG: Maternity Nursing: Dimensions of Change. Wadsworth Health Sciences Division, Monterey, Calif., 1985.

Bobak, IM and Jensen, MD: Essentials of Maternity Nursing: The Nurse and the Childbearing Family, ed. 2. CV Mosby, St. Louis, 1987.

Doenges, ME, Kenty, JR and Moorhouse, MF: Maternal/Newborn Care Plans: Guidelines for Client Care. FA Davis, Philadelphia, 1988.

Gilbert, ES and Harmon, JS: High-Risk Pregnancy and Delivery: Nursing Perspectives. CV Mosby, St. Louis, 1986.

Knor, ER: Decision Making in Obstetrical Nursing. BC Decker, Toronto, 1987.

Morgan, BS and Barden, ME: Unwed and Pregnant: Nurses' attitudes toward unmarried mothers. Matern Child Nurs J 10(2):114, 1985.

Neeson, JD and May, KA: Comprehensive Maternity Care: Nursing Process and the Childbearing Family. JB Lippincott, Philadelphia, 1986.

Ouimette, J: Perinatal Nursing: Care of the High-Risk Mother and Infant. Jones and Bartlett, Boston, 1986.

Panzarine, S, Elster, A, and McAnarney, ER: A systems approach to adolescent pregnancy. J Obstet Gynecol Neonatal Nurs 10(4):287, 1981.

Pritchard, JA, MacDonald, PC and Gant, NF: Williams Obstetrics, ed. 17. Appleton-Century-Crofts, Norwalk, Connecticut, 1985.

Reeder, SJ and Martin, LL: Maternity Nursing: Family, Newborn, and Women's Health Care. ed. 16. JB Lippincott, Philadelphia, 1987.

Smith, JE: The dangers of prenatal cocaine use. Matern Child Nurs J 13(3):174, 1988.

Whitney, N: A Manual of Clinical Obstetrics. JB Lippincott. Philadelphia, 1985.

Winslow, W: First pregnancy after 35: What is the experience? Matern Child Nurs J 12(2):92, 1987.

POST-TEST 8

CASE 1: A 14-year-old, G1PO with EDC tomorrow, arrives at the labor unit with her mother. Both women are extremely anxious because the antepartal clinic doctor sent them over immediately because the young girl is in labor. The clinical chart states upon vaginal examination she was found to be 3 cm dilated, 0 station, 50% effaced, and her blood pressure is 150/100. Previously her range was 100–120/60–80.

What interventions should the nurse take?

CASE 2: A 38-year-old nullipara at term experienced a normal course of pregnancy and labor up until now. She knew from the start that her baby may be too large for her pelvis but she wanted a trial of labor. After two hours of strong, every 2 minutes, 50–60 seconds contractions, she remained 8 cm and 0 station. Caput was palpated on the fetal head. Her physician explained the options to the woman, and upon joint decision, decided to do a cesarean delivery immediately. He obtained her signed consent. She accepted the decision well having previously learned that this may happen to her and realizing this may be the safest delivery method for her baby.

What nursing preparation is appropriate for this woman?

CASE 3: C.A. arrives on the labor unit of a large medical center complaining of vaginal bleeding and pain. She came by ambulance because she had no other transportation. She is a poor historian and gives no indication of having seen a doctor during her pregnancy. Her fundal height is consistent with approximately 35 weeks' gestation. She copes poorly with contractions that are 8 to 10 minutes and mild upon palpation. She denies taking drugs in the past three months but says she occasionally used street drugs before realizing she might be pregnant.

a. Identify what initial actions the nurse should take:

b. Identify what medical interventions are likely:

Answers

CASE 1: The following nursing interventions should be taken for this anxious young adolescent, pregnant for the first time, at term, in early labor, hypertensive for the first time, and accompanied by her anxious mother:

- Place her in a private room, encouraging the mother to stay with the laboring girl.
- Be calm, provide brief explanation of status.
- Explain need to stay in bed, lie on left side, have side rails up.
- Keep room quiet, softly lit and unstimulating.
- Place "preeclamptic tray" in room.
- Take initial history, including blood pressure, patellar reflex, clonus, discomforts, and behavioral response.
- Repeat blood pressure at least hourly.
- Assess each voiding for protein and amount. If catheter is inserted, assess urine at 1 to 2 hour intervals.
- Continuously monitor uterine contractions and fetal heart rate by electronic monitor.
- Inform physician of her current status.
- Anticipate order for intravenous line, blood type and cross-match.
- Assess her labor progress.
- Determine her prenatal education and preparation.
- Assist with relaxation and breathing techniques.
- Anticipate low pain threshold.
- Assist her, and her mother, to cope with labor, providing very basic information.
- Allow her to make decisions when possible.
- Respect her modesty.
- Immediately inform physician of progressive symptoms of PIH (see text).

CASE 2: The following nursing preparation is appropriate for this woman, experiencing a trial of labor that arrests in the transition phase due to cephalopelvic disproportion, and by joint decision, consents to a cesarean delivery:

- Anticipate that the cesarean delivery adds to her stress level and feeling of lack of control and possible feeling of failure.
- Discuss her expectations for during and immediately following the delivery.
- Seek information from her about how the nurse can best help her.
- Keep NPO.
- Following doctor's orders,
  - Obtain type and screen/cross-match, CBC, and serology.
  - Start intravenous using blood administration tubing.
  - Insert Foley catheter to dependent drainage and collect specimen for urinalysis.
- Collect valuables and remove polish, contacts, etc.
- Scrub and shave abdomen.
- Administer preoperative medications, if ordered.
- Notify involved members of the delivery team.
- Set up the delivery room.
- Physically and intellectually prepare the support person.
- Verify identification of woman.
- Transfer her to operating suite and position her securely on the table.

CASE 3: For C.A., a "walk-in" of approximately 35 weeks' gestation, who admits to using street drugs until 3 months ago, is coping poorly with mild, 8 to 10 minute

contractions, and now complains of vaginal bleeding and pains.
(a) The following nursing actions should be taken initially:

- Confine her to bed.
- Apply a perineal pad and assess it periodically.
- Have her inform the nurse of increased bleeding or uterine changes.
- Place her in left lateral position with head of bed elevated 20 to 30 degrees.
- Assess blood pressure, pulse, respirations and temperature at least hourly.
- Apply continuous electronic monitor for uterine contractions and fetal heart rate.
- Take history, including:
  Amount, color, consistency, and frequency (first time?) of bleeding.
  Presence of uterine pain between contractions.
- Mark fundal height with a pen.
- Perform Leopold's maneuvers noting in particular signs of malpresentation.
- Provide emotional support and encouragement.
- Discuss her knowledge of labor/delivery and provide the basics, as necessary.

(b) The following medical interventions can be anticipated:

- Order for IV, type and cross-match, hematocrit and hemoglobin, and analgesia as necessary.
- Order for ultrasound to determine source and extent of bleeding and fetal size.
- Delay vaginal exam until known diagnosis for bleeding.
- Do speculum exam.

9 FETAL WELL-BEING IN PRETERM AND POST-TERM GESTATION

Janet S. Malinowski

OBJECTIVES

Upon completing this chapter, you will be able to:

- Define preterm and post-term gestation.
- Relate three psychological effects that a preterm labor or a post-term labor are likely to have on a woman.
- Specify four physiologic hindrances to transition to extra-uterine life that occur in the preterm infant and four in the post-term infant.
- Explain and interpret at least three methods nurses use to determine the gestational age of a fetus.
- Indicate five measures that women can take to avoid preterm labor.
- Describe the rationale for, and the nursing interventions involved in, the following tests: ambulatory home monitoring, ultrasound, amniocentesis, nonstress test, contraction stress test/nipple stimulation test, fetal scalp pH sampling.
- State the nursing implications of administering betamethasone, ritodrine, terbutaline, isoxsuprine, magnesium sulfate, and ethanol.
- State five nursing measures to be instituted when preterm delivery is imminent.
- Compare physical features of a preterm infant with those of a post-term infant.
- Identify four physiological tasks of mothers of preterm infants.
- Discuss four ways that a nurse can facilitate parental-infant attachment following a preterm birth.

- Identify the components of the biophysical profile used to assess fetal well-being.
- Explain appropriate nursing interventions to be used during post-term labor.
- Identify the immediate care needed following delivery, based on the physiologic disadvantages of the post-term infant.

Delivery within 2 weeks of the predetermined due date is expected by both pregnant women and health professionals. There is a significant increase in infant morbidity and mortality when labor occurs before 38 weeks (preterm), as well as when labor has not occurred by 42 weeks (post-term). Preterm labor may start spontaneously or may be medically induced (started) because of concern about fetal well-being. Post-term labor usually is medically induced if it does not start spontaneously.

This chapter presents the reasons for concern and the interventions that can be used for preterm and post-term labors, including many methods used to determine fetal well-being. Probably the most relied-upon tool for fetal status is the assessment of fetal heart rate which was addressed in Chapter 3. The nurse plays a key role in providing information, emotional support, and physical care when fetal well-being is questioned.

PRETERM LABOR

Psychological Effects of Preterm Labor on the Mother

In order to appreciate the broad implications of a preterm labor, the nurse most consider the effects on both the fetus and the mother. Pregnancy is a time for maturation of the fetus and the mother. Forty weeks, plus or minus 2 weeks, are required for this to occur. If the fetus is delivered before 38 weeks' gestation, the chances of a healthy outcome are decreased because the baby is physically immature. For this reason the preterm infant is also called *premature*.

If the mother delivers before 38 weeks, she may not have had sufficient time to physically and mentally prepare for her new role. It is during the last trimester that the mother begins to *nest*—to do most of the preparation for the new baby's arrival. It is the time when she begins to *let go* of some habits and activities that conflict with caring for a new baby. Around the seventh month of pregnancy, she begins to think about possibly losing and hurting the baby. This is apparent in the overprotective shielding of self. As her due date approaches, these fears begin to subside. She actively wishes for termination of the pregnancy, separation from the fetus, and an ending to the symbiotic relationship that has existed between the fetus and herself. By the last few weeks of a full-term pregnancy, she is physically uncomfortable due to her large-sized abdomen, clumsiness, and fatigue.

The woman who goes into preterm labor may not have completed the preparatory processes. She may not be ready to break the close relationship that she has with the fetus. The result is that she may not be ready to take on the role of "mother" as quickly or as easily as a woman who has carried her baby to term. There is **self concept, disturbance in: role performance related to the untimely labor**. She is also justified in having concerns about or **anxiety [specify] related to the well-being of her preterm baby**.

• •

Review Question

State three ways in which a woman who experiences a preterm labor may not psychologically be prepared for her baby.

a. ____________________

b. ____________________

c. ____________________

Answer

Psychologically a woman may not be prepared for preterm labor because of the following:

a. She may not have completed nesting—preparing for the baby's arrival.
b. She may not have let go of the things in her life that conflict with caring for a new baby.
c. She may have great fears of losing or hurting her baby, especially in the seventh month of pregnancy.
d. She may wish to continue to carry her baby in utero rather than to be separated from a fetus that has become so much a part of her.

• •

Physiologic Hindrances of the Preterm Infant

Babies born prematurely (at a gestational age of less than 38 weeks, or before the completion of the 37th week, but at least 20 weeks) are called *preterm*. The closer babies are to term, the better their chances of survival. For many reasons preterm infants have difficulty maintaining physiologic homeostasis and, therefore, are constantly threatened by many stressors. The following facts are presented so that the reader will better appreciate the need for sound medical judgment in determining whether or not the fetus is mature enough to be delivered.

Preterm infants are hampered by difficult respirations. The medulla oblongata, the center of the brain controlling respirations, is poorly developed. The intercostal muscles and soft thoracic cage are weak. The involved alveolar capillaries are few in number, and oxygen utilization is inefficient owing to insufficient surfactant (which decreases surface tension) in the alveoli.

Preterm infants have poor control of body temperature owing to the immature thermal control center of the brain, poor peripheral circulation, large surface area with little fatty insulation, and low heat production.

Preterm infants experience a disturbance in the intake and utilization of food. They tire easily and have a weak suck. Their stomach capacity is small, and the existing enzymes are insufficient for complete digestion and absorption.

Preterm infants are unable to handle infections adequately. They have thin, fragile skin and mucous membranes that are poor barriers against infection. They have a low level of antibodies circulating in the plasma (immunoglobins), immature ability for phagocytosis (bacterial destruction), and an inability to localize infection.

Preterm infants have a tendency toward anemia and hemorrhage. Their thin, fragile capillaries are easily damaged. Their slow response to vitamin K_1 further complicates their rapidly falling hemoglobin level and decreased coagulation factors.

Preterm infants also are disadvantaged by a tendency toward fluid-electrolyte imbalance caused by an inability to excrete sodium and chloride and to concentrate urine. They also have inadequate stores of glycogen and calcium.

• •

Review Question

List four physiological hindrances found in the preterm infant.

a. ______________________________

b. ______________________________

c. ______________________________

d. ______________________________

Answer

A preterm infant has the following physiologic hindrances:

a. Respirations are difficult and inefficient.
b. Body temperature is poorly controlled.
c. Intake and utilization of food are disturbed—poor intake, poor use.
d. Response to infection is poor.
e. A strong tendency toward anemia and hemorrhage exists.
f. Fluid and electrolytes are unbalanced. The premature infant is unable to excrete, concentrate, and store them adequately.

• •

Methods of Determining Gestational Age

The admitting nurse on the labor/delivery unit is responsible (see Chapter 10) for recognizing whether the laboring woman is preterm or post-term. The nurse cannot totally rely on the stated due date. She needs to note if there are discrepancies in the calculations or measurements—especially Naegele's rule, fundal height, and gestational age reports from ultrasonic studies.

During routine antepartum care several techniques are performed by the nurse or physician to approximate the gestational age:

1. The *EDC* (estimated date of confinement or delivery) is determined by using Naegele's rule: Subtract 3 months from and add 7 days and 1 year to the first day of the woman's last (normal) menstrual period (LMP or LNMP).

   EXAMPLE:

   LMP = 5/10/89; EDC = 2/17/90.

   There are 40 weeks between 5/10/89 and 2/17/90.

   Several other methods are necessary to confirm gestational age because using the LMP may be erroneous for 20 to 40 percent of women.[1]
2. The time of *quickening* (the woman's first perception of fetal movement) is often determined during the assessment process. Fetal activity, felt as slight fluttering movements in the abdomen, begins sometime between 16 and 20 weeks following the LMP.[2,3] Gillieson and colleagues[4] found that quickening occurs earlier in the multigravida than in the primigravida. Because of the wide variability in occurrence and potential misinterpretation of intestinal peristalsis, quickening is no longer recommended as a determinant of EDC.
3. Using an ultrasonic device (for example, a Doppler), the *fetal heart rate* (FHR) can first be heard about 10 to 12 weeks. Using a fetoscope the FHR can first be heard at 17 to 19 weeks.[5]
4. The *fundal height* is measured from the upper border of the symphysis pubis to the top of the fundus. The fundus is usually midway between the symphysis pubis and umbilicus at 16 weeks. At 20 weeks the fundus is at or just below the umbilicus. After 20 weeks, the number of weeks' gestation is equal to the fundal height in centimeters, plus or minus 2 cm (for example, 24 weeks = 22 to 26 cm). This is commonly known as McDonald's rule. At 24 weeks the fundus is just above the umbilicus. A uterus larger than expected is significant because it may be due to multiple gestation, hydatidiform mole, hydramnios, or maternal diabetes. A large uterus can also indicate a large but healthy fetus. Conversely, a smaller-than-expected uterus may indicate intrauterine growth retardation (IUGR). IUGR may be associated with chronic intrauterine insufficiency, fetal anomalies, or a normal, small-size fetus.

Further diagnostic measures (ultrasound, x-ray, amniocentesis) may be necessary if there is uncertainty about the gestational period. Ultrasound (U/S) is preferred to x-ray because there are known fetal effects from radiation, but no known harmful effects from U/S.[6]

Gray-scale imaging *ultrasound* is done in the x-ray or radiology department because of the cumbersome equipment involved. At the time of assessment, the pregnant woman must have a full bladder so that the relationship of other structures, especially the placenta, can be viewed. Fluids may be forced orally or intravenously. The mother may complain of **comfort, alteration in: pain, acute from the full bladder related to the U/S procedure**. However, the U/S procedure is painless as a transducer arm repeatedly sweeps across the abdominal surface.

Real-time scanning U/S can be done with a portable machine at the hospital bedside. It projects images on a 12-inch television screen. The astute U/S technician or nurse will use the opportunity to point out major landmarks, including the placenta and umbilical cord, explaining their functions. By seeing her baby's image, the mother's fantasy of the baby becomes a reality. There is no need to fill the bladder for this procedure. With the mother in a supine position, an ultrasonic gel is used to coat her abdomen, and then a transducer scans the abdominal surface. There should be no pain involved.

Although radiographic studies (x-rays) may be performed in a small number of institutions, U/S usually is used to determine gestational age. Several measurements can be done:

1. *Crown-rump*, which is very accurate between 8 to 13 weeks' gestation.[1]
2. *Femoral calcification*, which is accurate up to 24 weeks' gestation.[7]
3. Bi-parietal diameter (BPD), which is most accurate in the second trimester, 95 percent accurate within ± 11 days from 17 to 26 weeks.[1] This method is a very common measurement used for determining gestational age.

U/S and x-ray also help to determine fetal weight and growth.

Placental maturity can be determined by U/S. The amount of calcium deposition and status of fibrous tissue are used to grade the placenta (see Table 9–1). When grade II placenta is present, amniocentesis may be unnecessary to determine lecithin/sphingomyelin (L/S) ratio.[11,12] (See next few paragraphs.) Caution is warranted in accepting the accuracy of this method for determining fetal maturity since some investigators have found that in high-risk pregnancies a mature L/S ratio is not always found with a grade III placenta.[13] It is apparent that there is inconsistency in interpreting fetal maturity using placental grading.

Amniocentesis involves a transabdominal puncture through the uterus and amniotic sac using a needle and syringe to remove amniotic fluid. One purpose of amniocentesis is to obtain laboratory speci-

Table 9–1. PLACENTAL GRADING

GRADE	FEATURES	GESTATIONAL AGE
0	Homogeneous tissue	Through week 27
I	Well-defined chorionic plate Mature L/S ratio 67% of time[8]	At least 28 weeks to term
II	Better-defined landmarks Mature L/S ratio 87.5% of time[8]	At least 28 weeks to term
III	Individual placental cotyledons visible Mature L/S ratio 100% of time[8]	May mean placental dysfunction[9,10]

mens that indicate fetal maturity. The specimens are assessed for L/S ratio, foam, creatinine, fat cells, and phospholipids (to name the most common assays). Another reason for amniocentesis in the third trimester is to test for Rh-hemolytic disease, amnionitis, and passage of meconium in the post-term pregnancy.[14]

Prior to the removal of amniotic fluid from the uterine cavity, the procedure must be explained to the mother and a consent form signed. (See Chapter 10.) Maternal **anxiety [specify] related to amniocentesis** is common. Studies show[15] that mothers fear injury to the fetus, the results of the tests, and the anticipated pain. Injury is possible although unlikely when the procedure is performed by a skilled physician. To prevent penetration of the placenta with the needle, sonographic localization of the placenta is recommended.[16,17] If the umbilical cord is punctured, "it will be manifested by a fall in maternal blood pressure and fetal *tachycardia*."[15] The results of the amniocentesis will influence the medical management, which can range from immediate delivery to postponement of the delivery. To alleviate the pain involved, local anesthetic is sometimes used at the site of entry into the abdomen. The discomfort is slight—comparable to having blood drawn. At other times, the anesthetic is omitted because the insertion of the needle is considered to be equally painful whether it is used for administering an anesthetic or for the amniotic procedure itself. Often physicians will give the woman a choice of whether to have local anesthetic.

Before and immediately after the amniocentesis, and at least 2 hours later, the fetal heart rate must be assessed. To avoid supine hypotension during the procedure, the mother lies on her side, propped with pillows or with her head and shoulders elevated. The nurse cleanses the abdomen with antiseptic (Betadine) solution using sterile technique. With a long 20- to 22-gauge needle, 20 to 50 ml of amniotic fluid is removed by the doctor. After the procedure is done, the Betadine solution is removed with pHisoHex and water, the area is dried, and the insertion site is bandaged. Blood pressure, fetal heart rate, and uterine activity are assessed. One risk of amniocentesis is the onset of labor. The amniotic fluid is sent to the laboratory for the following possible fetal maturity studies:

1. The *L/S ratio* can only predict fetal lung maturity. Gluck and associates[18,19] determined that the surfactant level is sufficiently mature when the L/S ratio is 2:1 which occurs between 33 to 37 weeks. With a 2:1 ratio there is enough *surfactant* (made up chiefly of lecithin) secreted by the fetal lungs to facilitate pulmonary gas exchange at the time of extrauterine breathing. Respiratory distress syndrome (RDS) is unlikely to develop. An exception is the infant of a diabetic mother, in which case a 2:1 ratio does not assure lung maturity. Some situations are thought to accelerate lung maturation; these include prolonged rupture of membranes[20-23] and pregnancy-induced hypertension.[15] In order for the amniotic fluid sample to be reliable for L/S ratio, it must be free of blood and meconium.
2. The *foam* or *shake test* is a simple, rapid test for lung maturity but is less precise than the L/S ratio. By mixing one part 90 percent ethanol with two parts amniotic fluid in a test tube, foam (bubbles) appears on the surface. If 15 minutes later a complete ring of foam remains, lung maturity is assumed. False-positive results are possible.
3. *Creatinine*, which indicates increased fetal muscle mass, is secreted by the fetal kidneys into the amniotic fluid. By at least 37 weeks' gestation there are 2 mg of creatinine per 100 ml of amniotic fluid. This indirectly measures fetal pulmonary maturity in the presence of a normal maternal plasma creatinine level.[24]
4. *Fat cells* from the fetal skin are also found in amniotic fluid. When stained with Nile blue, if more than 20 percent of the fluid is fat cells, the gestational age is thought to be 36 weeks or more.[25]
5. The surfactant *phospholipids* are measured in the process of doing a lung profile on the amniotic fluid. One of these lipids is *phosphatidyl glycerol* (PG), which is a lung stabilizer. When PG is present and the L/S ratio is 2:1 or greater, the diagnosis of lung maturity is more accurate. In the insulin-dependent-diabetic mother, without PG there is an increased incidence of neonatal lung immaturity, hypoglycemia, and size large for gestational age. In some parts of the country (e.g., in Louisiana), PG is done in place of L/S ratio. Because PG is thought to be unaffected by blood in the amniotic fluid, it may be more accurate.

• •

Review Questions

1. Methods of determining gestational age are listed in the chart below. Hypothetical findings are given. Fill in the third column with your estimate of the gestational age.

ESTIMATING GESTATIONAL AGE		ESTIMATE OF
Method	Finding	GESTATIONAL AGE
a. EDC compared with today's date	a. Preterm	a.
b. Quickening	b. Experienced 4 weeks ago	b.
c. Fetal heart rate	c. Not audible by fetoscope but audible by Doppler	c.
d. Fundal height	d. 27 cm	d.
e. Amniotic fluid via amniocentesis	e.	e.
1. L/S ratio	1. 2:1	1.
2. Foam test	2. + foam ring in 15 min	2.
3. Creatinine	3. 2 mg/100 ml fluid	3.
4. Fat cells	4. More than 20%	4.
5. Phospholipids	5. Present	5.

2. Circle the correct response: The nurse is responsible for assuring that the mother has a (full, empty) bladder at the time of an ultrasound done in the radiology department.

3. List at least five nursing interventions to be taken during an amniocentesis.
   a. ______________________________
   b. ______________________________
   c. ______________________________
   d. ______________________________
   e. ______________________________

Answers

1. a. If the finding is preterm, the gestational age is less than 38 weeks. Therefore, the EDC must be at least 2 weeks before today's date.
   b. If quickening occurred 4 weeks ago, gestation is 20 to 24 weeks, although quickening is not a reliable determinant of EDC.
   c. A fetal heart rate not audible by fetoscope indicates less than 17 to 19 weeks' gestation, but FHR audible by Doppler indicates at least 10 to 12 weeks' gestation.
   d. Fundal height of 27 cm indicates approximately 27 weeks' gestation.
   e. 1. An L/S ratio of 2 : 1 indicates 33 to 37 weeks' gestation.
      2. The presence of a foam ring after 15 minutes indicates the fetal lungs are probably mature.
      3. Two mg of creatinine in 100 ml of fluid indicates at least 37 weeks' gestation.
      4. More than 20 percent fat cells indicates 36 weeks' or more gestation.

5. Presence of phospholipids along with 2 : 1 L/S ratio provides considerable assurance that there is fetal lung maturity.

2. The nurse is responsible for assuring a *full* bladder at the time of an ultrasound done in the radiology department.

3. Nursing interventions during an amniocentesis include the following:
   a. Determine the mother's understanding of the procedure and its purpose and reinforce as necessary.
   b. Verify that a consent form has been signed.
   c. Check fetal heart rate before, immediately after, and at least 2 hours following the procedure.
   d. Position mother on her side with head and shoulders slightly elevated.
   e. Cleanse abdomen with antiseptic solution using sterile technique.
   f. Provide support to the mother as needed.
   g. Remove Betadine with pHisoHex and water, air dry, and apply bandage after the procedure is completed.

• •

Interventions to Arrest Preterm Labor

Although premature labor often is associated with conditions such as abruptio placentae, premature rupture of membranes, overdistended uterus, or poor nutrition, the triggering factor is still unknown. Table 9–2 lists factors associated with preterm labor.

Nonpharmacological Interventions. It is a nursing responsibility to assess for preterm labor risk factors. Women at risk for preterm labor are often advised to:

1. Increase their rest periods
2. Decrease strenuous activity at home and at work
3. Limit their traveling to less than 1 to 2 hours at a time
4. Modify sexual activity (use a condom during intercourse to prevent entry of seminal prostaglandins, avoid breast stimulation, orgasm, and/or intercourse)
5. Avoid stress[26]

The early symptoms of preterm labor may be so subtle that they are ignored or misinterpreted by both the pregnant woman and the physician or nurse. There may be no pain, or there may be pressure, cramping with or without diarrhea, or intermittent or constant pain. The discomfort may involve the uterus, lower back, thigh, or pelvic or intestinal region. There may be changes in the vaginal discharge.[27]

The effectiveness of ambulatory monitoring of uterine activity has been studied and found to have a significant impact on the early diagnosis of preterm labor.[28,29] Because women who experience preterm labor have a significantly greater frequency of contractions than those who labor at term, and the rise in frequency can be observed within 24 hours before the development of preterm labor, intermittent use of an ambulatory monitor may offer an effective

Table 9–2. RISK FACTORS FOR PRETERM LABOR*

PRESENT SOCIOECONOMIC STATUS

1. More than two children at home without domestic help.
2. Low-income or unskilled work.
3. Single parent.
4. Inadequate support systems.
5. Maternal age less than 18 or greater than 35 years.
6. No prenatal care.
7. Lack of education.
8. Poor nutrition.

MEDICAL/OBSTETRIC HISTORY

1. Previous preterm labor.
2. Previous preterm delivery.
3. Two or more spontaneous or induced abortions.
4. Period of less than 1 year between the last birth and conception of present pregnancy.
5. Uterine anomaly that prevents expansion (hypoplastic uterus, septate or bicornuate uterus, intrauterine synechiae, leiomyomas).
6. DES exposure in utero.
7. Incompetent cervix.
8. Prepregnancy maternal weight of less than 100 lb (45.5 kg).
9. Maternal height less than 5 ft (152.4 cm).

LIFE STYLE

1. Smoking more than 10 cigarettes per day, alcoholism, or drug usage.
2. Factors that can cause excessive fatigue and may trigger uterine contractions.
3. Any event or series of events precipitating unusual anxiety.

CURRENT PREGNANCY

1. Uterine overdistention—multiple pregnancy, polyhydramnios, fibroids.
2. Bleeding—placenta previa, abruptio placentae, vasa previa.
3. Malformation of the fetus or the placenta or severe intrauterine growth retardation.
4. Weight gain of less than 10 lb (4.5 kg) by 26 weeks' gestation.
5. Weight loss of 5 lb (2.25 kg) at any time during pregnancy.
6. Maternal illness or disease—high fever; acute pyelonephritis; bacteriuria; albuminuria; generalized peritonitis; acute systemic bacterial or viral infections.
7. Fetal manipulation, such as invasive transfusions or fetal surgery.
8. Premature rupture of the membranes.
9. Abdominal surgery after the first trimester.
10. Cervical cerclage.

*From Herron, MA and Dulock, HL: Preterm Labor. Series 2: Prenatal Care, Module 5, ed 2. White Plains, New York: The March of Dimes Birth Defects Foundation, 1987, pp 11–12, with permission of the copyright holder and the authors.

way to identify women about to experience preterm labor.[30] The implication is that the preterm birth rate can be reduced if treatment is begun early enough. This in turn means a decrease in the number of days of hospitalization for mother and baby. The self-monitoring device involved provides objective measurement of uterine activity. Four or more contractions in an hour represent excessive uterine activity and hastens the need for diagnosis of preterm labor.[31] The self-monitoring device is light-weight and is worn on a belt around the abdomen just below the umbilicus (Fig. 9–1). It contains a data storage recorder capable of rapidly transmitting the

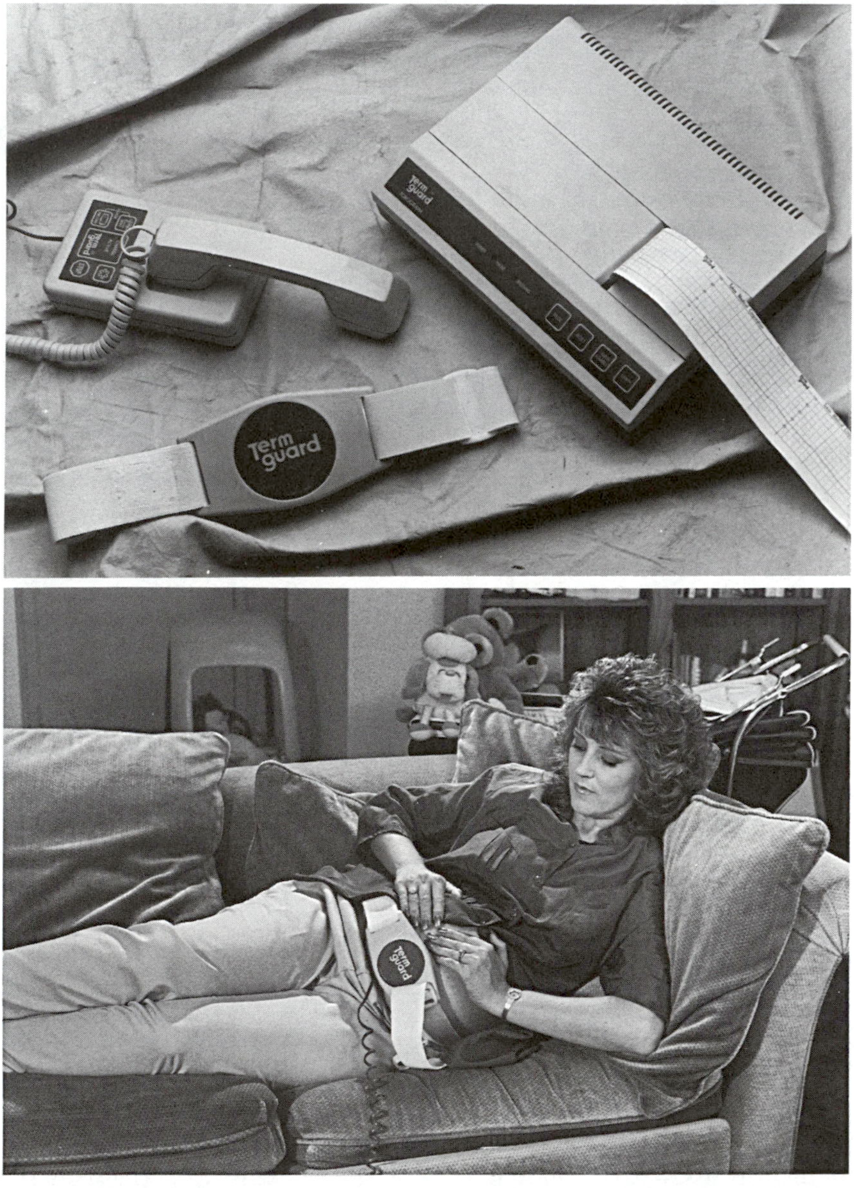

Figure 9–1. Ambulatory monitoring device for preterm uterine activity. (*Top*) Parts of the device. (*Bottom*) Device in use. (Courtesy of Tokos Medical Corporation)

uterine activity data over the telephone. A woman at risk for preterm labor wears the device at home, or while on break at work, for an hour 2 or 3 times a day. She is instructed about how to call in the data by phone at least twice a day to a center where the printout is interpreted by a nurse. Such a service is available 24 hours a day by means of an 800 number. Immediate therapy may be recommended based on interpretation of the data. This same phone service can be used for emotional support even when the findings are normal.

Rather than test the "contractions" by ambulating as is recommended in term gestation (see Chapter 5), the woman who experiences what is thought to be "preterm labor for more than 15 minutes while physically active should:

1. Empty her bladder,
2. Lie down,
3. Drink fluids (3 to 4 cups of juice or water),
4. Palpate for uterine contractions,
5. Rest for 30 minutes and gradually resume normal activity if symptoms subside, and
6. Call her health care provider if symptoms persist, even without palpable uterine contractions."[32]

If the membranes have ruptured, regardless of other symptoms, the woman is ordinarily advised to go to the hospital.

Sometimes uterine contractions, once begun, decrease spontaneously. Nonspecific measures that are used in the hospital that may reduce uterine activity include (1) bed rest in a lying-down position, which decreases hydrostatic forces on the cervix; (2) left-side lying position, which promotes placental perfusion; and (3) hydration with IV and oral fluids, which indirectly inhibits hormonal stimulation of uterine contractions.

• •

Review Questions

1. State five ways that women at risk for preterm labor might decrease the likelihood of its onset: (a) __________, (b) __________, (c) __________, (d) __________, and (e) __________

2. What should a woman who suspects preterm labor do before seeking medical advice? (a) __________, (b) __________, and (c) __________

3. Explain the purpose of ambulatory home monitoring: __________

Answers

1. In order to decrease the likelihood of the onset of preterm labor, a woman at risk should: (a) increase her rest periods, (b) decrease strenuous activity, (c) limit her traveling, (d) modify her sexual activity, and (e) avoid stress.

2. When a woman suspects she is having preterm labor, before seeking medical advice she should: (a) urinate, (b) rest lying down (preferably on her left side) for 30 minutes, and (c) drink a quart of liquid.
3. Because ambulatory electronic monitoring can detect preterm labor before it even starts, this method provides a means of starting treatment very early.

• •

Pharmacological Interventions. *Tocolytic agents,* drugs that arrest preterm labor, must be given early if they are to be effective. However, before attempts are made to prolong the pregnancy, there must be established certainty that prolongation is beneficial to the fetus and not detrimental to the mother. Tocolytics should be considered if the following criteria exist:

1. a live non-distressed fetus
2. a cervix dilated less than 4 cm
3. no medical or obstetric contraindications
4. no intrauterine infection

There are exceptions. For example, some women may be candidates despite their moderate pregnancy-induced hypertension or partial placenta abruption.

When the gestational period is less than 33 weeks, *betamethasone* (Celestone) may be given to the mother (12 mg IM every 12 hours × 2). Controversy exists, but the drug may be effective in accelerating fetal lung maturity if delivery does not occur prior to 48 hours following the first injection. If the baby is not delivered within 7 days, the treatment should be repeated.[33,34] Betamethasone may increase the potential for maternal pulmonary edema and mask signs of chorioamnionitis.[35] For the latter reason, the drug is usually not given when the membranes are ruptured. During administration of this drug, in addition to assessing for respiratory problems, the nurse should do frequent vital signs and keep accurate I&O records.

There are several groups of tocolytic agents: (1) beta-mimetics, (2) calcium antagonists, (3) prostaglandin synthetase inhibitors, and (4) ethanol. The beta-mimetics are most frequently used.

BETA-MIMETICS. The most commonly used *beta-mimetic* drugs are terbutaline, ritodrine, and isoxsuprine. This group of drugs stimulates the beta receptors in the myometrium and thereby inhibits uterine contractions. Because ritodrine is the only tocolytic drug approved by the FDA, a signed consent form is advised before administration of other drugs for arrest of preterm labor. Nursing responsibilities during the administration of any of the beta-mimetic drugs are similar.

Uterine activity and fetal heart rate must be continuously monitored and documented prior to, during, and for an hour after the IV treatment is discontinued. The status of the cervix (amount of dilatation and effacement) and membranes (whether intact or ruptured) must be initially assessed. The woman is placed in a left lateral position to promote placental perfusion. An IV of 200 to 500 ml (usually Ringers' lactate) is infused prior to starting the IV beta-mimetic, and laboratory tests are performed, including examination for bacteriuria. Antimicrobial therapy can alleviate urinary tract infection, which might be the precipitator of preterm labor. While the mother is receiving IV doses, lab work including K^+ and Ca^+ levels should be repeated every 12 hours. Sometimes a baseline electrocardiogram (ECG) is done. Emotional support to the laboring woman is important throughout this stressful therapy for preterm labor.

While the drug is infusing, the rate of administration is dependent on uterine response and the occurrence of side effects. Maternal blood pressure, pulse, and respirations may be assessed as often as every 10 minutes until the infusion rate is stabilized. Continuous electronic monitoring may be required. These vital signs should be recorded before increasing the infusion rate. After stabilization of the infusion rate, vital signs should be repeated every 30 minutes until 1 hour after discontinuance of the IV. The following side effects need to be considered:

- Hypotension commonly occurs with a widening pulse pressure (a greater decrease in the diastolic than in the systolic). The physician should be notified of a drop in blood pressure below 90/60. If severe hypotension occurs, Trendelenburg positioning, discontinuance of the tocolytic agent, and increased infusion of IV fluids may be needed.
- Tachycardia with palpitations and nervousness frequently occurs. A maternal pulse of 140 or more requires a decrease of the tocolytic. In the presence of chest tightness or pain, the IV must be discontinued and the physician notified.
- Respirations need to be assessed by auscultation for dyspnea because pulmonary edema is a possible complication of beta-mimetics.

Assessment should also be done for glycosuria (in urine) or glycosemia (in blood) since beta-mimetics stimulate an increased metabolism of glucose. The fetal heart rate may also increase. An FHR of greater than 180 bpm warrants decrease or discontinuance of the drug and immediate reporting of the rate to the attending physician. The woman remains NPO (or ice chips/clear liquids only) until 1 hour after cessation of contractions.

Intake and output must be recorded. The total intake should not exceed 1500 to 2000 ml in a 24-hour period.[36] This is extremely important since pulmonary edema, which is potentially fatal, is more likely to occur (although rare) if too much fluid is given. Discontinuance of the beta-mimetic drug is warranted in the presence of hypotension, cardiac arrhythmia (e.g., premature ventricular or nodal contractions, atrial fibrillation),[36] chest pain, or pulmonary edema. The nurse must be alert for hypoglycemia and hypokalemia in the newborn delivered within 5 hours of the discontinuance of beta-mimetics.

The details of administration of beta-mimetic drugs (and other tocolytic agents) are provided in Table 9–3. The beta-mimetic is

Table 9–3. TOCOLYTIC DRUG DOSAGE*

DRUG	MIXING DESIRED CONCENTRATION	DOSE/RATE	MAXIMUM RATE
Terbutaline			
IV	5 mg + 95 ml normal saline (yields 5 mg [50 μg]/100 ml concentration). Add to 500 ml Ringer's lactate.	Initial = 10 μg/min. Increase in increments of 5 μg/min until uterine contractions cease or unacceptable side effects appear.	50 μg/min.
SC	0.25 mg q 4 hr ½ hr before discontinuing IV or upon its completion.		
(o)	2.5 mg q 4–6 hr until tocolysis not needed.		
Ritodrine			
IV	150 mg. Add to 500 ml Ringer's lactate.	Initial = 0.1 mg/min. Increase in increments of 0.05 mg/min q 10 min until uterine contractions cease or unacceptable side effects appear. Usual effective dose = 0.15–0.35 mg/min. Continue for 12 hr after uterine contractions cease.	0.35 mg/min.
(o)		Begin ½ hr before discontinuing IV with 10 mg q 2 hr for 24 hr. Then 10–20 mg q 4 hr until tocolysis not needed.	

Isoxsuprine			
IV	80–160 mg. Add to 500 ml Ringer's lactate.	Initial = 0.1 mg/min. Increase in increments of 0.1 mg/min q 10 min until uterine contractions cease or unacceptable side effects appear. Usual effective dose = 0.25–0.5 mg/min. Continue IV for 12 hr after uterine contractions cease. Then decrease rate to $\frac{2}{3}$ dose for 4 hr, to $\frac{1}{3}$ for 4 hr, then discontinue.	0.9 mg/min.
(o)		Begin 1 hr before IV rate reduced. 5–20 mg q 3–4 hr until tocolysis not needed.	
Magnesium sulfate			
IV	4 g. Add to 250 ml Ringer's lactate.	Initial = 4 g infused over 20 min. Then maintain with 40 g/1000 ml at rate of 50 ml/hr (yield 2 g/hr). Desired serum level is 4–10 mg/ml. Continue 24–48 hr if effective.	
Ethanol			
IV	10% solution.	Initial = 7.5 mg/kg body weight/hr for 2 hr. Then 1.5 mg/kg body weight for 10 hr. Repeat with 1 or 2 more courses if uterine contractions recur.	7.5 mg/kg body weight/hr for 2 hr.

*Adapted from Oxorn, H: Oxorn-Foote: Human Labor & Birth, ed 5. Appleton-Century-Crofts, Norwalk, Connecticut, 1986, pp 738–742.

mixed in 500 to 1000 ml IV fluid, started at an initial rate, increased at the prescribed rate until either uterine contractions stop, intolerable side effects occur, or the maximum dose is reached. The effective dose is maintained for 12 to 24 hours following cessation of contractions; the IV rate is then tapered. Eventually an oral dose replaces IV administration. Many woman are sent home on the oral dose, but the importance of clear discharge instructions cannot be overemphasized. The prescribed dose and frequency must be followed. The mother should assess her pulse rate because mild tachycardia indicates an adequate drug level. She must know the signs of recurrent labor and appropriate actions to take.

The following information is specific to the various beta-mimetic drugs:

- *Terbutaline* (Brethine) is the one drug that can be given subcutaneously. This route may be used initially, as well as when tapering from IV to oral.
- *Ritodrine* (Yutopar) is much more expensive than terbutaline. This may be the primary reason why, although ritodrine is approved by the FDA, terbutaline is used more frequently in some areas.
- *Isoxsuprine* (Vasodilan) has two major problems: frequent and quite severe hypotension[37] and marked tachycardia[38] in the mother and fetus.

CALCIUM ANTAGONISTS. Calcium antagonists are occasionally used as tocolytic agents. They are not beta-mimetics. Calcium antagonists include magnesium sulfate and nifedipine.

- *Magnesium sulfate* relaxes uterine smooth muscle by displacing calcium. It is also therapeutic as a tocolytic because it decreases arteriole pressure and increases uterine blood flow.[39] It is contraindicated in women with cardiac or renal disorders. Flushing, increased warmth, and increased heart rate are possible side effects. This is the same drug frequently used in pregnancy-induced hypertension (see Chapter 8). The same signs of toxicity must be assessed: hypotension, respirations less than 12 per minute, absent knee jerk, and less than 30 ml per hour of urinary output. Its effects on the fetus/neonate may be decreased beat-to-beat variability and respiratory depression. The drug is given intravenously.
- *Nifedipine* is an experimental drug that has had promising results in its limited use.[40] Further study is needed to prove its safety and effectiveness. It is chewed and swallowed.

• •

Review Questions

1. What criteria should exist for use of tocolytic agents?
   a. ______________________ c. ______________________
   b. ______________________ d. ______________________

2. **Bethamethasone is given to ____________________**

3. **During the administration of ritodrine, terbutaline, or isoxsuprine, similar nursing interventions are appropriate. Identify six of them.**
   a. ____________ d. ____________
   b. ____________ e. ____________
   c. ____________ f. ____________

4. **What signs of toxicity must the nurse watch for when magnesium sulfate is administered?**
   a. ____________ d. ____________
   b. ____________ e. ____________
   c. ____________

Answers

1. Criteria for use of tocolytic agents include: (a) live nondistressed fetus, (b) cervix dilated less than 4 cm, (c) no medical or obstetrical contraindications, and (d) no intrauterine infection.

2. Bethamethasone is given to *accelerate fetal lung maturity.*

3. During the administration of ritodrine, terbutaline, or isoxsuprine, the following nursing interventions are appropriate:
   a. Have the mother assume a left-side lying position in bed.
   b. Monitor uterine contraction status.
   c. Monitor fetal heart rate — specifically watch for tachycardia.
   d. Monitor blood pressure for hypotension and pulse for tachycardia.
   e. Increase IV rate gradually (according to hospital protocol) if uterine contractions continue.
   f. Assess for maternal pulmonary edema and glycosuria/glycosemia.
   g. Continue medication by other than IV route following cessation of contractions.
   h. Provide emotional support.

4. When administering magnesium sulfate, the following signs of toxicity must be noted: (a) hypotension, (b) respirations less than 12 per minute, (c) absence of knee jerk, and (d) urine output less than 30 ml per hour.

• •

PROSTAGLANDIN SYNTHETASE INHIBITORS. These drugs, which include *indomethacin* and *aspirin*, are known to inhibit premature labor. Because of the untoward effects of indomethacine on the fetal cardiovascular system, it is currently contraindicated[41] or limited to investigative study.[42] Theoretically aspirin should act as a tocolytic agent, but it is not clinically recommended at this time.[42]

ALCOHOL. For many years alcohol was, and in a few places still is, used to arrest preterm labor. It is rarely used since the advent of other effective drugs and better knowledge of adverse effects of alcohol on the fetus. *Ethanol* is thought to arrest labor by inhibiting the release of oxytocin (which is theorized to play a dominant role in the initiation and maintenance of labor). It is administered intravenously. Shortly after the initiation of the medication, the woman becomes intoxicated, experiencing nausea, vomiting, headache, restlessness, and sometimes respiratory depression. Her physical safety becomes a prime concern for the hospital staff. She is kept in bed with the side rails up and padded, and she is not left alone. She is kept NPO, since aspiration of vomitus is likely. Her respiratory status needs to be evaluated carefully. The FHR needs to be monitored frequently as ethanol readily crosses the placenta. Usually 24 hours after discontinuation of the medication, the ill effects from the medication cease.

Appropriate Nursing Measures When Preterm Delivery Is Imminent

The medical staff does not always conclude that a preterm labor should or can be arrested. Often an attempt to stop preterm labor is unsuccessful. Therefore, it is always important that the nurse working in the labor and delivery area be aware of her responsibilities if a preterm infant should be born. The situation may warrant that the pregnant mother be transported to a tertiary center so that a "skilled" health care team and the necessary equipment will be available immediately at the time of delivery.

This is a critical time for the hospital staff and the fetus and also for the expectant parents, who deserve much emotional support. They need to be informed of all changes in status and all procedures being done. At times emergency measures will be necessary, and only brief statements can be given. Further explanation should be given as soon as time permits. The pediatrician and nursery must be notified of the imminent delivery and resuscitation equipment must be assembled. These are precautionary measures that parents usually find comforting, as it is further proof that all that can be done will be done for their baby. The nurses must be aware that a small infant may not require complete dilatation of the cervix. The mother must be discouraged from bearing down, since this might cause damage to the soft tissues of the fetal head (if it is the presenting part). Only those medications that are absolutely necessary for the mother must be administered, because most agents cross the placenta to the baby. Parents are usually more accepting of this approach if they are told the reason for it. General anesthesia is not used because it quickly crosses the placenta to the baby. A local anesthetic is preferred because it has no side effects on the baby. A rather large episiotomy is usually performed by the physician to decrease the pressure of the pelvic floor on the baby's fragile head.

Once birth occurs, only procedures that are absolutely necessary should be done to the newborn, since injury and infection easily occur. Efforts must be made to establish respirations, and the baby should be moved to a source of warmth, humidity, and oxygen. The ideal position for the baby is on his back (supine) with the shoulders elevated so that the abdomen is lower than the thorax and the airway is clear. A folded towel or diaper placed under the shoulders and back helps to expand the thoracic cavity. After briefly sharing the baby with his parents, he is usually transferred to a special-care nursery.

• •

Review Question

List five interventions the nurse should initiate in the event of a preterm delivery.

a. ____________________
b. ____________________
c. ____________________
d. ____________________
e. ____________________

Answer

Anticipatory care that should be provided for the preterm infant in the labor and delivery area includes the following:

a. Notify the pediatrician and nursery.
b. Assemble resuscitation equipment.
c. Avoid all medications for the mother.
d. Anticipate delivery without complete dilatation.
e. Discourage mother from bearing down.
f. Perform only those procedures necessary on the infant—establish respirations, provide warmth, humidity, and oxygen.
g. Position baby to facilitate respirations.
h. Transfer baby to special-care nursery if necessary, after the parents have seen the baby.

• •

Variations in Physical Features of the Preterm Infant

The preterm infant is not only at risk for physical well-being but also for acceptance by his parents. The parents of the preterm infant may need assistance in claiming the infant as their own and in proclaiming him worthy of their love. They need to be allowed to see and touch their baby as soon as possible and as long as conditions permit. These first few minutes (and hours) of close contact with their baby may be crucial for optimal development later in life. Unless the parents come in contact with their newborn, they are justified in thinking he will not survive.

The preterm baby has many characteristics that differ from those seen in the term infant. Many of these characteristics are not usually noticed by the mother (and father), but some of them might create anxiety. The nurse should know the normal signs of the preterm infant and should inform the mother of those that seem appropriate. The cardinal signs of the preterm infant are:

1. *General appearance.* The preterm infant lies flat in a frog-legged position with shoulders, elbows, and knees all touching the mattress. The head is turned to one side. He is inactive with few spontaneous movements. Movements that do occur may be jerky and exaggerated.
2. *Skin.* The skin is very transparent, shiny, and red owing to superficial blood vessels. Vernix caseosa begins to form at 5 months and increases until 36 weeks when it begins to slough off.
3. *Lanugo.* At 20 weeks lanugo first appears on the face and shoulders. It vanishes from the face around 28 weeks and small amounts are on the shoulders through 32 to 37½ weeks.
4. *Plantar creases.* These begin to form on the anterior part of the soles by 34 weeks. More creases develop as the baby approaches term.
5. *Breasts.* Breast tissue, nipples, and areolae begin to form at 34 weeks. They are 1 cm and raised at term gestation.
6. *Ears.* They are pliable with little cartilage. When manipulated, they do not return to their original position.
7. *Genitalia.* The male has a small penis. The scrotal sac appears undergrown with little pigmentation and few rugal folds. The testes are undescended or in the canal. The female has a gaping vulva because of poorly developed labia majora. The labia minora and clitoris are prominent and thick, and viscid mucoid discharge is lacking or very scanty. There is no bloody discharge.

Except for posture, no mention has been made of the preterm's neurologic reflexes. Refer to Ballard or Dubowitz for these (see Bibliography).

•   •

Review Question

Give one normal characteristic for the preterm infant for each of the following:
General appearance: ______
Skin: ______
Lanugo: ______
Plantar creases: ______
Breasts: ______
Ears: ______
Genitalia: ______

Answer

See list in paragraph above the question.

•   •

Psychological Tasks for Mothers of Preterm Infants

The nurse must realize the potential crisis that preterm labor and possible delivery of a preterm infant has for a mother. Throughout this chapter it has been stressed that the infant has many challenges for survival. Most mothers are aware of some of them and this knowledge naturally creates anxiety. At the time of the preterm infant's birth, the mother and father are faced with working through four psychological tasks.

1. The smaller and more immature the infant, the greater the possibility of death or permanent disability—much more so than with the term infant. Even if the infant survives, a period of grieving normally occurs. There is **grieving, anticipatory related to loss of the "perfect" baby, the potential loss of the baby**.
2. The mother must also admit that she has not carried this baby the normal length of time. This is likely to create guilt feelings, which she must acknowledge. There is **self-concept, disturbance in: self-esteem related to failure to deliver at term**.
3. Assuming that the baby survives, the mother needs to begin to relate to her baby—to see, touch, care for it. There is potential for **self-concept, disturbance in: role performance related to mother's lack of knowledge about how to meet the needs of a preterm infant**.
4. She needs to gain a realistic understanding of how her baby differs in its needs and approaches from that of a term infant. There is a **knowledge deficit [about care of the preterm infant] related to lack of preparation**.

• •

Review Question

What are the four psychological tasks that a mother of a preterm infant must work through?

a. ____________________
b. ____________________
c. ____________________
d. ____________________

Answer

The mother of a preterm infant must:

a. Prepare for possible loss of the infant.
b. Acknowledge failure to deliver a normal full-term infant.
c. Initiate a process of relating to the baby.
d. Understand the special needs of a preterm infant.

• •

Ways a Nurse Can Facilitate Parental-Infant Attachment

Nursing interventions can assist the parents to accept their new baby. First, a trusting relationship between the parents and nurse is necessary. The nurse should accept that both parents, but especially the mother, may have negative feelings about the premature birth experience. The nurse should encourage the parents to express these feelings freely and, when necessary, encourage them to seek help with these feelings. The nurse should communicate the infant's progress to the parents, make it possible for them to see and touch their infant frequently, and allow them to care for the infant when possible. When they do something to comfort the baby, they should be praised. Positive reinforcement will encourage further parental-infant interaction. They may wonder why the baby startles in such an exaggerated fashion and why he doesn't grasp a parent's finger. They need to be assured that these are the normal responses of an immature infant. It is a healthy response for parents to ask many questions about their baby and these questions warrant answers that the parents can understand. The baby who appears as attractive as possible and who is treated with warmth by the nurses will be more acceptable to the parents. Even though it will require a longer period of time for these parents to identify with and claim their baby, if they can gain confidence in their ability to care for their baby while in the hospital, the parental-infant relationship will be a much more satisfactory one at home.

•　　•

Review Question

Identify four ways a nurse can promote parent-infant attachment following a preterm birth.

a. ____________________
b. ____________________
c. ____________________
d. ____________________

Answer

A nurse can promote parental-infant attachment in the following ways:

a. Establish a trusting relationship with the parents.
b. Accept and help them work through their negative feelings about the preterm birth.
c. Keep the parents informed about the status of their infant.
d. Allow them to be with their infant when possible.
e. Encourage their positive interactions with the baby.
f. Allow them to ask questions and provide them with answers.
g. Help them to gain confidence in caring for their baby.

•　　•

Death of a Preterm Infant

Before concluding this section on the preterm infant, at least brief consideration needs to be given to the preterm infant who dies, since this is a possible outcome. Parents need to know about the death of their infant as soon as possible. At first, disbelief will be evident. They should be encouraged to see their baby, since an unseen baby is imagined to be far worse than he actually is. Many parents find it helpful to touch or hold their baby, to take a picture of him, and to give him a name. These measures help make the situation real for them. They will experience distress, irritability, and feelings of guilt and anger. A funeral service provides an opportunity for them to work through the grieving process. Preoccupation with thoughts about their baby will continue for several weeks. During this time the couple needs to support each other, by talking about the death with each other and with professionals—the physician, nurse, social worker, or clergy. Support groups and literature on perinatal grieving may also be helpful. Normal activities should gradually be resumed. Although no person or object will ever replace the child they have lost, by 6 to 8 months the couple normally has worked through the largest part of the grieving process.

POST-TERM LABOR

Effects of Post-Term Labor on Mother and Infant

Pregnancy that goes beyond 42 weeks is termed *post-dates, prolonged gestation,* or *post-term.* Like preterm labor, it takes its toll on both mother (and father) and fetus. It is important that the gestational period of a pregnancy be properly dated during the second trimester if the EDC is thought to be unreliable.

By 42 weeks the mother has been ready to have her baby for weeks. She is fatigued and frustrated. The repeated question "Haven't you had your baby yet?" doesn't help. She begins to lose self-confidence and becomes critical of her own abilities. Around week 42 her doctor usually recommends a series of tests to determine the fetal status and to verify that she is post-term. A previously well-functioning placenta could now begin to show signs of insufficiency in meeting the needs of the fetus. As the mother realizes this she begins to fear for the well-being of her baby. At what post-term age the fetus will become compromised is not predictable. Some fetuses continue to grow without degeneration in their biologic functioning. Some become so large that vaginal delivery becomes difficult. Those who stop growing and lose weight are called *postmature* or *dysmature.*

The post-term infant normally has the following readily identifiable characteristics:

- *General appearance*: arms and legs fully flexed; large.
- *Skin*: thick, pink, parchment like due to the lack of vernix; may peel.
- *Lanugo*: little if any.
- *Plantar creases*: deep indentations over more than one third of anterior sole.
- *Breasts*: tissue, nipples, areolae well-developed.
- *Ears*: well-defined, firm pinna.
- *Genitalia*: pigmented. Male: numerous rugae, 1 or 2 testes descended. Female: labia majora covering minora and clitoris, bloody discharge possible.

(Note that a comparable list of characteristics is given for the preterm infant earlier in this chapter.)

The post-term infant may also have signs of *postmature syndrome* (which are found in other dysmature situations; for example, severe pre-eclampsia in which blood flow to the fetus is decreased). Signs of postmaturity include:

- Thin and scrawny, with loose fitting skin due to decreased placental perfusion and use of his own glucose stores.
- Skin, nails, and cord often stained with meconium, passed during episodes of anoxia in utero.
- Wide-eyed and alert but worried appearing, symptomatic of chronically compromised placental function.

Review Questions

1. At what time is a fetus classified as post-term? ________________

2. What psychological effects might a prolonged gestation have on a mother?
   a. ________________
   b. ________________
   c. ________________

3. In addition to post-term characteristics, a postmature infant has the following characteristics:
   a. Owing to use of his own glucose stores, he appears________________
   ____
   b. His ________________ are often meconium stained.
   c. Chronically compromised placental function causes him to look ________________

Answers

1. Greater than 42 weeks' gestation is classified as post-term.
2. The psychological effects on the mother of prolonged gestation include: (a)

fatigue and frustration, (b) loss of self-confidence, self doubt, and (c) fear about the well-being of the fetus.

3. a. Owing to use of his own glucose stores, the postmature infant appears *thin and scrawny with loose fitting skin.*
   b. His *skin, nails, and cord* are often meconium stained.
   c. Chronically compromised placental function causes him to look *wide-eyed and alert but worried.*

• •

Assessment for Postmaturity and Fetal Well-Being

Many of the procedures done to determine the gestational age of the preterm fetus apply here also, that is, time of quickening and hearing of the first fetal heart rate, fundal height, BPD via U/S, and amniotic fluid analysis for determining the gestational age or fetal growth. Other observations are made to assess placental function and fetal well-being. They include estriol levels, fetal activity tests (including nonstress tests), biophysical profiles, contraction stress tests, and fetal scalp sampling for pH.

SERUM and URINARY ESTRIOL LEVELS are one indicator of fetal well-being, but alone are not diagnostic. Estriol is a product of estrogen metabolism, which is dependent upon maternal-placental-fetal unit functioning. Estriol levels normally increase with gestational age. The significance of a dropping level is that a source of its production (e.g., fetal adrenal and pituitary glands, fetal liver, or placenta) is not functioning properly. Katagiri and colleagues found that if the estriol level is 40 to 45 percent of the mean of the last three tests, there is fetal distress.[43]

The estriol levels can be assessed from either serum or urine specimens. Maternal serum estriol levels are usually less burdensome for the mother, and give reliable results.[44] Collection of 24-hour urine requires more than one 24-hour collection because each individual varies in her excretion of estriol in each voiding. It is the nurse's role to provide the woman with a container(s) suitable for collection, a refrigeration source (if the lab requires such), and clear instructions about how to collect every voiding in that 24-hour period. The woman should be told that more than one 24-hour collection is routinely necessary.

Maternal estriol levels used to be a popular method of determining fetal well-being. Owing to the many drawbacks of the method (i.e., serial studies needed, difficult to interpret, time-consuming to get results, expensive), more efficient methods (discussed in the next few pages) are almost always used.

FETAL ACTIVITY is an indicator of fetal well-being or compromise. Vigorous activity indicates well-being; cessation or marked decrease indicates compromise and requires immediate evaluation.[45] In post-term pregnancies, placental deterioration is likely to result in decreased fetal activity. Each fetus has its own normal activity level, which remains relatively constant throughout pregnancy until near term when a gradual decrease occurs. There is no clinical significance in the number of movements per day unless the daily rate is very low.[46,47] Sadovsky found that mothers feel approximately 87 percent of the movements, which he classified as strong, weak, or rolling,[48] and that 80 to 90 percent of fetal movements can be electronically recorded.[49] A pregnant woman experiencing decreased fetal activity should be instructed to document the activity. Some practitioners recommend that all pregnant women document fetal activity, assessing for any significant decrease. Several methods may be used. The simplest involves the mother lying recumbent on her side for 30 to 60 minutes and counting fetal movements. In a resting state she is more perceptive of fetal activity. More than one session is necessary for accuracy, but when it is done is not important. Factors, such as fetal rest periods of approximately 20 minutes, and maternal ingestion of alcohol, sedatives, and nicotine (cigarettes) must be considered because they may decrease fetal activity. Rayburn states that three or fewer perceived fetal movements per hour on two consecutive days is reason for serious concern.[50]

Using the Cardiff count-to-10 method developed by Pearson, the woman begins to count fetal movements at the same time every day (e.g., 10 A.M.) and continues for up to 12 hours. She records on a chart each time she feels fetal movement. Upon feeling 10 movements, which usually takes 1 to 2 hours, she stops counting and should start again at 10 A.M. the next day. The time to be concerned is at the end of the 12-hour period (10 P.M.). If 10 movements have not been felt by then, the care provider should be immediately notified. "A decrease or cessation of fetal movements to less than three in twelve hours (<3/12 hrs) while the fetal heart beat still can be heard is an alarm signal requiring delivery . . . within 12 to 48 hours before fetal death" occurs.[48] Immediate follow-up should involve real-time ultrasound that documents fetal activity and other fetal well-being studies.[50] **Noncompliance [with instructions to inform the physician of significant decrease in fetal activity] related to perceived lack of seriousness of problem** can result in loss of the baby.

NONSTRESS TEST (NST), FETAL ACTIVITY ACCELERATION DETERMINATIONS (FAD), or FETAL ACTIVITY TEST (FAT) is a form of fetal activity test done in an outpatient setting or on the labor unit. It is noninvasive and nonhormonal, with no potential side effects other than increased stress level in the woman. Ordinarily, an external electronic monitor (described in Chapter 3) is used to record the FHR and fetal activity. The mother may be instructed to press a button on the fetal monitor at the time she feels fetal movement in order to record the movement on the monitor's graph. Monitoring may need to be continued beyond 20 or 30 minutes, because the lack of activity for that time may be due to the quiet fetal sleep state. Normally the baseline for the FHR varies from 5 to 15 bpm, and the rate ranges between 120 and 160. The results of NST are as follows:

- A healthy fetus experiences an FHR acceleration with fetal movement (a *negative* or *reactive result*). Two or more accelerations of 15 bpm lasting 15 seconds per 10-minute period are required. This indicates good central nervous system control over the heartbeat. Repetition of this test can safely be delayed for 1 week.
- Little or no FHR acceleration despite tactile stimulation of the maternal abdomen results in a *positive* or *nonreactive result.* A fetus with a positive test result is a candidate for biophysical profile and/or CST.
- Questionable acceleration or weak, infrequent movements yield *inadequate* or *suspicious result,* and the test should be repeated in 24 to 48 hours.

An alternative to the NST is to auscultate fetal heart rates with a fetoscope for 5 minutes intermittently (i.e., listen 5 minutes, pause 5 minutes). In a study conducted by nurse-midwives,[51,52] it was found that they could confidently detect accelerations and that by combining this technique with a fetal activity record, they could assess fetal well-being with a success rate comparable to that of an NST.

BIOPHYSICAL PROFILE (BPP) is a series of assessments of fetal well-being. It is more sensitive and reliable than the single variable of fetal activity and heartbeat accelerations assessed in the NST. The fetal biophysical profile assesses the following variables:[53–55]

1. the standard *nonstress test*—presence of at least two accelerations of the fetal heart rate by at least 15 bpm for at least 15 seconds in response to documented activity
2. *fetal breathing movements*—presence of at least one episode for at least 30 (or 60) seconds during a 30-minute period; involves contraction of the diaphragm and expansion of the abdominal wall
3. *gross fetal body movement*—presence of at least three separate rolling movements of the trunk and fetal limbs lasting longer than 3 seconds within a 30-minute period
4. *fetal tone*—presence of one episode of flexion, extension, and return to flexion of an extremity or hand
5. *volume of amniotic fluid*—presence of one pocket of amniotic fluid measuring at least 1 cm in vertical and horizontal planes

All but the NST are observed by using real-time ultrasound. All the variables can be assessed while the pregnant woman assumes a semi-Fowler position or reclines in a lounge chair. Specially trained nurses or technicians perform the profile. A normal fetal response indicates the involved portion of the central nervous system is functioning normally. If there is depression of the CNS, the biophysical actions will be decreased or cease to exist.

Each variable is given a 2 for a normal finding and a 0 for an abnormal one. Some institutions also assign a 1. A total score of 8 to 10 indicates a normal outcome (Table 9–4). Currently an abnormal score is 4 or less, although reclassification to "equivocal" = 4 or 6 and "abnormal" = 0 or 2 is more consistent with the clinical find-

Table 9–4. BIOPHYSICAL PROFILE

SCORE	INTERPRETATION	INTERVENTION
0–2	Abnormal	Repeat total profile; if results the same, deliver.
4–6	Equivocal	Expect intervention if oligohydramnios present.
8–10	Normal	None.

ings. There is a high morbidity rate with scores of 0 to 2, but fetal improvement is known to occur if the mother's condition improves in the presence of scores of 4 to 6. Therefore, active intervention is not indicated for 4 or 6 except in the presence of oligohydramnios. In the case of a score of 0 or 2, a repeat total profile is warranted, and if the findings are confirmed, delivery should take place.[56] In many institutions, the biophysical profile is recommended as the immediate intervention after a nonreactive NST. If the biophysical profile is 8 or more, the nonreactive NST is ignored but repeated at the appropriate interval. When the biophysical profile is not available, a contraction stress test is normally done.

CONTRACTION STRESS TEST (CST), OXYTOCIN CHALLENGE TEST (OCT), STRESS TEST, PLACENTAL SUFFICIENCY TEST, FETAL RESERVE TEST or NIPPLE STIMULATION CONTRACTION TEST are all names for the same test. Weekly or semiweekly CSTs are done in the hospital to determine the ability of the post-term fetus to tolerate the stress of uterine contractions stimulated by oxytocin infusion or nipple stimulation. Since poor placental perfusion due to an aging placenta is common in the post-term pregnancy, uterine contractions can cause late FHR decelerations, which are evidence of uteroplacental insufficiency. The test is also done on mothers who are hypertensive and diabetic. Contraindications to CST include a history of cesarean delivery with a classic (vertical) type incision, placenta previa, and threatening preterm labor.

Prior to the test the woman must sign a legal consent form and be forewarned that the procedure could stimulate labor. She is encouraged to eat a light meal before (since food in the stomach decreases bowel sounds which otherwise interfere with the FHR recording) and to void (preventing interruption of the test). She is placed in a semi-Fowler position, tilted slightly to her left. An external electronic monitor is applied and interpreted in 10 to 30 minutes. If spontaneous contractions occur every 3 minutes, oxytocin is not necessary. If oxytocin infusion or nipple stimulation is done, her blood pressure is assessed every 10 to 15 minutes to determine any changes that might affect the FHR. In the presence of reassuring FHR, stimulation is given until three contractions occur in a 10-minute period. The printout is also observed for the resting tone of the uterus and the FHR baseline. In the presence of late or variable decelerations, the stimulation should be discontinued immediately and in the case of oxytocin infusion, the primary IV left infusing; the mother should lie on her left side and the physician should be notified immediately.

The results of a CST are as follows:

- Consistent late deceleration with most contractions is a *positive test.* Termination of the pregnancy without labor may be necessary.
- Inconsistent decelerations is a *suspicious test.* The CST should be repeated in 24 hours.
- Three contractions in 30 minutes without late decelerations is a *negative test.* The test need not be repeated for a week in some instances.

The physiology, contraindications, and methodology of nipple stimulation are presented in Chapter 5 where it is discussed as a possible labor stimulant. Stimulation of the onset of labor may not be a desired outcome of the test.

FETAL SCALP SAMPLING FOR pH is a test for hypoxia. A frequent problem of post-term gestation is hypoxia caused by inadequate utero-placental sufficiency. Fetal hypoxia resulting in acidosis (a low pH, <7.20) is suspected in the presence of an abnormal FHR pattern (late or variable decelerations, bradycardia or tachycardia, minimal variability). There is a good correlation between immediate newborn condition (i.e., Apgar score) and fetal blood pH. An Apgar of less than 6 is usually consistent with a pH of less than 7.20. Although this is a test for fetal well-being, it is the only test discussed in this chapter that is done during labor. Like some of the other tests, it is used in a variety of situations where fetal well-being is questioned.

Because obtaining a fetal blood sample is done when there is a suspicion of fetal distress during labor, the mother is likely to be anxious before the procedure even begins. The nurse, as the main source of emotional support, should stay with the mother and explain what is being done, since the doctor(s) is usually absorbed in the technical aspects of the procedure. As the mother lies supine (or on her left side), the mother's perineum is illuminated and cleansed and a cone-shaped instrument is inserted vaginally through her cervix. (Membranes must be ruptured.) A small light in the cone permits visualization of the fetal presenting part (scalp or buttocks), which is cleansed with a sterile swab, dabbed with silicone, and pricked with a blade. The blood is collected on a reagent strip and inserted in a portable machine for immediate analysis. More than one sample will be necessary for reliable results. Continuous tissue pH monitoring is available but so far rarely used. In the presence of a borderline pH (7.20 to 7.25) another blood sample is often taken within 15 to 30 minutes. Values below 7.20 during stage I and below 7.15 in stage II usually result in termination of the labor by operative delivery (low forceps or cesarean).

• •

Review Question

Briefly summarize the information you would give to a woman before the following tests:

a. Nonstress test
   Purpose: ____________________
   Procedure: ____________________
   ____
   ____
   Frequency: ____________________
   ____

b. Biophysical Profile
   Purpose: ____________________
   Procedure: ____________________
   ____
   ____
   Frequency: ____________________
   ____

c. Contraction stress test
   Purpose: ____________________
   Procedure: ____________________
   ____
   ____
   Frequency: ____________________
   ____

d. Fetal Scalp pH
   Purpose: ____________________
   Procedure: ____________________
   ____
   ____
   Frequency: ____________________
   ____

Answer

a. Nonstress test
   Purpose: To assess fetal well-being—the response of the FHR to fetal activity.
   Procedure: An external electronic monitor is placed on the abdomen and the FHR and fetal activity recorded; time involved is usually more than 30 minutes.
   Frequency: The frequency of repeated tests depends on the test results.

b. Biophysical Profile
   Purpose: To assess fetal well-being using five variables—NST, fetal breathing movements, gross fetal body movement, fetal tone, and volume of amniotic fluid.
   Procedure: A standard NST and specific ultrasonic measurements are done.
   Frequency: It is often done immediately after a non-reactive NST. If the profile score is 0 or 2, it should be immediately repeated.

c. Contraction Stress Test
   Purpose: To assess fetal well-being—the response of the FHR to uterine contractions stimulated by IV oxytocin or nipple stimulation.
   Procedure: With external electronic monitor in place, IV oxytocin is administered

or nipple(s) stimulated until the effect of uterine contractions on the FHR can be determined. Time involved is usually dependent on the time it takes for the uterus to contract 3 times in 10 minutes.

Frequency: A suspicious test result requires repitition in 24 hours. A negative test result indicates that the test need not be repeated for a week in some instances.

d. Fetal Scalp pH

Purpose: To assess for fetal acidosis.

Procedure: A speck of blood is obtained from the fetal presenting part by the physician.

Frequency: Depending on the results, the procedure may need to be repeated within 15 to 30 minutes.

• •

Nursing Measures during Post-Term Labor

Post-term labor may occur spontaneously or with the aid of stimulants (refer to Chapter 5). Although the mother is undoubtedly relieved that the pregnancy finally is ending, the fetus is about to undergo his most stressful time. Normally, uterine contractions temporarily decrease the amount of oxygenation the fetus receives. If there is any placental insufficiency, the fetus is most frequently compromised during uterine contractions. Careful monitoring of the FHR with a continuous electronic monitor is necessary. Intolerance of uterine contractions is evidenced by persistent late decelerations and decreased baseline variability (refer to Chapter 3) and warrants medical intervention. The nurse should encourage the mother to be on her side or in a semi-Fowler position to facilitate fetal oxygenation. Oxytocin stimulation, if used, should be regulated to produce contractions of less than 90 seconds' duration with a minimum of 30 to 60 seconds' relaxation between contractions. Intravenous fluids should be administered. Helping the woman to decrease her pain perception is very important, since all medications should be avoided if possible. In the presence of fetal distress, oxygen should be administered to the mother via a face mask. Fetal scalp sampling for pH may be done and the results influential about what type and when the delivery is done. If delivery has not occurred after 12 to 18 hours of good labor, a cesarean delivery is often performed, regardless of the fetal pH, in order to decrease fetal morbidity and mortality.

• •

Review Question

When preparing a mother for her post-term labor, what five (or more) items would you share with her about the care she would expect to receive?

a. ______________________________

b. ______________________________

c. ______________________________
d. ______________________________
e. ______________________________

Answer

Information a nurse should share with a woman anticipating a post-term labor includes:

a. If labor does not start on its own, it will be stimulated, probably by IV oxytocin.
b. Continuous electronic monitoring will be done.
c. She will be discouraged from lying on her back but encouraged to be in semi-Fowler or side-lying position.
d. IV fluids will be given.
e. Medication will be avoided if possible.
f. If the fetus shows the need for it, oxygen will be given.
g. Fetal scalp sampling for pH will be done if necessary.
h. If necessary a cesarean delivery may be performed.

• •

Immediate Care of the Post-Term Infant

In addition to routine newborn care (i.e., establishing airway, drying skin, providing warmth, identifying mother and baby, instilling eye prophylaxis), the post-term infant has special needs. The nurse is responsible for notifying the pediatrician and anesthetist when delivery is imminent. In the presence of meconium staining, tracheal suctioning should be done immediately following birth. Suctioning is necessary since aspiration of meconium-stained amniotic fluid is likely to have occurred in utero or at the time of birth. Since the amount of amniotic fluid decreases following 38 weeks, the fluid is often thick and pea-souplike. If aspirated it would clog the air passages and irritate the lungs, causing meconium aspiration syndrome and respiratory distress. Pneumonitis and/or pneumothorax could result. Oxygen may also be necessary especially in the presence of bradycardia.

The nurse usually assesses the post-term infant for hypoglycemia by means of a Dextrostix. Low levels should be validated by laboratory blood glucose values. If there is no standing order for these, an order should be sought. A Dextrostix reading of less than 45 indicates a low blood sugar level, which requires immediate administration of oral or IV glucose solution. Frequent feedings may be necessary. Some post-term infants may have little subcutaneous fat and a large body surface. Therefore, they are subject to cold stress. Special care must be taken to prevent heat loss and to provide heat to these infants. Although post-term infants are at risk while in labor, by taking these measures, they often function well after delivery.

• •

Review Questions

1. Identify four physiologic disadvantages that the post-term infant is likely to have that warrant nursing interventions:
   a. ______________________________
   b. ______________________________
   c. ______________________________
   d. ______________________________
2. What nursing actions are necessary for the infant who shows signs of the above physiologic conditions?
   a. ______________________________
   b. ______________________________
   c. ______________________________
   d. ______________________________

Answers

1. Physiologic disadvantages that a post-term infant is likely to have that warrant interventions are: (a) clogged air passages and irritated lungs owing to meconium aspiration, (b) bradycardia, (c) hypoglycemia, and (d) cold stress.
2. The nursing actions necessary for the infant who shows signs of the above physiologic conditions include:
   a. Provide for pediatrician and anesthetist to be present at delivery so that tracheal suctioning can be immediately performed if needed.
   b. Give oxygen as necessary.
   c. Check for low blood sugar with Dextrostix. Seek order, if there is no standing order, for oral or IV glucose solution if results are less than 45.
   d. Provide warmth and prevent heat loss.

• •

CONCLUSION

Throughout this chapter, ways to assess and promote fetal well-being have been discussed. In the presence of preterm or post-term labor, this is no simple task. Numerous assessment techniques—ultrasound, laboratory tests, electronic monitors, physical assessment—may be involved.

The nurse plays a vital role in the assessment process—not only in doing some of the actual assessments but also in making accurate evaluations. Many times the nurse must make immediate decisions about when to do a nursing intervention independently and when to seek medical assistance. As the contents of this chapter indicate, these decisions are based on numerous factors. The basics of nursing care for women in preterm and post-term labor have been addressed.

REFERENCES

1. Sabbagha, R, Tamura, R, and Socol, M: The use of ultrasound in obstetrics. Clin Obstet Gynecol 25(4):736, 1982.

2. Pritchard, JA, MacDonald, PC, and Gant, NF: Williams Obstetrics, ed 17. Appleton-Century-Crofts, Norwalk, Connecticut, 1985, p 218.
3. Oxorn, H: Oxorn-Foote: Human Labor & Birth, ed 5. Appleton-Century-Crofts, Norwalk, Connecticut, 1986, p 41.
4. Gillieson, M, et al: Placental site, parity and date of quickening. Obstet Gynecol 64:44, 1984.
5. Pritchard, JA, MacDonald, PC, and Gant, NF: Williams Obstetrics, ed 17. Appleton-Century-Crofts, Norwalk, Connecticut, 1985, p 211.
6. Ouimette, J: Perinatal Nursing: Care of the High-Risk Mother and Infant. Jones & Bartlett, Boston, 1986, p 44.
7. Ouimette, J: Perinatal Nursing: Care of the High-Risk Mother and Infant. Jones & Bartlett, Boston, 1986, p 45.
8. Granuum, P, Berkowitz, R, and Hobbins, S: The ultrasonic changes in the maturing placenta and their relation to fetal pulmonic maturity. Am J Obstet Gynecol 133(8):915, 1979.
9. Kazzi, G, et al: The relationship of placental grade, fetal lung maturity, and neonatal outcome in normal and complicated pregnancies. Am J Obstet Gynecol 148(54):54, 1984.
10. Quinlan, R, et al: Changes in placental ultrasonic appearance. II. Pathologic significance of Grade III placental changes. Am J Obstet Gynecol 144(4):471, 1982.
11. Dudley, DKL: Assessment of the fetus in utero. In Oxorn, H: Oxorn-Foote: Human Labor & Birth, ed 5. Appleton-Century-Crofts, Norwalk, Connecticut, 1986, p 590.
12. Ouimette, J: Perinatal Nursing: Care of the High-Risk Mother and Infant. Jones & Bartlett, Boston, 1986, p 46.
13. Quinlan, RW and Cruz, AC: Ultrasonic placental grading and fetal pulmonary maturity. Am J Obstet Gynecol 142(1):110, 1982.
14. Ouimette, J: Perinatal Nursing: Care of the High-Risk Mother and Infant. Jones & Bartlett, Boston, 1986, p 51.
15. Ouimette, J: Perinatal Nursing: Care of the High-Risk Mother and Infant. Jones & Bartlett, Boston, 1986, p 52.
16. Pritchard, JA, MacDonald, PC, and Gant, NF: Williams Obstetrics, ed 17. Appleton-Century-Crofts, Norwalk, Connecticut, 1985, p 268.
17. Dudley, DKL: Assessment of the fetus in utero. In Oxorn, H: Oxorn-Foote: Human Labor & Birth, ed 5. Appleton-Century-Crofts, Norwalk, Connecticut, 1986, p 582.
18. Gluck, L, et al: The interpretation and significance of the lechithin/sphingomyelin ratio in amniotic fluid. Am J Obstet Gynecol 120(1):142, 1974.
19. Kubovick, M, Hallman, M, and Gluck, L: The lung profile I. Normal pregnancy. Am J Obstet Gynecol 135(1):57, 1979.
20. Berkowitz, RL, et al: The relationship between premature rupture of the membranes and the respiratory distress syndrome: An update and plan of management. Am J Obstet Gynecol 131:503, 1978.
21. Richardson, DJ, et al: Acceleration of fetal lung maturation following prolonged rupture of the membranes. Am J Obstet Gynecol 118:1115, 1974.
22. Sell, EJ and Harris, ZR: Association of premature rupture of membranes with idiopathic respiratory distress syndrome. Obstet Gynecol 49:167, 1977.
23. Worthington, D, Maloney, AHA, and Smith, GL: Fetal lung maturity. I. Mode of onset of premature labor; influence of premature rupture of the membranes. Obstet Gynecol 49:275, 1977.

24. Pritchard, JA, MacDonald, PC, and Gant, NF: Williams Obstetrics, ed 17. Appleton-Century-Crofts, Norwalk, Connecticut, 1985, p 275.
25. Dudley, DKL: Assessment of the fetus in utero. In Oxorn, H: Oxorn-Foote: Human Labor & Birth, ed 5. Appleton-Century-Crofts, Norwalk, Connecticut, 1986, p 588.
26. Herron, MA and Dulock, HL: Preterm Labor, ed 2. March of Dimes Birth Defects Foundation, Series 2 Prenatal Care, Module 5, White Plains, New York, 1987, p 16.
27. Herron, MA, Katz, M, and Creasy, RK: Evaluation of a preterm birth prevention program: Preliminary report. Obstet Gynecol 59(4):452, 1982.
28. Katz, M, Gill, PJ, and Newman, RB: Detection of preterm labor by ambulatory monitoring of uterine activity for the management of oral tocolysis. Am J Obstet Gynecol 154(6):1253, 1986.
29. Morrison, JC, et al: Prevention of preterm birth by ambulatory assessment of uterine activity: A randomized study. Am J Obstet Gynecol 156(3):536, 1987.
30. Katz, M, Newman, RB, and Gill, PJ: Assessment of uterine activity in ambulatory patients at high risk of preterm labor and delivery. Am J Obstet Gynecol 154(1):44, 1986.
31. Gill, PJ and Katz, M: Early detection of preterm labor: Ambulatory home monitoring of uterine activity. J Obstet Gynecol Neonatal Nurs 15(6):439, 1986.
32. Herron, MA and Dulock, HL: Preterm Labor, ed 2. March of Dimes Birth Defects Foundation, Series 2 Prenatal Care, Module 5, White Plains, New York, 1987, p 15.
33. Gilbert, ES and Harmon, JS: High-Risk Pregnancy and Delivery: Nursing Perspectives. CV Mosby, St. Louis, 1986, p 327.
34. D'Alton, M: Preterm labor. In Oxorn, H: Oxorn-Foote: Human Labor & Birth, ed 5. Appleton-Century-Crofts, Norwalk, Connecticut, 1986, p 746.
35. Angellini, DJ, Knapp, CMW, and Gibes, RM (eds.): Perinatal/Neonatal Nursing: A Clinical Handbook. Blackwell Scientific Publications, Boston, 1986, p 184.
36. Benedetti, TJ: Maternal complications of parenteral B-sympathomimetic therapy for premature labor. Am J Obstet Gynecol 145(1):1, 1983.
37. D'Alton, M: Preterm labor. In Oxorn, H: Oxorn-Foote: Human Labor & Birth, ed 5. Appleton-Century-Crofts, Norwalk, Connecticut, 1986, p 738.
38. Pritchard, JA, MacDonald, PC, and Gant, NF: Williams Obstetrics, ed 17. Appleton-Century-Crofts, Norwalk, Connecticut, 1985, p 752.
39. Petri, RH: Tocolysis using magnesium sulfate. Sem Perinatol 5:266, 1981.
40. Ulmsten, U, Anderson, KE, and Wingerup, L: Treatment of premature labor with the calcium antagonist nifedipine. Arch Gynecol 229:1, 1980.
41. Ouimette, J: Perinatal Nursing: Care of the High-Risk Mother and Infant. Jones & Bartlett, Boston, 1986, p 284.
42. D'Alton, M: Preterm labor. In Oxorn, H: Oxorn-Foote: Human Labor & Birth, ed 5. Appleton-Century-Crofts, Norwalk, Connecticut, 1986, p 744.
43. Katagiri, H, et al: Estriol in pregnancy: IV. Normal concentrations, diurnal and/or episodic variations and day-to-day changes of unconjugated and total estriol in late pregnancy plasma. Am J Ob Gynecol 124(3):272, 1976.

44. Miller, C, et al: Maternal serum unconjugated estriol and urine estriol concentrations in normal and high-risk pregnancy. Obstet Gynecol 49(3):287, 1977.
45. Sadovksy, E and Yaffe, H: Daily fetal movement recording and fetal prognosis. Obstet Gynecol 41(6):845, 1973.
46. Clark, J and Britton, K: Factors contributing to clinical nonuse of the Cardiff count-to-ten fetal activity chart. J Nurs-Midw 30(6):321, 1985.
47. Ouimette, J: Perinatal Nursing: Care of the High-Risk Mother and Infant. Jones & Bartlett, Boston, 1986, p 43.
48. Sadovsky, E, Polishuk, W, and Mahler, Y: Correlation between electromagnetic recording and maternal assessment of fetal movement. Lancet 1:1141, 1973.
49. Sadovsky, E and Polishuk, W: Fetal movements in utero. Obstet Gynecol 50:49, 1977.
50. Rayburn, W: Antepartum fetal assessment: Monitoring fetal activity. Clin Perinatol 9(2):231, 1982.
51. Paine, LL, Payton, RG, and Johnson, TRB: Auscultated fetal heart rate accelerations. I. Accuracy and documentation. J Nurs-Midw 31(2):71, 1986.
52. Paine, LL, et al: Auscultated fetal heart rate accelerations. II. An alternative to the nonstress test. J Nurs-Midw 31(2):76, 1986.
53. Manning, FA, et al: Biophysical profile scoring. Am J Obstet Gynecol 140:289, 1981.
54. Dudley, DKL: Assessment of the fetus in utero. In Oxorn, H: Oxorn-Foote: Human Labor & Birth, ed 5. Appleton-Century-Crofts, Norwalk, Connecticut, 1986, pp 608–613.
55. Simkins, S: Fetal Biophysical Profile. Presentation at NAACOG/Henry Ford Hospital Conference, Livonia, MI, September 11, 1987.
56. Dudley, DML: Assessment of the fetus in utero. In Oxorn, H: Oxorn-Foote: Human Labor & Birth, ed 5. Appleton-Century-Crofts, Norwalk, Connecticut, 1986, pp 608–613.

BIBLIOGRAPHY

Angelini, DJ, Knapp, CMW, and Gibes, RM (eds): Perinatal/Neonatal Nursing: A Clinical Handbook. Blackwell Scientific Publications, Boston, 1986.

Ballard, JL, Novak, KK, and Driver, M: A simplified score for assessment of fetal maturation of newly born infants. J Pediatr 95(5):769, 1979.

Campbell, B: Overdue delivery: Its impact on mothers-to-be. Matern Child Nurs J 11(3):170, 1986.

Dubowitz, LM, Dubowitz, V, and Goldberg, C: Clinical assessment of gestational age. J Pediatr 77:1, 1970.

Gill, PJ and Katz, M: Early detection of preterm labor: Ambulatory home monitoring of uterine activity. J Obstet Gynecol Neonatal Nurs 15(6):439, 1986.

Herron, MA and Dulock, HL: Preterm Labor, ed 2. March of Dimes Birth Defects Foundation, Series 2 Prenatal Care, Module 5, White Plains, New York, 1987.

Gilbert, ES and Harmon, JS: High-Risk Pregnancy and Delivery. CV Mosby, St. Louis, 1986.

Knuppel, RA and Drukker, JE: High-Risk Pregnancy: A Team Approach. WB Saunders, Philadelphia, 1986.

Manning, F, Platt, L, and Sipos, L: Antepartum fetal evaluation: Development of a fetal biophysical profile. Am J Obstet Gynecol 136:787, 1980.

NAACOG: OGN nursing practice resource: Preterm labor and tocolytics. NAACOG No. 10, September 1984.

Ouimette, J: Perinatal Nursing: Care of the High-Risk Mother and Infant. Jones & Bartlett, Boston, 1986.

Oxorn, H: Oxorn-Foote: Human Labor & Birth, ed 5. Appleton-Century-Crofts, Norwalk, Connecticut, 1986.

Pearson, J: Fetal movements: A new approach to antenatal care. Nurs Mir 144:49, 1977.

Pritchard, JA, MacDonald, PC, and Gant, NF: Williams Obstetrics, ed 17. Appleton-Century-Crofts, Norwalk, Connecticut, 1985.

9 POST-TEST

1. On the time line below, *circle* the numerals (representing weeks' gestation) that pertain to preterm and post-term and *label* them.
   32 33 34 35 36 37 38 39 40 41 42 43 44
   ____

2. In the chart below, list the psychological effects a nonterm labor might have on a woman.

PRETERM	POST-TERM
a. ____________	a. ____________
b. ____________	b. ____________
c. ____________	c. ____________

3. Specifiy which physiologic hindrances tend to occur in the preterm infant and which in the post-term infant. Indicate PRE and POST in the blanks.
   a. _____ Difficult respirations due to surfactant level in lungs
   b. _____ Loose fitting skin, deprived looking
   c. _____ Parchment like, peeling skin
   d. _____ Weak suck
   e. _____ Hemorrhage
   f. _____ Meconium staining
   g. _____ Poor resistance to infection

4. Explain three methods nurses use to determine the gestational age of a fetus and state the normal findings:
   a. ____
   ____
   ____
   b. ____
   ____
   ____
   c. ____
   ____
   ____

5. List the following physical features in a preterm infant and a post-term infant.

	PRETERM	POST-TERM
a. Position		
b. Vernix		
c. Plantar creases		
d. Pinna of ears		
e. Majora/minora		

6. State five measures that women can take to avoid preterm labor.
   a. ______
   b. ______
   c. ______
   d. ______
   e. ______

7. Explain why the nurse assesses the fetal heart rate or uterine activity in the following procedures:
   a. Ambulatory home monitoring: ______
   b. Amniocentesis: ______
   c. Nonstress test: ______
   d. Contraction stress test: ______

8. Match the drugs in Column I with the appropriate statement in Column II. More than one drug can be used for each statement.

COLUMN I	COLUMN II
a. Betamethasone	______ May increase potential for maternal pulmonary edema
b. Ethanol	______ Decreased blood pressure and tachycardia frequently occur
c. Ritodrine	______ Physical safety is a prime concern
d. Terbutaline	______ Is approved by FDA as tocolytic agent
e. Isoxsuprine	______ Can be given subcutaneously
f. Magnesium sulfate	______ Is at toxic level when knee jerk reflex is absent

9. *Circle* True or False and explain your answer.
   When preterm delivery is imminent, the nurse should:
   a. T F Inform the mother of the disadvantages her baby will have.
   ______

b. T F Provide the mother with enough medication so that she is comfortable both mentally and physically.

____

____

____

c. T F Inform the mother that the baby may be taken to the nursery where he can be given a warm environment and can be closely watched.

____

____

____

d. T F Let the mother know that both the nursery and the pediatrician have been informed that her baby is on the way.

____

____

____

e. T F The mother should be discouraged from bearing down even following complete dilatation.

____

____

____

10. A preterm infant's mother must work through the psychological tasks listed below. At the same time a maternal-infant bond needs to be promoted. Indicate how a nurse can promote a favorable bond, considering the tasks the mother must go through.

PSYCHOLOGICAL TASKS	NURSING INTERVENTIONS
a. Feel grief and guilt	a.
b. Initiate relationship with baby	b.
c. Understand baby's needs	c.

11. List the components of the biophysical profile used to assess fetal well-being.

a. ____________________ d. ____________________

b. ____________________ e. ____________________

c. ____________________

12. **Explain why the following measures are carried out during a post-term labor/delivery:**
    a. **Continuous electronic monitoring:** ______________________

    ____

    ____

    b. **Tracheal suctioning of newborn:** ______________________

    ____

    ____

    c. **Dextrostix test:** ______________________

    ____

    ____

Answers to Post-Test

1. The circled numerals represent the weeks' gestation.

(32 33 34 35 36 37) 38 39 40 41 (42 43 44)

2. The psychological effects a nonterm labor might have on a woman are:

PRETERM
a. Has not completed nesting
b. Has not let go of incompatible practices
c. Not ready to separate from fetus
d. Fears losing or hurting baby

POST-TERM
a. Fatigued, frustrated
b. Lacking self-confidence
c. Fearful of fetal well-being

3. Physiologic handicaps that tend to occur in PREterm and POST-term:
   a. PRE Difficult respirations due to surfactant levels
   b. POST Loose fitting skin, deprived looking
   c. POST Parchment like, peeling skin
   d. PRE Weak suck
   e. PRE Hemorrhage
   f. POST Meconium staining
   g. PRE Poor resistance to infection

4. Methods nurses use to determine gestational age:
   a. To determine the EDC using Naegele's rule, subtract 3 months and add 7 days and 1 year to date of onset of LMP. LMP = 4/10/89; EDC = 1/17/90.
   b. Auscultate the fetal heart rate. Expect to first hear it with a Doppler device at 10 to 12 weeks, and for the first time with a fetoscope at 17 to 19 weeks.
   c. Measure the fundal height from the upper border of the symphysis pubis to the top of the fundus. At 16 weeks, it is midway between pubis and umbilicus; at 20 weeks, at umbilicus; at 24 weeks, just above umbilicus.

5. Physical features of preterm and post-term infants:

	PRETERM	POST-TERM
a. Position	Frog-legged, extended	Fully flexed
b. Vernix	Maximum at 36 weeks	Lacking

(continued)

	PRETERM	POST-TERM
c. Plantar creases	Some on anterior sole	Deep; over more than ⅓ of anterior sole
d. Pinna or ears	Pliable, floppy	Firm
e. Majora/minora	Minora prominent	Majora covering minora

6. Measures that women can take to avoid preterm labor include:
   a. Increase their rest periods.
   b. Decrease strenuous activity at home and at work.
   c. Limit their traveling to less than 1 to 2 hours at a time.
   d. Modify their sexual activity (use a condom; avoid breast stimulation, orgasm, and/or intercourse).
   e. Avoid stress.
7. The rationale for fetal heart rate or uterine activity assessment in the specified procedures is the following:
   a. Ambulatory home monitoring: The occurrence of subtle uterine activity is detectable by this method of monitoring. As a result, early diagnosis is possible in women at risk for preterm labor.
   b. Amniocentesis: Because injury of the fetus, cord, or placenta may occur due to penetration with the needle used to withdraw the amniotic fluid, assess for fetal heart rate decrease or cessation.
   c. Nonstress test: NST specifically looks for accelerations in FHR upon fetal movement. A healthy fetus experiences an FHR acceleration with each fetal movement. Lack of accelerations warrants further assessment.
   d. Contraction stress test: CST specifically looks for the FHR response to uterine contractions. It is abnormal for the fetus to experience late decelerations, which is fairly common in the post-term fetus.
8. (a) Betamethasone, (c) Ritodrine, (d) Terbutaline, and (e) Isoxsuprine may increase the potential for maternal pulmonary edema.
   (c) Ritodrine, (d) Terbutaline, and (e) Vasodilan frequently cause decreased blood pressure and tachycardia.
   (b) Ethanol makes physical safety a prime concern.
   (c) Ritodrine is approved by the FDA as a tocolytic agent.
   (d) Terbutaline can be given subcutaneously.
   (f) Magnesium sulfate is at a toxic level when the knee jerk reflex is absent.
9. a. F Since the disadvantages of the baby are not known until they are actually assessed, the mother's anxiety needs to be acknowledged and the baby shared with her as soon as possible after birth.
   b. F Only those medications that are absolutely necessary for the mother must be administered because most agents cross the placenta to the baby.
   c. T Mother should be told that the baby may need immediate care in the nursery.
   d. T Mother should be assured that the pediatrician and nursery have been notified of the baby's imminent delivery.
   e. T Bearing down might damage the soft tissue of the preterm baby's head.

10.

MATERNAL PSYCHOLOGICAL TASKS	NURSING INTERVENTIONS
a. Feel grief and guilt	a. Accept/work through mother's negative feeling
b. Initiate relationship with baby	b. Allow mother to be with baby
c. Understand baby's needs	c. Allow for and answer mother's questions

11. The components of the biophysical profile for fetal-well being are:
    a. the standard nonstress test
    b. fetal breathing movements
    c. gross fetal body movement
    d. fetal tone
    e. volume of amniotic fluid

12. During a post-term labor/delivery, the following measures are done:
    a. Continuous electronic monitoring: Assess for signs of placental insufficiency (late decelerations in FHR) with contractions.
    b. Tracheal suctioning of newborn: In the presence of meconium-stained amniotic fluid, aspiration could cause respiratory distress.
    c. Dextrostix test: Hypoglycemia is common in post-term infants and requires early diagnosis and treatment (early, frequent glucose feedings).

10 LEGAL CONSIDERATIONS

Janet S. Malinowski

OBJECTIVES

Upon completing this chapter, you will be able to:

- ▶ Explain how general principles of law apply to nursing.
- ▶ Describe the implications of standards of care.
- ▶ Discuss who, in the health care team, is liable and for what.
- ▶ Using the steps of the nursing process, identify common errors that have legal implications, and remedies to avoid them.
- ▶ Recall two reasons for carrying the various forms of malpractice insurance.
- ▶ Explain nurses' roles and responsibilities related to patient rights and informed consent.
- ▶ Describe documentation strategies that discourage legal actions.
- ▶ Discuss the components and procedures of a malpractice lawsuit.

Today's consumer has high expectations of the health care profession. Consumers are generally better educated and expect quality care. This is also the decade of more legal actions and higher malpractice insurance rates for labor/delivery nurses than ever before in the history of nursing. Not only are there fast moving, complex physiologic occurrences during the birth process, but there are numerous professionals involved and machinery available which can be misinterpreted, improperly used and/or malfunctioning. Therefore, nurses must be concerned about their accountability (to whom, for what, when), how they can protect themselves, and how they can sufficiently prepare themselves to deal with the legal environment.

The purpose of this chapter is not to provide legal advice, but to serve as an educational tool so the reader will be less vulnerable to professional liability. Although reference is made to the nurse, the reader should keep in mind that the courts generally make little distinction between the liability of the registered nurse, the LPN/LVN, and nursing students.[1]

OVERVIEW OF GENERAL LAW APPLIED TO NURSING

Law may take the form of a constitution, a statute, an administrative regulation, or a court decision interpreting these forms of law. Most nurses are familiar with constitutional law. The Constitution guarantees people certain fundamental liberties. For example, the Fourth Amendment, prohibiting unlawful search, means that a nurse cannot search a patient's belongings without permission. The other forms of law may not be as familiar.

Statutes are usually broad, general laws that describe legal boundaries. Statutes enable or grant power. They are more fully defined by other sources of law, such as regulations. Statutes are laws enacted by state or federal legislative bodies. Nurse practice acts are statutes. The nurse practice act of a state usually delegates to the state board of nursing authority to set admission standards and to control (grant, suspend, and revoke) licenses. Mandatory licensure law exists in all states but Texas,[2] Oklahoma, and District of Columbia where permissive law exists.[3] Permissive law permits practicing nursing as long as the unlicensed person does not call herself a registered nurse. Mandatory licensure requires that, in order to practice as a registered nurse, one must meet established standards and become licensed. The nursing practice statute also grants the licensing board authority to issue rules and regulations which more fully define nursing practice.

Regulations provide the rules. They are more specific and detailed than statutes. Regulations are enacted by administrative agencies, made up of experts, for the purpose of implementing statutes. State boards of nursing establish regulations which tell nurses how to function in a manner consistent with the legally permissible scope of practice. Examples of regulations include minimum standards and continuing education requirements.

Law, as described so far, and "common law" regulate the conduct of human beings in a legally binding manner. *Common law* is not the result of legislative action but is made by a judge. It arises out of decisions in specific cases. In the remainder of this chapter, the reader will find examples of *trial decisions* involving obstetrical nurses. These decisions apply to individual cases and illustrate the types of cases that are tried. Only cases which have been tried by an Appellate Court become law by way of *case law* decision. Case law sets precedent, is authorative, and, therefore, eligible for citation as law to a court, a hospital, or a client. The reader should note the description used for each example, that is, trial decision versus case law. (The case law examples used have been verified by Attorney Norman D. Tucker of Sommers, Schwartz, Silver and Schwartz, P.C., in Southfield, Michigan.)

Each state has its own common laws, independently developed by its own courts' decisions. Most common law is "negative" since it usually arises out of actions of negligence or license sanction and tells us what is bad or suboptimal. Several examples of trial decisions are cited that illustrate the decisions made on particular issues. Occasionally common law in the form of case law is helpful in defining practice. As evident in the *Sermchief v. Gonzales* case, a court can be persuaded to interpret nursing practice acts broadly. The conclusion in this case is that nursing function is not limited to that specified but must be within the limits of the individual nurse's skill and education based on the standard of care.

Example of Case Law. In *Sermchief v. Gonzales*, nurses with postgraduate training in OB/Gyn were charged with unauthorized practice of medicine, and the physicians involved, with aiding and abetting them. No one was injured or harmed from the nurses taking histories; performing breast and pelvic exams; doing Pap smears, GC cultures and blood serology; giving contraceptive information and devices; dispensing certain designated medications; and providing counseling and education. All nursing functions were covered by written standing orders and protocols that the involved physicians had signed. The Missouri Supreme Court concluded that, under their Nurse Practice Act, professional nurses can assume responsibilities consistent with their "special education, judgement, and skill based on knowledge and application of principles derived from the biological, physical, social and nursing sciences." [660 S.W. 2d 683 (S.Ct. Mo. 1983)]

In the courts, case law[4] or decisional law,[5] such as that cited above, originates as a result of *litigation* (a lawsuit). This law is then accepted as a precedent in the same jurisdiction for subsequent case decisions.

A distinction has already been made between statutory and common law. Statutory law is based on legislative decision; common law is from judicial decisions. Nurses should also realize that there are two major classifications of common law—criminal and civil. *Criminal law* deals with conduct considered offensive to society (for example, murder, burglary, illegally dispensing narcotics). The penalty is usually imprisonment. *Civil law* addresses private legal rights and interests. The unsuccessful party in a civil case usually pays money to the successful party.

The branch of civil law that deals with wrongs committed by and against private persons is called the *law of torts*. In all torts, the person(s) who has been wronged has a legal right to institute a

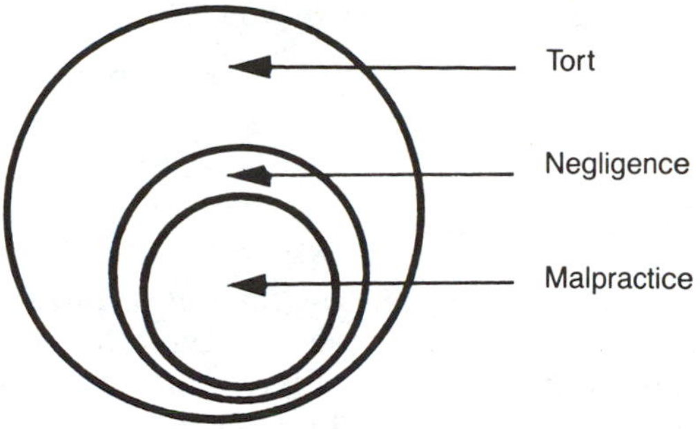

Figure 10–1. The circles symbolically represent the fields of tort law, negligence law, and malpractice law.

lawsuit against the person(s) who caused the wrong. Tort may be *intentional* (for example, invasion of privacy, assault and battery) or *unintentional,* such as negligence. According to law, a person who fails to act in a reasonable and prudent manner is *negligent.*

Negligence is a general term that applies to all negligent acts. For example, when a person (nurse or someone else) fails to be cautious when driving and injures another person, the driver is negligent. When a person engaged in performing professional skills does a negligent act, *malpractice* occurs. The relationship of tort law, negligence, and malpractice is illustrated in Figure 10–1. Malpractice may be due to a number of factors, such as lack of training, carelessness due to stress or fatigue, or failure to follow the standard of care for any number of reasons. This action may ultimately result in a lawsuit.

• •

Review Questions

Fill in the blanks.

1. Statutes that are of great importance to the nursing profession are ____________________.
2. Regulations for nursing, explaining precise methods for implementing statutes, are formulated and enforced by state ____________________.

Circle the correct response:

3. Negligence is a (criminal, civil) offense.
4. Malpractice (is, is not) a form of negligence.

Answers

1. *Nurse practice acts* are statutes of great importance to nursing.
2. State *boards of nursing* formulate and enforce regulations for nursing.

3. Negligence is a *civil* offense.
4. Malpractice *is* one form of negligence.

• •

Negligence

Malpractice is negligence committed by a professional. Most cases involving nurses involve allegations of negligence. A nurse, as an individual, is negligent, or at fault, when she does something wrong or does not do something that should be done. In order for there to be malpractice, the nurse must be considered legally liable to the patient.

Four elements are required to establish liability—duty, breach of duty, causation, and injury. The nurse must be involved in *giving care (duty)* to the specific patient. Ordinarily, one thinks of assigned patients only. But Fiesta[6] states that "the nurse has a duty (even if only a minimal duty to assist a patient when an emergency arises) to all patients in the hospital. The nurse's failure to respond to a patient's request for assistance in an emergency is clearly practicing below a reasonable standard of care."

A *breach of duty* occurs when the nurse fails to comply with the standard of care. The nurse may fail to act (an act of omission), perform an unauthorized act, or have authority to act but perform the authorized act in an improper manner. In order for there to be malpractice, as a *result of the breach* there must be injury to the patient (*causation*). The patient must experience physical, emotional and/or financial *injury*.

Causation must be direct or proximate. For example, a nursing action may be deemed a cause of a newborn's brain damage. A *direct cause* may be the nurse's attempt to delay the delivery by putting firm pressure on the presenting fetal head at the time of imminent delivery. A *proximate or contributing cause* may be the nurse's lack of recognition of problems, misinterpretation of the fetal monitor strip, or failure to communicate the presence of nonreassuring fetal heart rate patterns. In turn, the physician can use the nurse's failure (to contact him) as an excuse for his not taking definitive action. The Hiatt case law example at the end of this chapter involves a nurse who was negligent by failing to notify the physician in time and, therefore, the nurse was considered a proximate cause to the injury.

WHO IS LIABLE?

Nurses are personally liable if a patient is injured due to the nurse's incompetence or carelessness when performing nursing skills and duties. Nurses in critical care areas, such as labor/delivery, are responsible for having sufficient knowledge so they can make reasonably correct decisions, including understanding the monitors and other electronic devices used. Incompetence in these areas may result in a civil liability. In contrast, gross negligence—disregard for human life—is viewed as criminal by the law.[7]

Floating—moving around to different areas to counteract nursing shortages—increases nurses' chances of liability suits, although job retention may depend on their willingness to float. It is a logical expectation that the nurse must explain significant deficits, if any, in her abilities so that nursing management can make appropriate float assignments. Orientation should be provided by the hospital as necessary. Another possible solution is to use the "float" for only task-oriented functions.

Understaffing is another problem nurses often face. It puts the hospital at risk since the Joint Commission on Accreditation of Hospitals (JCAH) standard requires that there be sufficient personnel to meet the physical needs of the patients. "A special staffing ratio is established for labor and delivery: the number of nursing personnel on duty each shift will be one half the average number of deliveries per day, based on the previous fiscal year."[8] A nurse who views an assignment as unsafe and is unable to meet the patient's needs is obligated to notify the supervisor of the situation. If upon the supervisor's evaluation there is found to be inadequate staffing, the supervisor must make this known to hospital administration promptly and emphatically, preferably in writing. Careful documentation of the endangering incidents should be kept.[9]

Supervisory nurses are responsible for the consequences of their own acts as well. The supervisor must properly evaluate the patient's nursing needs and the assigned nurse's capabilities.[10,11] When aware of a hazardous situation, the supervisor must take action when possible to avoid an injury.[11] The supervisor who elects to cover a unit during the absence of the originally assigned nurse must be competent to carry out the latter's duties.[12]

Although the nurse injures the patient, the hospital is also responsible to the injured person. The employer is liable for wrongful acts of any of its employees. The hospital can be held liable even if it provided a comprehensive, competent orientation, assigned the nurse based on her abilities, and provided sufficient supervision.[13] This hospital (institutional or corporate) liability is due to a master-servant or *respondeat superior* rule. The injured person may sue both the hospital and the nurse. An exception exists when the nurse is a private duty nurse or hired by an independent contractor. These nurses are responsible for their own wrongs and the hospital in which they are working is not liable.[14]

• •

Review Questions

1. When paraphrasing the four elements needed to establish nursing liability (that is, duty, breach of duty, causation, and injury), it is correct to say that if a patient is injured, the nurse is liable if: ____ ____.

Circle correct response:

2. The hospital (is, is not) ordinarily liable for its patient's injury.

Answers

1. If a patient is injured, the nurse is liable if, *during her/his responsibility for patient care, the nurse caused injury through negligence.*
2. The hospital *is* ordinarily liable for its patient's injury.

• •

STANDARD OF CARE

A standard, as it will be used throughout this chapter, is the basis for judging quality. In nursing, as well as in the legal profession, the standard, or quality, of care, is of utmost importance. Standards should provide a tool for evaluating and ultimately improving one's individual or institutional performance. Standards are not meant to be punitive. Standards define not only what should be done, but what should not be done. Standards define appropriate practice as recognized by authorities in the field.

There are both external and internal sources of standards. Several of the external standards were previously mentioned—namely, nurse practice acts, board of nursing regulations. Many standards are published by professional organizations, such as:

- Standards for Nursing Service for the Joint Commission for Accreditation of Hospitals (JCAH),
- The Organization for Obstetric, Gynecologic, and Neonatal Nurses (NAACOG) standards, competencies and guidelines, and
- American Nurses' Association (ANA) Standards of Maternal-Child Health Nursing Practice.

The standards set by these national organizations are recognized in the legal community as the "respected minority" rule. They must be adhered to if prudent care is to be given. An extensive list of professional associations that provide standards for maternal-child nursing is available in some publications, for example, Bobak and Jensen (1987, A-3). Another external source of standards is nursing literature in the form of current periodicals, technical bulletins, and textbooks. Realizing that there are so many sources of standards, one must anticipate they will be inconsistent and at times conflict. It behooves the nurse to use her best judgment, seeking a collective opinion when possible, to decide on which standards must be followed.

Internal (hospital) standards of care must be based on accepted external standards. The internal standards may be higher, but not lower. Internal standards include the hospital's job descriptions, policies and procedures (including specific actions and rationales), and standard care plans. Caution must be taken by the nurse to individualize the plan as necessary for each patient and to recognize that a nurse's training, knowledge, and experience may vary the job expectations. These internal standards should be part of orientation to the hospital, and it is a professional responsibility of the nurse to periodically review these standards.

Individual hospitals promulgate (make known as official) policies and procedures. These "standards" serve as an important source of information in lawsuits. Therefore, hospitals should save them for future reference. The policies determine what nurses (and other health care personnel) may do in that institution. The procedures provide details about how tasks are to be performed. In order for a nurse to practice within the law, she must be knowledgeable about hospital policies and procedures, follow them, and vertify that they reflect the current "state of practice," as well as national standards of care. It is no longer appropriate to have a "community standard of care," which implies that different geographic areas may practice differently. The trend today is to recognize national, not community, standards.

When physicians were first held to national standards, it was because of the board specialties, and the fact that the certification was national as opposed to merely state licensure. Today many labor/delivery nurses are being certified by organizations such as NAACOG and ANA. These certified nurses can no longer be content to limit their performance of nursing to ordinary care; they must be knowledgeable about the state of practice of obstetrical nursing throughout the country. The courts are beginning to recognize with nurses, as they did almost two decades ago with physicians, that when nurses specialize in a particular area, they are held to a higher standard of care. The following case sets precedent for similar circumstances, such as certified obstetrical nurses.

Example of Case Law. In *Whitney v. Day*, the Michigan Supreme Court recognized that there may be differences in the duties and obligations a nurse may owe a patient depending on her expertise, knowledge, and training. The Certified Registered Nurse Anesthetist (CRNA) involved was sued as a result of a cardiac arrest during surgery. The Court noted that CRNAs are licensed nurses, but also certified after 18 months of study in their speciality. The Court indicated that the nurse anesthetist would be held to a standard of care ordinarily possessed by nurses of similar education and training, and not the standard of an ordinary nurse. [100 Mich App 707 (1980)]

"REASONABLE NURSE" STANDARD

Standards of care for nurses are what an average nurse would do when acting under the same or similar circumstances. The concept of *the reasonably prudent nurse* is applicable here. An individual nurse's behavior should be consistent with that of other "reasonable" nurses. This concept gives strong support for nurses to: (1) ask their colleagues how they would approach a particular patient situation, (2) participate in formal and informal peer review of practices, and (3) attend professional meetings, such as NAACOG.

General standards of nursing practice apply to all nurses. Whenever a nurse gives a medication to a patient, the nurse is accountable for knowledge about the drug's proper use—its actions, common side effects, safe administration, etc. Specialty standards apply only to nurses who work in the particular area under consideration.

In labor, assessment is not done every 4 hours or once a shift, although that might be appropriate on a general medical unit. The frequency of assessment is dependent on the phase of labor and normalcy of fetal and maternal response. There are times when a vaginal examination should be done in labor (for example, the woman is complaining of a strong urge to push) and times when careful consideration must first be given to the possible complications that might result (for example, the woman is vaginally bleeding, or the membranes have been ruptured for several hours).

It is the nurse's responsibility to be informed about the current standards; for example, she should know what is included in a competent assessment. She cannot rely on what she learned in her basic nursing education but must update her knowledge base by informal and formal continuing education.

When a nurse (or other health care professional) does not follow the standard of care, she commits a breach of duty or breach of the standard of care. The most frequent basis for liability of nurses is the negligent tort, but negligence alone is not enough to bring forth a lawsuit. There must be injury caused by the negligence. The source or cause of the injury may be difficult for the legal profession to prove but a focal point of the investigation is what standards of care were not followed. The best evidence of the care actually given is found in the medical record. A second source of information is the testimony of the witnesses. (Documentation in the medical record and the use of witnesses in the lawsuit are discussed later in this chapter.)

• •

Review Questions

1. List three external and three internal sources of nursing standards:
   External: (a) ________________, (b) ________________, (c) ________________.
   Internal (hospital): (a) ____________________, (b) ____________________
   (c) ________________.

2. In order to practice as a reasonable nurse, the nurse should:
   a. ____
   b. ____

3. **Define what a standard of care for a nurse is:** ______________________________

4. **Identify the significance of a breach of standards:** ______________________________

Answers

1. Sources of nursing standards include the following: External—*nurse practice acts, Board of Nursing regulations, professional organizations* (e.g., JCAH, ANA, NAACOG) *official statements, nursing literature;* internal sources—*hospital job descriptions, policies and procedures,* and *standard care plans.*
2. A reasonable nurse should know what the accepted standards of care are, know that the hospital employing her has standards consistent with those accepted, and follow hospital policies and procedures.
3. A standard of care is *what an average nurse would do when acting under the same or similar professional circumstances.*
4. *Non-compliance with the standard of care* is the most frequent basis for nursing liability.

• •

POTENTIAL LIABILITY IN EACH STEP OF THE NURSING PROCESS

Assessment. The nurse is responsible for patient assessment. It is especially important that the labor/delivery nurse identify the risk factors during the assessment process. Errors occur when the nurse fails to gather information completely and correctly, fails to interpret the significant data, and/or fails to communicate the methods and information gathered.

Example of Trial Decision. In *Herrup v. South Miami Hospital Foundation, Inc.*, nurses failed to assess contractions and fetal heart rate every 30 minutes per hospital and national standards. Although an external monitor was available and ordered by the physician, it was not used. When the previously normal heart rate was reassessed 1½ hours later, fetal distress was noted. Though arrangements were made to do an emergency cesarean, the fetal heart rate stopped. The stillborn was delivered vaginally. [No. 83-37139, Fla. Dade Cty Cir. Ct. (October 24, 1984), reported in 28 ATLA L REP 88 (March 1985)]

Example of Trial Decision. In *Patel v. South Fulton Hospital,* the mother came to the hospital with ruptured membranes. Fetal heart rates were first taken 5½ hours after arrival. They were found to be absent. The nurses were charged with failure to monitor this patient sufficiently. [No-C-65704, Fulton Cty. Superior Ct. Georgia. (October 5, 1984), reported in 28 ATLA REP 42 (February 1985)]

Plan. Based on the data collected, the nurse must formulate an appropriate plan—one that is consistent with the standards of care. The plan must include the physician's orders. Errors usually do not involve the plan itself but instead an inappropriate act or act of omission that follows.

In a case where the laboring woman is a diabetic, the doctor may order a blood sugar be drawn. Not only must the lab work be done, but the nurse must realize that, during the course of labor, the blood sugar will vary and the plan must include repeated blood sugar assessment. Such an omission may have detrimental effects on mother and baby. Therefore, the nurse should seek an order for repeated blood sugars as necessary.

Example of Trial Decision. In *Trevino v. United States*, despite diagnosed marginal separation of the placenta, the nurse instructed the laboring mother to continue walking. She continued to bleed profusely, yet 1½ hours later the nurse gave her an enema. The nurse still failed to use continuous fetal monitoring and bedrest. Delivery was complicated by the physician's unsuccessful attempt with vacuum extraction when the cervix was not fully dilated. A brain-damaged infant resulted. [No. V84-179T (W.D. Wash.), reported in 28 ATLA L REP 465 (December 1985)]

Intervention. It is the nurse's duty to implement the plan derived from the nursing assessment, as well as interpret and carry out the physician's orders. The prime concern is that the intervention be consistent with the standard of care.

Medication errors are frequent sources of liability related to nursing interventions. Physician's orders that are ambiguous or apparently erroneous first need to be clarified by the prescribing physician. In situations where inappropriate orders remain, hospitals usually have established policies for nurses to follow—for example, notify the nursing supervisor who then contacts a medical officer.

In labor an order may be correct when originally written but inappropriate as the patient's condition changes. This happens frequently with oxytocin and narcotic orders which require nursing judgment as to the appropriateness of their administration. "The physician should provide guidance and delegate this responsibility only to nurses who are able to make the required judgments."[15]

Fetal monitoring is a prime example of where intervention errors are made. A poor monitor tracing is unacceptable. Frequent reassessment is required despite the presence of continuous electronic monitoring. An internal fetal monitor is desirable when the feedback from an external is questionable. Based on the assessment of certain fetal heart rate and contraction patterns—for example, variable and late decelerations, uterine hyperstimulation—nursing intervention is required. (See Chapter 3 for details.) All relevant information must be communicated. (See later section on documentation.) Timely notification of the physician is imperative, providing enough information so a valid management decision can be made.

Example of Trial Decision. In *Capaccia v. Newman*, the obstetrician ordered IV drip oxytocin for a post-term mother. Although external monitoring was done, the nurse failed to discontinue the infusion when the physician left the unit (hospital policy) and to notify the physician of fetal tachycardia, meconium-stained amniotic fluid, and rapid cervical dilatation that resulted from hyperstimulated contractions. The baby sustained anoxic brain injury. [No. 21831/81, New York Supreme Court (October 26, 1984), reported in 28 ATLA L REP 89 (March 1985)]

Example of Trial Decision. In *May v. Wm. Beaumont Hospital*, nurses failed to implement the orders for fetal monitoring and IV therapy. The non–English speaking mother complained of severe pain through her interpreter. Because the nurse and attending physician assumed she was not in labor, they did not place her in bed and ignored her. She delivered while standing up. The baby fell head first to the floor, sustaining trauma resulting in mental retardation. [No. 81-230-540-NO. Mich. Oakland County Cir. Ct. (April 23, 1985) reported in 28 ATLA L REP 419 (November 1985)]

Evaluation. The nurse is responsible for review and documentation of the effect of the interventions to assure they are completed properly. Revision of the plan and, as a result, further assessment and nursing intervention are often necessary. Nurses must evaluate more than their own care. Courts expect nurses to evaluate the appropriateness of the medical management and to report their concerns to their nursing supervisor (or whatever the established hospital policy is).[16]

Example of Trial Decision. In *James v. Kennebec Valley Medical Center of Maine*, the physician induced labor without an infusion pump and monitored fetal heart rate every 15 minutes with a stethoscope because data from the external monitor was unreadable. The baby suffered hypoxic brain damage. The nurses were charged with negligence for improperly evaluating the appropriateness of this ordered approach. [No. 80-CV649 Kennebec Cty. Supreme Ct. (February 4, 1985) reported in 27 ATLA L REP 183 (May 1985)]

Nurses should be particularly aware of the following errors that frequently "appear in charts that come to litigation:

- incomplete initial history and physical
- failure to observe and take appropriate action
- failure to communicate changes in a patient's condition
- incomplete and/or inadequate documentation
- failure to use/interpret fetal monitoring appropriately."[17]

Example of Case Law. In *Goff v. Doctor's General Hospital from San Jose*, the nurse assessing in the postpartum area failed to take any definitive action with regard to the patient's continued bleeding. She did not take blood pressures, temperatures, pulses, or respirations. She also did not call the attending physician because from her experience she did not feel he would come to the hospital. The Court found that the nurse was negligent in her failure to assess the patient, failure to contact the attending physician, and if she felt he would not come to the hospital if contacted, then she had an obligation to notify her supervisor. The significance of this decision by the California District Court of Appeals is that a nurse is responsible for assessing the patient and calling the physician. If it is apparent to her that the patient is not properly cared for, she has an independent obligation to the patient to do what is necessary to obtain that appropriate care and treatment. The decision has implications beyond the particular patient's case. The Court stated that it "is elementary that knowledge received during the course of their employment as nurses is in legal effect binding upon their employer, the defendant hospital." Broadly speaking this places an obligation on nurses to report inadequacies, abuses (including substance), or deficiencies of a particular hospital employee, or physician, that could reasonably be anticipated to affect patient care. [33 P.2d 29 (1958)]

• •

Review Question

For each of the identified steps of the nursing process, list general remedies to avoid common nursing errors:

Assessment:

a. ______

b. ______

c. ______

Plan:

a. ______

b. ______

Intervention:

a. ______

Evaluation:

a. ______

b. ______

c. ______

Answer

General remedies to avoid common nursing errors include:

Assessment:

a. Collect data using correct method and frequency (follow standard of care)
b. Interpret significant data (for example, identify high risk factors)
c. Communicate methods of assessment and gathered information in chart, and to physician as necessary

Plan:

a. Base plan on data collected (follow standard of care), and
b. Incorporate doctor's orders

Intervention:

a. Carry out plan of care following standard of care

Evaluation:
a. Review and document effect of interventions
b. Revise plan as necessary
c. Communicate inappropriate medical management

• •

MALPRACTICE INSURANCE

Professional liability insurance is the same as malpractice insurance. Although a nurse's best defense against malpractice suits is always to practice in a reasonably prudent manner consistent with the standards of care, this is an era of lawsuits. Obstetrics is a frequent target area. The fact that labor/delivery nurse malpractice insurance premiums increased seven-fold in 1987 by a major carrier is evidence of that.[18]

It is the nurse's responsibility to determine what protection is provided since hospitals vary in the insurance coverage they provide. The nurse also needs to evaluate the need for additional personal coverage. Consideration should be made of the riskiness of the area and the degree of independence involved. The greater the risk and independence, the greater the need for personal insurance.

There are several purposes of nursing malpractice insurance. Among the purposes are: (1) provision of an award of damages against the nurse up to the specified limits of the policy, and (2) payment of the lawyers' fees to defend the nurse.

The scope of the policies vary as to the cost, amount of coverage, what they cover and do not cover, and when the company must be notified of a claim. Usually the insurance carrier has 28 days to file an answer to a claim. Failure to file an answer within that period of time may result in a default judgment entered against the nurse and in denial of coverages.[19] The specifics are available from the agent, as well as from the printed policy.

A very important factor to note is what kind of policy it is. An *occurrence policy* covers incidents occurring when the policy is in effect regardless of when the claim is made. This type of policy provides a more complete protection than claims-made alone. The nurse with an occurrence policy should not discard the policy because it may be the only evidence that she was insured at the time of the legal incident. A *claims-made policy* covers claims made only during the year(s) the nurse subscribed to the policy. With an added "tail," the coverage can be extended to claims made after the expiration of the policy on incidents that occurred during the time the policy was in effect. This option is something to think about when terminating the policy for any reason.

Several considerations should be made when deciding whether to acquire a personal malpractice policy:

1. If a lawsuit is lost and there is no insurance covering it, personal assets may be confiscated to satisfy the award.

2. If the hospital is not willing to defend the nurse's actions, the nurse will probably not be covered by the hospital policy.
3. The nurse could be sued by the hospital's insurer if the nurse is found guilty.
4. Having personal and hospital coverage may mean some duplication but may be preferable to not having a portion covered. Personal insurance may ensure coverage beyond that of the hospital —for example, beyond working hours, away from the hospital.
5. The cost of litigation may be increased if more than one insurance company (hospital's and individual's) is involved.
6. Since it is very unusual for the nurse to be sued without the hospital also being sued, and lawyers tend to sue only agents who are insured and for the amount for which they are insured, some authorities suggest that perhaps nurses do not need to carry their own insurance.

Ultimately, the decision of whether or not to have personal liability is an individual one, but worth serious consideration.

• •

Review Questions

1. List two reasons that favor carrying malpractice insurance:
   a. ____________________
   b. ____________________

Circle the correct option in the parentheses.

2. An advantage of (occurrence, claims-made) policy is that if a claim is made ten years after the occurrence, the nurse insured at that earlier time is covered.

3. Having both hospital and personal coverage is (useless, an absolute safeguard, a personal decision).

Answers

1. Reasons for carrying malpractice insurance include:
   a. It provides the award of damages against the nurse.
   b. It pays lawyers' fees to defend the nurse.

2. *Occurrence* policies cover suits that occurred in the year(s) when the policy was in effect.

3. Having both hospital and personal coverage is a *personal decision.*

• •

PATIENT'S RIGHTS AND CONSENT

As a patient advocate, the nurse must deal with patient's rights and consent. The basic principle of all patients' consents is the right to agree to be, or not to be, touched. Ordinarily, nurses don't ask directly for this privilege, but they imply it and the patient responds positively or negatively in verbal or nonverbal behaviors. A second principle is that the patient must be allowed to make an informed choice. This is consistent with holistic health concepts that emphasize education and self-care. Patients and nurses collaborate, freely exchanging information, permitting the patient to make a decision about the patient goals.

Today's labor/delivery nurse is also expected, although not always held liable, to apply the principles inherent in two fairly recent documents which address patient rights. The Patient's Bill of Rights was adopted by the American Hospital Association in 1972. Many states have passed acts and/or established rules and regulations based on the Patient's Bill. The other document is the Pregnant Patient's Bill of Rights which greatly influences today's obstetrical care.

The *Patient's Bill of Rights* makes explicit statements about the patient's right to information from the physician about:

- The complete and current diagnosis, treatment and prognosis in understandable terms, along with the name of the responsible physician. When it is inadvisable to tell the patient, information should be given to the appropriate significant other.
- Information needed to give informed consent before starting the procedure and/or treatment. Included should be the specific procedure/treatment, significant risks involved, and probable length of incapacitation. Alternatives should be discussed if the patient requests them.
- Medical consequences of actions if the patient refuses the treatment.

JCAH[21] supports these statements and adds that, if the hospital plans to do experimentation affecting the care/treatment, the patient has the right to refuse to participate, as well as to refuse treatment.

The nurse should know who the employing hospital delegates as responsible for obtaining informed consents. Usually it is the medical staff and individual physicians, as delineated in the hospital policies and procedures. "Whatever the procedure in regard to the signing and execution of a consent form, the nurse who attempts to explain the nature of a procedure, the risks involved, or the alternatives available is exposing himself or herself to considerable risk through the lack of knowledge required to properly explain these points to the patient."[22] The nurse may witness the patient signing a consent form, clarify what the physician said, and answer the patient's questions. Specific informed consent questions should be referred back to the physician.

The patient who is 18 years of age or older (the age of majority in most states) may legally give consent. An exception is the mentally incompetent patient. In the case of a minor, as defined by state law, a parent, adult family member, or court-appointed guardian consents to medical treatment. An "emancipated minor" is one who is no longer subject to his parents' control or regulation through no longer living at home, being self-supporting and/or is/has been married. In some states, an emancipated minor is allowed some consent privileges, including those involving childbirth. All states have legislation regarding minors' consent to treatment for venereal disease, substance abuse, pregnancy and termination of pregnancy, as well as prescription of contraceptives. Despite the fact that in some states, a minor may obtain treatment on his own, it is usually wise for the health care provider to suggest that the minor discuss the situation with the parents or guardians. The ultimate exception to seeking signed consent is an emergency when immediate care (for example, urgent cesarean delivery) is needed to save a life or prevent serious impairment.

The *Pregnant Patient's Bill of Rights and Responsibilities*[23] recognizes that, in addition to those identified in the AHA document, the pregnant patient represents two patients and that they, therefore, have additional rights. In summary, the rights are knowledge of:

- Prescribed drugs and procedures including alternatives, effect on fetus, proven safety, brand and generic drug names, name and qualifications of person administering, and whether procedure is medically indicated or elective
- Benefits of minimal preoperative medications
- Right to voluntarily consent or refuse therapy
- Right to a labor partner of choice, least stressful position in labor and birth, rooming-in and feed baby on demand
- Person who delivered baby, any known/suspected long-term problems
- Accessibility of hospital records and storage of them until age of majority

These rights serve to help the patient make informed decisions about her care and that of her baby's, as well as to protect the health care team and hospital against litigation founded on resentment or misunderstanding by the mother. Along with the rights, the pregnant patient has (not legally enforceable) responsibilities which are identified. They include:

- Seek good obstetrical care.
- Become knowledgeable about birth process, hospital's policies and regulations, self and baby care.
- Collaborate with physician/midwife about birthing plans, including finances.
- Notify physician or hospital in case of change.
- Following birth, provide evaluation of care received.

It is recognized that these statements apply to a normal obstetrical experience and that, in complicated situations, the expectant couple must rely more on the expertise of the health care team. See Chapter 7 for more specific application of these rights and responsibilities.

• •

Review Questions

1. List two basic principles regarding patient's rights and consent:
   a. ______________________________
   b. ______________________________

2. The Patient's Bill of Rights identifies specific information the patient should receive from the physician before signing a consent form. They include:
   a. ______________________________
   b. ______________________________
   c. ______________________________

3. Since it is the physician's responsibility to gain the patient's consent for a procedure/treatment he is to perform, the nurse's role should be limited to:
   a. ______________________________
   b. ______________________________

4. Indicate with a check mark (✓) which of the following patients can legally sign a consent form:

   _____ clear thinking adult
   _____ mentally ill adult
   _____ parent/guardian of a minor
   _____ emancipated minor defined by state law

5. The Pregnant Patient's Bill of Rights identifies several rights and responsibilities. List five of each:

RIGHTS	RESPONSIBILITIES
a. ____________	a. ____________
b. ____________	b. ____________
c. ____________	c. ____________
d. ____________	d. ____________
e. ____________	e. ____________

Answers

1. Basic principles regarding patient's rights and consent are:
   a. Patient must consent to be touched.
   b. Patients must be allowed to make a knowledgeable choice.

2. The Patient's Bill of Rights identifies that the patient should receive the following information from the physician:
   a. An understandable explanation of diagnosis, treatment, and prognosis.
   b. Plans and expected outcomes of procedure and/or treatment.
   c. Consequences of not being treated.

3. The nurse's role in the consent process should be limited to:
   a. Witnessing the signing of the consent form by the patient.
   b. Clarifying what the physician said and answering questions.
4. The following patients can legally sign a consent form: a clear thinking adult, the parent/guardian of a minor, and an emancipated minor as defined by state law.
5. Consult the preceding paragraphs for the lists of rights and responsibilities identified in the Pregnant Patient's Bill of Rights.

• •

DOCUMENTATION: STRATEGIES TO DISCOURAGE LEGAL ACTIONS

The medical chart, including monitor strips, is a permanent record stored by the medical records department of the hospital and available to lawyers upon request if certain legal criteria are met. The chart provides retrospective facts about the details of a patient's care. The chart is heavily relied upon to verify if there is compliance with standards of care when litigation occurs. At this time the nurse rarely recalls anything about the case which may have occurred several years ago. The nurse is totally dependent upon the information recorded on the chart.

The chart, of course, serves many useful purposes at the time it is being written. It stores the assessment data, plans of care, and evaluation of the outcomes. It provides communication between responsible caretakers—nurses, doctors, other interdisciplinary team members, on current and other shifts. Dr. Emanuel Friedman, pioneer of labor curves, was known to say, "An observation not recorded is an observation not made." The assumption is that anything not charted was not done.

Documentation should reflect the patient's status, including the patient's needs, capabilities, limitations, and problems. Critical areas in labor/delivery include the identification of labor status, maternal vital signs, fetal heart rate, and high risk factors. Consideration must be given to abnormalities found in the prenatal history.

Timing is important. Upon admission, a detailed data base is needed. The physician must be immediately informed of the findings and orders obtained. Routine observations at a minimum are a must even if the condition is normal or unchanged. (See Chapter 1 for specifics.) Because exact times are often critical in labor/delivery, the same clock (usually on the labor room wall) should be used in the labor area. Ideally, the delivery area clock is synchronized with that used in labor. Documentation should be done as soon as possible in order to assure accuracy and to keep the communication with other team members current. A clearly identified "late entry" is better than no entry at all. It should be placed on the next available line. The one time it is inappropriate to add late entries is after receiving a subpoena from the legal system for that chart.

When a continuous electronic monitor is used, documentation can be put directly on the strip. This is especially desirable when nonreassuring fetal heart rates are evident and when Pitocin is being administered. It is important that the documentation indicates that the nursing interventions are in response to the data collected—for example, patient turned to left side (as late deceleration is seen), Pitocin rate discontinued (as resting period between contractions is 0 to 20 seconds). Although it should not be necessary to repeat in the nursing progress notes those which appear on the monitor strip, most hospitals recommend repeated documentation because fetal monitor strips are often lost, not retrievable, or illegible. The nurse should be careful to record in a firm, readable penmanship, especially on the strip. *A good habit is to initial the strip every time you enter the room so it is obvious that you are aware of what it says.*

Documentation on the chart should be legible, correct in spelling and grammar, and in ink. Black ballpoint ink is preferred since duplication is likely. Abbreviations used must be accepted by the employing hospital. ROM is usually acceptable even though in other than labor/delivery it may mean "range of motion." Although FOB is not nationally approved as "father of baby," it is recognized in some hospitals as other than "foot of bed." All pages should be stamped with the patient identification. The date must appear near the top of the sheet and each entry must contain the time and initials (or name) of the writer. Signature boxes are acceptable so that initials can be used elsewhere on that page.

Flow sheets provide for evaluation and comparison of findings. Repetition of data found in other areas of the chart, such as the flow sheet, is not necessary unless there is a change in the patient's condition. For example, routinely fetal heart rates are charted in their specified column. Upon rupture of membranes, in sequential order in the remarks column, there should be indication of what method was used (AROM or SROM), if artificial by whom, and a record of the immediate fetal heart rate. Documentation of the patient's responses should also follow the administration of medications, change of position, and so forth.

All relevant information should be charted. Include what your senses tell you—what is heard, seen, felt, and smelled. Procedures may be charted as done "per protocol" when protocols are available in that hospital. The nurse is cautioned to make certain that the protocol is consistent with established standards. (Incident reports are separate from the chart and ordinarily are not referred to in the chart notations.) Be specific—try to avoid words like "apparently." Describe meconium-stained fluid in detail—"brown like motor oil" or "slightly brown." When seeing a newborn with suspected other than term gestation, provide specific descriptive characteristics of SGA, IUGR or LGA (see Chapter 9). Provide details, especially when there is deterioration of the patient's condition. Indicate each action taken in the response. Be clear about whether the nurse called the physician or the physician called the nurse. Include what information was communicated. Be more specific than "informed of progress." Also include when efforts failed to reach the physician and what action was then taken. In an emergency, one nurse may assume responsibility for the charting, but each professional is responsible for seeing that his or her contributions to care are complete and accurately charted.

Do not skip lines and do not leave blank spaces at the end of a note. Draw a line to the end of the line if necessary. These actions prevent someone from adding a note. When an entry continues on the next page, sign at the end of the first page and continue to the second, repeating the date and time so that there is no question about the sequence of events. When an error is made, cross it out with a single line so the error is still readable. Over it write your initials. Immediately after the error, put the correct information. Never alter a record—for example, an Apgar score. If pressured to change the score, notify the supervisor or the person above her in the chain of command if she is pressuring. It is best to have the other person (physician, anesthetist, etc.) put down their impressions as a separate set of scores and for each person to initial his or her own scores.

• •

Review Question

List five documentation strategies which may discourage legal actions:

a. ______________________________

b. ______________________________

c. ______________________________

d. ______________________________

e. ______________________________

Answer

Documentation strategies which may discourage legal action include:

- Chart detailed admission assessment.
- Document initial communication with doctor and orders.
- Follow routine, if not more frequent, observation patterns and chart findings.
- Specify exact times in notations.
- Keep chart current.
- Clearly indicate that nursing interventions are in response to critical data collected.
- Chart in sequence that interventions/responses occurred.
- Do "late entry" as necessary placing it on the first available blank line.
- Use black ink and write legibly.
- Chart all relevant information.
- Be specific in descriptions.
- Be clear about who called whom, when, and what information was communicated.
- Do not leave blank space in narrative portion of chart.
- Neatly line out and initial your errors.

• •

COMPONENTS AND PROCEDURES OF A MALPRACTICE LAWSUIT

In a malpractice suit, nurses can play several roles. Nurses assume the role of a *defendent*, or *factual witness*, when identified as participants in the provision of care to the injured patient. They are called to testify about the facts of the care involved in the case. They do not receive pay. *Expert witnesses*, hired by both defense and plaintiff sides, provide opinions about what standards of care applied in the specific case and where violations occurred. Nurses who are experienced and well educated in the relevant area of nursing are qualified to serve as witnesses and are paid for their work. In the rare instance, a *character witness* speaks about the professional competence of the nurse(s) named in the suit.

A lawsuit begins with the filing of a *complaint* in court. The state's *statute of limitations* places a time restraint on when the complaint must be made. A typical deadline is 2 or 3 years beyond the eighteenth birthday of the person claiming birth trauma. The *plaintiff*, injured patient, or family member offering the complaint, is interviewed by one or more attorneys and possibly some experts including a nurse. They are looking for the four essential elements: duty, breach of duty, causation, and injury. If the conclusion is that the case is worthy of litigation, they seek signed consents in order to obtain all pertinent medical records. The records are eventually reviewed by experts—nurses, obstetricians, neonatologists, and others.

If the attorneys conclude that malpractice has occurred, the case is officially filed in the courthouse and a notice or summons is presented to the defendants. A *summons* is a court order that directs a legal officer to notify the defendant that a suit is filed and informs the defendant of what the general responsibilities are. At this point all defendants (nurses, hospital, doctors, etc.) involved are encouraged to notify their insurance carriers, if they have not already done so. (Many times the hospital risk management department was informed of the injury shortly after it occurred and at that time the insurance company was contacted. When a risk management program is in effect, a settlement may take place without legal action.)

The next step in the lawsuit is *discovery* to determine what evidence the opposing side will present if the case goes to trial. Discovery is done by several methods. Some methods involve questions that must be answered as completely and accurately as possible. The answers are given under oath. *Interrogatories* are lists of written questions sent from one party in the suit to the other. *Depositions* involve orally asked questions by all involved law firms. A complete transcript of the deposition is made by a court recorder. Extensive preparation should be done by all participants. A nurse should be thoroughly knowledgeable about the case and the standards that prevailed at the time, and coached by her attorney about the tactics to use during the deposition.

An arbitration panel or board is used in some states to assist in screening cases for their merit. Regardless of the outcomes, the suit can proceed to a trial by jury. Some suits are dismissed.

Some suits are settled during the discovery period. Negotiations between attorneys on both sides are involved. The amount of compensation is based on the estimated amount of damage suffered, with consideration given to the long-term expenses.

If no settlement has occurred, the next step is *trial* by a jury made up of community members. The jury hears the testimonies of the plaintiff, defendants, and expert witnesses and then weighs the credibility of both sides. The judge informs the jury of how law should be applied. The jury then decides if negligence occurred and what damages should be awarded. The losing party has a right to *appeal* in certain instances. At any point before the jury's decision, either side may settle the case and remove it from the jury.

• •

Review Question

Match the term with the correct definition:

a. Character witness
b. Expert witness
c. Defendant
d. Plaintiff
e. Complaint
f. Statute of limitation
g. Summons
h. Discovery
i. Interrogatories
j. Deposition
k. Arbitration
l. Trial by jury
m. Appeal

1. ____ Injured patient or family member offering complaint
2. ____ Time constraint for filing of complaint
3. ____ Official notification about suit and responsibilities
4. ____ One who provides opinions about implications of standards of care
5. ____ Written questions posed by the opposing side
6. ____ One who speaks to the professional competence of another person
7. ____ Participant in care to the injured
8. ____ Orally posed questions and answers

Answer

1. d, 2. f, 3. g, 4. b, 5. i, 6. a, 7. c, 8. j.

• •

Example of Case Law: In order to prove a case against the defendant nurse, the general rule is that the patient must provide expert testimony from another physician or nurse that what the defendant nurse did on a particular occasion was not consistent with the standard of care of the average nurse, with the same or similar education or experience, under the same or similar circumstances. Exceptions exist when the nurse's actions are so flagrant the Court feels even a layperson would know that what was done was inappropriate.

In *Hiatt v. Groce*, the nurse's actions were so harsh and insensitive to the patient's and family's needs, the Court went farther than normal in making this case law precedent. The laboring patient's husband went repeatedly to the nursing desk asking the nurse in charge to call the attending physician since the husband strongly suspected that labor was progressing rapidly. On each occasion, the nurse was reading a magazine and was very slow to respond to the patient. When she did see the patient, she made comments to the effect, "She's piddling around. It will be quite some time before she has the baby . . . this hospital has never lost a father yet so you just go back there and sit down." The nurse waited too long, and she ultimately delivered the infant as the mother experienced vaginal and labial tears which henceforth hindered her sexual activity.

Although the defendant nurse had multiple experts who testified in her support, the Court found it was not necessary for the plaintiff, under these circumstances, to present expert testimony. The jury, after listening to the facts and circumstances, was permitted to decide in favor of the plaintiff without any expert testimony on behalf of the plaintiff. [523 P.2d 320 (1974)]

CONCLUSION

Although the whole legal process might seem overwhelming, the nurse should realize that even in a situation worthy of a lawsuit, first someone must be willing to make the claim. Nurses who maintain a good relationship with their patients before and after incidents are less likely to be sued. When a possible lawsuit incident occurs, the risk management department should be promptly notified. That department should initiate steps to minimize the chances of a lawsuit. The best way to prevent a lawsuit is for the nurse to recognize her limitations, to practice within the level of preparation, and to give quality comprehensive nursing care based on the standards of care.

REFERENCES

1. Bernzweig, EP: The Nurse's Liability for Malpractice: A Programmed Course, ed 4. McGraw-Hill, New York, 1987, p xiii.
2. Auvenshire, MA and Emriquez, MG: Maternity Nursing: Dimension of Change. Monterey, California, Wadsworth, Inc., 1985, p 99.
3. Creighton, H: Law Every Nurse Should Know, ed 5. WB Saunders, Philadelphia, 1986, p 9.
4. Auvenshire, MA and Emriquez, MG: Maternity Nursing: Dimension of Change. Monterey, California, Wadsworth, Inc., 1985, p 98.
5. Creighton, H: Law Every Nurse Should Know, ed 5. WB Saunders, Philadelphia, 1986, p 2.

6. Fiesta, J: The Law and Liability: A Guide for Nurses. John Wiley & Sons, New York, 1983, p 25.
7. Creighton, H: Law Every Nurse Should Know, ed 5. WB Saunders, Philadelphia, 1986, p 100.
8. Northrop, CE and Kelly, ME: Legal Issues in Nursing. CV Mosby, St. Louis, 1987, p 353.
9. Bernzweig, EP: The Nurse's Liability for Malpractice: A Programmed Course, ed 4. McGraw-Hill, New York, 1987, p 86.
10. Bernzweig, EP: The Nurse's Liability for Malpractice: A Programmed Course, ed 4. McGraw-Hill, New York, 1987, p 84.
11. Rhodes, AM and Miller, RH: Nursing and the Law. Aspen, Rockville, Maryland, 1984, p 163.
12. Creighton, H. Law Every Nurse Should Know, ed 4. WB Saunders, Philadelphia, 1986, p 119.
13. Rhodes, AM: Establishing liability for negligence. Matern Child Nurs J 11(2):127, 1986.
14. Creighton, H: Law Every Nurse Should Know, ed 5. WB Saunders, Philadelphia, 1986, p 65.
15. Rhodes, AM and Miller, RD: Nursing and the Law. Aspen, Rockville, Maryland, 1984, p 151.
16. Chagnon, L and Easterwood, B: Managing the Legal Risks of OGN Nursing. NAACOG Continuing Education Program, Phoenix, May 30, 1987.
17. Chagnon, L and Easterwood, B: Managing the risks of obstetrical nursing. Matern Child Nurs J 11(5):303, 1986.
18. Author's personal experience.
19. Author's personal correspondence.
20. Standards for Nursing Service of the Joint Commission for the Accreditation of Hospitals, 1981, xiv, xv.
21. Rocereto, LR and Maleski, C: The Legal Dimension of Nursing Practice. Springer, New York, 1982, p 8.
22. Haire, D: The Pregnant Patient's Bill of Rights and Responsibilities. International Childbirth Educations Association, Inc., Committee on Health Law and Regulation, Minneapolis, Minnesota, 1975.

BIBLIOGRAPHY

American Nurses' Association Executive Committee and the Standards Committee of the Division on Maternal-Child Health Nursing Practice: Standards of Maternal-Child Health Practice. American Nurses' Association, Kansas City, 1973.

Auvenshire, MA and Emriquez, MG: Maternity Nursing: Dimension of Change. Monterey, California, Wadsworth, Inc., 1985.

Bernzweig, EP: The Nurse's Liability for Malpractice: A Programmed Course, ed 4. McGraw-Hill, New York, 1987.

Bobak, IM and Jensen, MD: Essentials of Maternity Nursing: The Nurse and the Childbearing Family. CV Mosby, St. Louis, 1987.

Chagnon, L and Easterwood, B: Managing the Legal Risks of OGN Nursing. NAACOG Continuing Education Program. Phoenix, May 30, 1987.

Chez, BF: Perinatal Technology and Nursing Malpractice. NAACOG National Conference. Phoenix, June 3, 1987.

Creighton, H: Law Every Nurse Should Know, ed 5. WB Saunders, Philadelphia, 1986.

Cwik, M: Nursing's Role in Perinatal Risk Management. NAACOG National Conference. Phoenix, June 3, 1987.

Dietrich, MS: The Nurse in the Changing Health Care Environment: Legal Issues. Mercy College & Michigan League for Nursing Conference, Detroit, March 17, 1988.

Drane, JF: Competency to give an informed consent—A model for making clinical assessments. JAMA 252(10):925, 1984.

Fiesta, J: The Law and Liability: A Guide for Nurses. John Wiley & Sons, New York, 1983.

Haire, MF: Common Obstetric Malpractice Exposures: Risks and Remedies. Presentation at National Conference of Obstetric Nursing, Dearborn, Michigan, April 21, 1987.

Hogue, E: Nursing and Legal Liability: A Case Study Approach. National Health Publishing, 1985.

Murchison, I, Nichols, TS, and Hanson, R: Legal Accountability in the Nursing Process. CV Mosby, St. Louis, 1982.

NAACOG: Practice Competencies and Educational Guidelines for Nurse Providers of Intrapartum Care. NAACOG, Washington, DC, 1988.

NAACOG Section Conference. Legal Issues in Obstetrical, Gynecological, and Neonatal Nursing. Flint, Michigan, April 24, 1985.

NAACOG: Standards for Obstetric, Gynecologic, and Neonatal Nursing, ed 3. NAACOG, Washington, DC, 1986.

NAACOG: Professional Liability Series. NAACOG, Washington, DC, 1987.

Northrop, CE and Kelly, ME: Legal Issues in Nursing. CV Mosby, St. Louis, 1987.

Rhodes, AM and Miller, RD. Nursing and the Law, ed 4. Aspen Systems Corporation, Rockville, Maryland, 1984.

Rocereto, LR and Maleski, CM: The Legal Dimensions of Nursing Practice. Springer, New York, 1982.

Vice, L: Monitoring the Fetal Heart: Level II as the Beat Goes On. Medical Media Associates Conference, Ann Arbor, October 27, 1986.

Willson, JR and Peters, D: Malpractice in Obstetrics: Legal Aspects. Michigan Conference on Maternal and Perinatal Health, Dearborn, Michigan, March 20 and 21, 1985.

10 POST-TEST

Fill in the blanks:

1. In nursing, the legal statutes which set boundaries are the ______________ and the regulations established by ______________. Regardless of whether the wrong doing is intentional or ______________, a nurse who fails to act in a reasonable and prudent manner is ______________. If this occurs during the performance of the professional role, ______________ occurs. This violation of the patient's legal rights is contrary to ______________ law and may result in a lawsuit or ______________________________.

2. Standards of care are the basis for: ____.

   Broadly speaking, sources of standards of care include:
   a. __________________________________
   b. __________________________________
   c. __________________________________
   d. __________________________________

3. Each ______________ is responsible for his or her own professional actions. In order to be determined liable, the nurse (or other) must be ______________ for the patient, fail to ______________ and, as a result, __________________________________.

4. Give two reasons for carrying malpractice insurance:
   a. __________________________________
   b. __________________________________

5. Regarding patient's rights, the OB nurse is responsible for being knowledgeable about the contents of two documents, namely, (1) ______________ and (2) ______________ and ensuring that they are ______________. The nurse must follow ______________ policy regarding who obtains the signed consent. The nurse's role may be to ______________ the patient's signing (determined by ______________ law), ______________ must sign for the minor patient. An exception is the ______________ minor.

6. The following are situations based on real litigations where facts are given and the nursing errors and remedies need to be briefly identified.
   Situation A:
   Facts: Part of the initial assessment includes gathering EDC which patient says is 8/18. The chart confirms the EDC but adds that LMP was 10/25/87.
   Errors/Remedies:

   Situation B:
   Facts: During pitocin stimulation, nurse does hourly assessments and finds dilatation of 9 cm (increase of 2 in past hour), +1 station, bradycardic fetal heart rate baseline, reoccurring late decelerations, frequent contraction rest intervals of less than 30 seconds. The nurse charts: 9 cm, +1, contractions q 2, 60–90 secs, monitor recording.
   Errors/Remedies:

   Situation C:
   Facts: During paracervical administration, nurse charts: 5:00 AM Paracervical given by Dr. Smith, 50 cc. GH 6:00 AM (next entry)
   Errors/Remedies:

7. Fill in the blanks to correctly describe the components and procedures of a lawsuit: The ______________ files a ______________ within the time stated in the ______________. The perspective case is then reviewed by lawyers and experts to determine its validity. Following the official filing of the litigation case, a ______________ informs all involved ______________ of their general responsibilities regarding the case. During the ______________ stage, written ______________ and/or oral ______________ are used to gather the facts. ______________ —determination of the extent of damage (award)—can occur at any time. If it has not already occurred, there is a ______________ by jury at which time plaintiff, defendants and experts testify. In certain circumstances, their decision can be ______________.

Answers to Post-Test

1. In nursing, the legal statutes which set boundaries are the *nurse practice acts* and the regulations established by *state boards of nursing*. Regardless of whether the wrong doing is intentional or *unintentional*, a nurse who fails to act in a reasonable and prudent manner is *negligent*. If this occurs during the performance of the professional role, *malpractice* occurs. This violation of the patient's legal rights is contrary to *civil* law and may result in a lawsuit or *litigation*.

2. Standards of care are the basis for determining what a nurse should or should not do under similar circumstances. Sources of standards of care include: (a) state nursing practice acts and board of nursing regulations, (b) professional nursing organizations' standards, (c) nursing literature, and (d) hospital documents (job descriptions, policies and procedures, standard care plans).

3. Each *individual* is responsible for his or her own professional actions. In order to determine liability, the nurse (or other) must be *caring* for the patient, fail to *comply with the standard of care*, and as a result, *injury occurs to the patient*.

4. Two reasons for carrying malpractice insurance are:
   a. It provides financial award to patient for the damages.
   b. It pays the legal fees.

5. Regarding patient's rights, the OB nurse is responsible for being knowledgeable about the contents of the *Patient's Bill of Rights* and *Pregnant Patient's Bill of Rights and Responsibilities*, and ensuring that they are *implemented*. The nurse must follow *hospital* policy regarding who obtains the signed consent. The nurse's role may be to *witness* the patient's signing and answer *patient's questions*. In the case of a minor (determined by *state* law), *parent, adult family member, or guardian* must sign for the patient. An exception is the *emancipated* minor.

6. *Situation A:*
   Errors/Remedies: LMP and EDC do not correlate using Naegele's rule or OB wheel. Since LMP of 10/25 → EDC of 8/1 or 2, this is a 42 weeks' gestation (post-dates)—a high-risk factor. The nurse is responsible for noting this, verifying that the EDC was not changed based on ultrasound, and if not, communicating the facts to the physician. The charting must indicate both the communication of facts and assessment more frequent than routine, using continuous electronic monitoring.
   Situation B:
   Errors/Remedies: The assessment interval is too infrequent. It should be every 15 to 20 minutes. The recorded data is incomplete and lacks needed description. Nursing interventions are inappropriate in the presence of fetal stress and hyperstimulation. The Pitocin needed to be turned off, mother positioned on her left side, oxygen given and the physician immediately notified of the situation (if he is not at the bedside, indicate on chart).
   Situation C:
   Errors/Remedies: Charting lacks identification of drug used, as well as consideration of its effect on maternal comfort and BP, and fetal heart rate. Assessments are too infrequent. As charted, the dose is excessive. The nurse should not chart how much was actually poured but the amount given to the patient.

7. The *plaintiff* files a *complaint* within the time stated in the *statute of limitations*. The perspective case is then reviewed by lawyers and experts to determine its validity. Following the official filing of the litigation case, a *summons* informs all involved *defendants* of their general responsibilities regarding the case. During the *discovery* stage, written *interrogatories* and/or oral *depositions* are used to gather the facts. *Settlement*—determination of the extent of damage (award)—may occur at any time. If this does not occur, there is a *trial* by jury at which time plaintiff, defendants and experts testify. In certain circumstances, their decision can be *appealed*.

APPENDIX A: LIST OF NURSING DIAGNOSES

Note: The following nursing diagnoses are listed in the order in which they appear in this book. They are usually stated as real problems. They could also be potential problems.

Chapter 1: AN OVERVIEW OF LABOR AND DELIVERY

Stage I

Knowledge deficit [of premonitory signs of labor] related to lack of exposure. (p. 16)
Anxiety [specify] related to uncertainty about the onset of labor. (p. 22)
Fear (of pain) related to labor; delivery; examinations; needles. (p. 22)
Fear (of long labor) related to inability to tolerate the pain. (p. 22)
Fear (of abandonment during labor) related to lack of understanding of usual routines. (p. 22)
Fear (of internal injury or tears) related to intrusive procedures; body size. (p. 23)
Fear (of losing self-esteem) related to doubtfulness of her ability to cope; loss of control during labor. (p. 23)
Fear (of embarrassment: nudity; urinating and defecating in bed; messiness from amniotic fluid and vaginal discharge; possibility of using foul language) related to uncertainty about acceptance of others. (p. 23)
Fear (of helplessness) related to inability to control onset or progress of labor; inability to control what others do to her during labor and deliver. (p. 23)
Fear (that baby might not survive labor/delivery process) related to lack of confidence in caretaker; predictive signs (fetal distress, early gestation). (p. 23)
Fear (that baby might be injured during delivery) related to use of forceps/vacuum extractor; relatively large size of baby. (p. 23)
Fear (that baby will have gross deformities) related to family history;

advanced maternal age; maternal drug ingestion; unfounded myths. (p. 23)
Fear (that baby will not come out at all) related to size of baby in relation to size of pelvis. (p. 23)
Anxiety [specify] related to unfamiliar surroundings. (p. 24)
Infection, potential for related to inadequate primary defenses. (p. 24)
Cardiac output, alteration in: decreased (maternal) related to dorsal recumbent position. (p. 24)
Hyperthermia related to infection; dehydration. (p. 24)
Injury, potential for; (fetal) trauma related to decreased oxygenation. (p. 25)
Activity intolerance related to excessive expenditure of energy during contractions. (p. 25)
Fluid volume deficit, potential related to inadequate fluid intake. (p. 25)
Comfort, alteration in: pain, acute related to bladder distention. (p. 25)
Comfort, alteration in: pain, acute related to contraction frequency; contraction intensity; maternal position; tension. (p. 26)
Coping, ineffective individual related to rapid labor progression. (p. 27)
Comfort, alteration in: pain, acute related to increased rectal pressure; strong contractions. (p. 28)

Stage II

Comfort, alteration in: pain, acute related to stretching of the vagina; diaphoresis; heat production; bladder distention; strong uterine contractions. (p. 30)
Cardiac output, alteration in: decreased related to dorsal recumbent position; analgesia; anesthesia. (p. 30)
Gas exchange, impaired (fetal) related to head compression; decreased placental perfusion; maternal anesthesia; malpresentation. (p. 30)
Skin integrity, impairment of: potential related to uncontrolled expulsion of fetus. (p. 30)
Fluid volume deficit, potential related to decreased oral intake; diaphoresis; blood loss; vomiting; hyperventilation. (p. 30)

Stage III

Fluid volume deficit, potential related to bleeding from placental separation. (p. 31)
Injury, potential for; (newborn) trauma related to improper positioning. (p. 32)
Family process, alteration in related to separation of parents and newborn. (p. 32)
Comfort, alteration in: pain, acute related to fundal massage; perineal repair. (p. 32)

Stage IV

Fluid volume deficit, potential related to excess blood loss; distended bladder causing fundal relaxation. (p. 33)

Comfort, alteration in: pain, acute related to perineal trauma; uterine contractions; exhaustion. (p. 33)

Family process, alteration in related to separation of parents and newborn. (p. 33)

NEWBORN

Gas exchange, impaired (newborn) related to cold stress; excess mucus, ineffective respiratory effort; intrauterine hypoxia. (p. 35)

Hypothermia related to change in environment; body size; inadequate subcutaneous fat; absence of shiver response. (p. 35)

Injury, potential for; trauma (to newborn) related to eye prophylaxis; hemorrhage; cold stress; resuscitation. (p. 35)

EMERGENCY DELIVERY

Anxiety [specify] related to delivery in an unplanned environment. (p. 37)

Injury, potential for; trauma (to mother) related to lacerations; hemorrhage; infection. (p. 37)

Comfort, alteration in: pain, acute related to fear; anxiety; hysteria; lack of medical support; rapid labor progression. (p. 37)

Injury: potential for; trauma (to fetus/newborn) related to rapid uncontrolled delivery of head; cord compression; inappropriate care; contamination; prematurity. (p. 37)

Chapter 2: MECHANISMS OF LABOR

Anxiety [specify] related to more painful and longer than usual labor. (p. 65)

Comfort, alteration in: pain, acute related to descent of occipital posterior fetal head down maternal back bones, extended period of uterine contractions. (p. 65)

Injury, potential for; trauma (to maternal birth canal [perineum, urethra and anus]) related to abnormal occipital posterior fetal position, larger than usual fetal diameters presenting, and possible use of forceps to assist in delivery. (p. 65)

Injury, potential for; trauma (to fetus) related to longer than usual labor, precipitating fetal distress and difficult delivery. (p. 65)

Injury, potential for; trauma (to fetus [intracranial hemorrhage, central nervous system damage, fractures, anoxia from compression of umbilical cord]) related to the numerous manipulations and progressive size of the fetal diameters during vaginal delivery of fetus in breech presentation. (p. 67)

Injury, potential for; trauma (to mother [genital tract lacerations, hemorrhage]) related to the vaginal delivery of a breech presentation. (p. 67)

Chapter 3: MATERNAL-FETAL MONITORING

Coping, ineffective individual related to painful hypertonic contractions. (p. 95)
Fluid volume deficit related to exertion involved in abnormal labor. (p. 95)
Activity intolerance related to nonproductive labor. (p. 95)
Injury, potential for; trauma (to fetus) related to abnormal contractions. (p. 95)
Comfort, alteration in: pain, acute related to ineffective management of uterine contraction pain. (p. 97)
Tissue perfusion, alteration in: cardiopulmonary related to interruption in placental blood flow. (p. 98)

Chapter 4: GRAPHING LABOR CURVES

Injury, potential for, trauma (to fetus) related to hypoxia. (p. 135)
Injury, potential for, trauma (to mother) related to vigorous uterine contractions. (p. 135)
Comfort, alteration in: pain, acute related to uterine contractions. (p. 135)
Anxiety [specify] related to unexpected, rapid labor. (p. 135)
Anxiety [specify] related to changes in expected pattern of labor. (p. 145)
Diversional activity, deficit related to prolonged labor. (p. 145)
Knowledge deficit [of normal labor/delivery process] related to lack of information (or inadequate preparation, or lack of previous experience). (p. 145)
Infection, potential for, related to invasive procedures. (p. 145)
Fluid volume deficit, potential related to excessive fluid loss. (p. 145)
Coping, ineffective individual related to prolonged painful labor. (p. 146)
Urinary retention [acute] related to pressure of fetal presenting part. (p. 146)
Bowel elimination, alteration in: constipation related to pressure of fetal presenting part. (p. 146)
Injury, potential for; trauma (to fetus) related to prolonged labor. (p. 146)
Injury: potential for; trauma (to mother) related to prolonged labor. (p. 146)

Chapter 5: LABOR STIMULATION

Self-concept, disturbance in: self-esteem related to mis-(self-)diagnosed labor. (p. 159)
Comfort, alteration in: pain, acute (i.e., cramping and slight vaginal bleeding) related to stripping of membranes. (p. 160)

Bowel elimination, alteration in: constipation related to pressure of fetal presenting part. (p. 161)
Anxiety [specify] related to exposure during defecation. (p. 161)
Self-concept, disturbance in: self-esteem related to exposure during defecation. (p. 161)
Anxiety [specify] related to enema procedure. (p. 162)
Comfort, alteration in: pain, acute related to a full rectum. (p. 162)
Sexuality patterns, altered related to labor stimulation by means of nipple stimulation. (p. 164)
Anxiety [specify] related to labor stimulation by means of nipple stimulation. (p. 164)
Anxiety [specify] related to the artificial rupture of membrane procedure. (p. 166)
Injury, potential for; (fetal) trauma related to rupture of membranes. (p. 166)
Infection, potential for, related to the rupture of membranes. (p. 167)
Injury, potential for; (maternal and/or fetal) trauma related to injudicious administration of oxytocin. (p. 173)
Knowledge deficit [about induction of labor] related to lack of exposure. (p. 175)
Anxiety [specify] related to interruption in normal labor process. (p. 175)
Comfort, alteration in: pain, acute (abrupt onset of uterine contractions) related to oxytocin-induced contractions. (p. 175)
Hyperthermia related to prostaglandin's effect on the hypothalamus. (p. 177)

Chapter 6: MANAGEMENT OF PAIN WITH DRUGS

Comfort, alteration in: pain, acute related to lack of knowledge about the labor process. (p. 190)
Coping, ineffective individual related to inadequate or ineffective support during labor. (p. 190)
Activity intolerance related to inadequate rest during labor. (p. 190)
Comfort, alteration in: pain, acute related to inadequate use of distraction techniques. (p. 190)
Comfort, alteration in: pain, acute related to ineffective application of cutaneous stimulation. (p. 190)
Comfort, alteration in: pain, acute related to generalized muscle tension during labor. (p. 191)
Comfort, alteration in: pain, acute related to inadequate support with guided imagery. (p. 191)
Comfort, alteration in: pain, acute related to continued perception of uterine contractions. (p. 191)
Injury, potential for; (maternal/fetal/newborn) related to drugs received during labor. (p. 191)
Breathing pattern, ineffective related to narcotic agonists. (p. 196)

Gas exchange, impaired related to maternal narcotic agonists received during labor. (p. 198)
Thought processes, alteration in related to use of mixed agonists/antagonists. (p. 200)
Sensory-perceptual alteration: visual, auditory, gustatory, olfactory related to use of mixed agonists/antagonists. (p. 200)
Activity intolerance related to use of sedatives. (p. 202)
Injury, potential for; (maternal) trauma related to regional anesthesia. (p. 204)
Injury, potential for: trauma related to paracervical anesthesia. (p. 213)
Cardiac output, alteration in: decreased (maternal and fetal) related to administration of anesthetics. (pp. 216–217)
Airway clearance, ineffective related to aspiration of stomach contents. (p. 218)
Gas exchange, impaired related to inhalation anesthesia. (p. 219)

Chapter 7: CONTEMPORARY APPROACHES TO THE LABOR PROCESS

Anxiety [specify] related to lack of exposure. (p. 239)
Knowledge deficit (of implications of VBAC) related to lack of exposure. (p. 239)
Knowledge deficit (of prepared childbirth methods) related to lack of experience. (p. 243)
Comfort, alteration in: pain, acute related to lack of information about labor process. (p.243)
Comfort, alteration in: pain, acute related to generalized muscle tension during labor. (p. 256)
Knowledge deficit (of cutaneous stimulation and other relaxation techniques) related to lack of exposure; unfamiliarity with information resources. (p. 256)
Coping, ineffective individual related to inadequate support during labor. (p. 260)
Family process, alteration in related to birth of new baby. (p. 260)
Family process, alteration in related to lack of involvement in birth process. (p. 260)

Chapter 8: SELECTED MATERNAL COMPLICATIONS

Knowledge deficit [about the birth process] related to lack of exposure, unfamiliarity with sources of information, cognitive limitation, and/or lack of interest in learning in the adolescent. (p. 275)
Coping, ineffective individual (adolescent) related to situational and maturational crisis of labor. (p. 275)
Self-concept, disturbance in: role performance related to biophysi-

cal, psychosocial, intellectual, and cultural factors of adolescent pregnancy. (p. 275).

Family process, alteration in related to situational and developmental transition/crisis involved in adolescent giving birth. (p. 275)

Social isolation related to adolescent pregnancy. (p. 275)

Comfort, alteration in: pain, acute related to low pain threshold during labor. (p. 275)

Anxiety [specify] related to situational and maturational crises, threat to self-concept, threat of death, and unmet needs. (p. 275)

Injury, potential for; (fetal) trauma related to maternal malnutrition, physiologic immaturity, and inadequate health care. (p. 275)

Knowledge deficit [of labor process] related to lack of prenatal care of substance abuser. (p. 279)

Infection, potential for (in numerous sites) related to substance abuse. (p. 279)

Nutrition, alteration in: less than body requirements related to substance abuse. (p. 279)

Injury, potential for; trauma related to drug abuse and impaired mental processes. (p. 279)

Coping, ineffective individual related to dependence and/or denial of substance abuse. (p. 280)

Family process, alteration in related to substance abuse. (p. 280)

Communication, impaired: verbal related to withdrawal symptoms of substance abuse. (p. 280)

Anxiety [specify] related to well being of herself and her baby. (p. 281)

Knowledge deficit [of cause of bleeding and therapy involved] related to lack of exposure, lack of recall. (p. 281)

Infection, potential for related to open sinuses at placental site and/or nearness of placenta to cervix. (p. 284)

Fluid volume deficit, potential related to altered blood flow at placental site. (p. 284)

Tissue perfusion, alteration in: cardiopulmonary related to hypovolemia. (p. 284)

Parenting, alteration in: potential related to physical status of hemorrhaging mother. (p. 288)

Urinary elimination, alteration in patterns related to pregnancy-induced hypertension as evidenced by diuresis and excess fluid retention. (p. 294)

Anxiety [specify] related to fear of unknown and lack of predictable outcomes in presence of pregnancy-induced hypertension. (p. 294)

Coping, ineffective individual/family: compromised related to stress of pregnancy-induced hypertension. (p. 294)

Fluid volume, alteration in: excess related to decreased urine production. (p. 294)

Self-care deficit: bathing/hygiene, dressing/grooming, toileting related to absolute bedrest status. (p. 294)

Comfort, alteration in: pain, acute related to uterine contractions in presence of anxiety, possible abruptio placenta, and oxytocin infusion. (p. 294)
Injury, potential for; trauma related to sedation (from medications administered), eclamptic episode(s), aspiration of gastric or oral secretions. (p. 294)
Knowledge deficit [of intrapartal hypertension] related to lack of exposure, cognitive limitation. (p. 294)
(Fetal) Gas exchange, impaired related to inadequate uteroplacental perfusion as evidenced by vasospasms, and/or decreased uterine relaxation. (p. 294)
(Fetal) Gas exchange, impaired related to placental abruption or oxytocin infusion as evidenced by decreased or inadequate uterine relaxation between contractions. (p. 294)
Injury, potential for; trauma (to the mother and baby) related to reasons for and procedure involved in cesarean. (p. 296)
Self-concept, disturbance in: self-esteem related to cesarean birth implying failure in ability to birth "normally." (p. 296)
Fear (of unknown) related to condition of self/fetus, pain, procedures, and outcomes. (p. 296)
Knowledge deficit [about reasons for cesarean, procedures, methods of relaxation and pain relief] related to lack of exposure, lack of recall (pp. 296–297)
Coping, ineffective individual related to being tired from labor or lacking sleep. (p. 297)
Cardiac output, alteration in: decreased related to excessive blood loss, positional changes, anesthetic/analgesic reactions. (p. 298)
Skin integrity, impairment of: potential related to knicks in skin from shaving process. (p. 299)
Anxiety [specify] related to cesarean procedure. (p. 299)

Chapter 9: FETAL WELL-BEING IN PRETERM AND POST-TERM GESTATION

Self concept, disturbance in: role performance related to untimely (preterm) labor. (p. 311)
Anxiety [specify] related to well-being of her preterm baby. (p. 311)
Comfort, alteration in: pain, acute from full bladder related to ultrasound procedure. (p. 314)
Anxiety [specify] related to amniocentesis. (p. 315)
Grieving, anticipatory related to loss of "perfect" baby, potential loss of baby. (p. 331)
Self-concept, disturbance in: self-esteem related to failure to deliver at term. (p. 331)
Self-concept, disturbance in: role performance related to mother's lack of knowledge about how to meet needs of preterm infant. (p. 331)

Knowledge deficit [about care of preterm infant] related to lack of preparation. (p. 331)

Noncompliance [with instructions to inform physician of significant decrease in fetal activity] related to perceived lack of seriousness of problem. (p. 336)

Chapter 10: LEGAL CONSIDERATIONS

(none)

APPENDIX B: LIST OF NURSING DIAGNOSES

According to Doenges' Diagnostic Divisions Using NANDA Approved Nursing Diagnoses*

Note: "ch." refers to chapter number, and "p." refers to page reference in this book.
"RT" is the abbreviation used for "related to."

Activity/Rest

Activity Intolerance
- RT excessive expenditure of energy during contractions, ch. 1, p. 25
- RT nonproductive labor, ch. 3, p. 95
- RT inadequate rest during labor, ch. 6, p. 190
- RT use of sedatives, ch. 6, p. 202

Diversional activity, deficit
- RT prolonged labor, ch. 4, p. 145

Circulation

Cardiac output, alteration in: decreased
- RT dorsal recumbent position, ch. 1, p. 24 and p. 30
- RT analgesia, anesthesia, ch. 1, p. 30
- RT administration of anesthetics, ch. 6, pp. 216–217
- RT excessive blood loss, positional changes, anesthetic/analgesic reactions, ch. 8, p. 298

Tissue perfusion, alteration in: cardiopulmonary
- RT decreased placental perfusion (interruption in placental blood flow), ch. 3, p. 98
- RT hypovolemia, ch. 8, p. 284

Elimination

Bowel elimination, alteration in: constipation
- RT pressure of fetal presenting part, ch. 4, p. 146; ch. 5, p. 161

Urinary elimination, alteration in patterns

---

*Doenges, M and Moorhouse, M: Nurse's Pocket Guide: Nursing Diagnoses with Interventions, ed. 2. FA Davis, Philadelphia, 1988.

RT pregnancy-induced hypertension as evidenced by diuresis and excess fluid retention, ch. 8, p. 294

Urinary retention [acute]

RT pressure of fetal presenting part, ch. 4, p. 146

Emotional Reactions

Anxiety [specify degree as Mild, Moderate, Severe]

RT uncertainty about the onset of labor, ch. 1, p. 22

RT unfamiliar surroundings, ch. 1, p. 24

RT delivery in an unplanned environment, ch. 1, p. 37

RT more painful and longer than usual labor, ch. 2, p. 65

RT unexpected, rapid labor, ch. 4, p. 135

RT changes in expected pattern of labor, ch. 4, p. 145

RT exposure during defecation, ch. 5, p. 161

RT enema procedure, ch. 5, p. 162

RT labor stimulation by means of nipple stimulation, ch. 5, p. 164

RT artificial rupture of membrane procedure, ch. 5, p. 166

RT interruption in normal labor process, ch. 5, p. 175

RT lack of exposure, ch. 7, p. 239

RT situational and maturational crises, threat to self-concept, threat of death, unmet needs, ch. 8, p. 275

RT the well being of herself and her baby, ch. 8, p. 281

RT fear of unknown and lack of predictable outcomes in presence of pregnancy-induced hypertension, ch. 8, p. 294

RT cesarean procedure, ch. 8, p. 299

RT well-being of preterm baby, ch. 9, p. 311

RT amniocentesis, ch. 9, p. 315

Coping, ineffective individual

RT rapid labor progression, ch. 1, p. 27

RT painful hypertonic contractions, ch. 3, p. 95

RT prolonged painful labor, ch. 4, p. 146

RT inadequate or ineffective support during labor, ch. 6, p. 190

RT inadequate support during labor, ch. 7, p. 260

RT situational and maturational crisis of (adolescent in) labor, ch. 8, p. 275

RT dependence and/or denial of substance abuse, ch. 8, p. 280

RT stress of pregnancy-induced hypertension, ch. 8, p. 294

RT being tired from labor or lacking sleep, ch. 8, p. 297

Fear

(of pain) RT labor: delivery; examinations; needles, ch. 1, p. 22

(of long labor) RT inability to tolerate pain, ch. 1, p. 22

(of abandonment during labor) RT lack of understanding of usual routines, ch. 1, p. 22

(of internal injury or tears) RT intrusive procedures; body size, ch. 1, p. 23

(of losing self-esteem) RT doubtfulness of ability to cope; loss of control during labor, ch. 1, p. 23

(of embarrassment: nudity; urinating and defecating in bed;

messiness from amniotic fluid and vaginal discharge; possibility of using foul language) RT uncertainty about acceptance of others, ch. 1, p. 23
(of helplessness) RT inability to control onset or progress of labor; inability to control what others do to her during labor and delivery, ch. 1, p. 23
(that baby might not survive labor/delivery process) RT lack of confidence in caretaker; predictive signs (fetal distress, early gestation), ch. 1, p. 23
(that baby might be injured during delivery) RT to use of forceps/vacuum extraction; relatively large size of baby, ch. 1, p. 23
(that baby will have gross deformities) RT family history; advanced maternal age; maternal drug ingestion; unfounded myths, ch. 1, p. 23
(that baby will not come out at all) RT size of baby in relation to size of pelvis, ch. 1, p. 23
(of unknown) RT condition of self/fetus, pain, procedures, outcomes, ch. 8, p. 296

Grieving, anticipatory
RT loss of the "perfect" baby, potential loss of baby, ch. 9, p. 331

Self-concept, disturbance in: self-esteem
RT mis-(self-)diagnosed labor, ch. 5, p. 159
RT exposure during defecation, ch. 5, p. 161
RT cesarean birth implying failure in ability to birth "normally," ch. 8, p. 296
RT failure to deliver at term, ch. 9, p. 331

Food/Fluid

Fluid volume, alteration in: excess
RT decreased urine production, ch. 8, p. 294

Fluid volume deficit, potential
RT inadequate fluid intake, ch. 1, p. 25
RT decreased oral intake; diaphoresis; blood loss; vomiting; hyperventilation; ch. 1, p. 30
RT bleeding from placental separation, ch. 1, p. 31
RT excess blood loss; distended bladder causing fundal relaxation, ch. 1, p. 33
RT exertion involved in abnormal labor, ch. 3, p. 95
RT excessive fluid loss, ch. 4, p. 145
RT altered blood flow at placental site, ch. 8, p. 284

Nutrition, alteration in: less than body requirements
RT substance abuse, ch. 8, p. 279

Hygiene

Self-care deficit: bathing/hygiene, dressing/grooming, toileting
RT absolute bedrest status, ch. 8, p. 294

Neurologic

Communication, impaired: verbal
RT withdrawal symptoms of substance abuse, ch. 8, p. 280
Sensory-perceptual alteration: visual, auditory, gustatory, olfactory
RT use of mixed agonists/antagonists, ch. 6, p. 200
Thought processes, alteration in
RT use of mixed agonists/antagonists, ch. 6, p. 200

Pain

Comfort, alteration in: pain, acute
RT bladder distention, ch. 1, p. 25
RT contraction frequency; contraction intensity; maternal position; tension, ch. 1, p. 26
RT increased rectal pressure; strong contractions, ch. 1, p. 28
RT stretching of the vagina; diaphoresis; heat production; bladder distention; strong uterine contractions, ch. 1, p. 30
RT fundal massage; perineal repair, ch. 1, p. 32
RT perineal trauma; uterine contractions; exhaustion, ch. 1, p. 33
RT fear; anxiety; hysteria; lack of medical support; rapid labor progression, ch. 1, p. 37
RT descent of occipital posterior of fetus down maternal back bones, extended period of uterine contractions, ch. 2, p. 65
RT ineffective management of uterine contraction pain, ch. 3, p. 97
RT uterine contractions, ch. 4, p. 135
RT stripping of membranes, ch. 5, p. 160
RT full rectum, ch. 5, p. 162
RT oxytocin-induced contractions, ch. 5, p. 175
RT lack of knowledge about labor process, ch. 6, p. 190 and ch. 7, p. 243
RT inadequate use of distraction techniques, ch. 6, p. 190
RT ineffective application of cutaneous stimulation, ch. 6, p. 190
RT generalized muscle tension during labor, ch. 6, p. 191 and ch. 7, p. 256
RT inadequate support with guided imagery, ch. 6, p. 191
RT continued perception of uterine contractions, ch. 6, p. 191
Rt low pain threshold during labor, ch. 8, p. 275
RT uterine contractions in presence of anxiety, possible abruptio placenta, and oxytocin infusion, ch. 8, p. 294
RT ultrasound procedure, ch. 9, p. 314

Relationship Alterations

Coping, ineffective family: compromised
RT stress of pregnancy-induced hypertension, ch. 8, p. 294
Family process, alteration in
RT separation of parents and newborn, ch. 1, p. 32 and p. 33

RT birth of new baby, ch. 7, p. 260
RT lack of involvement in birth process, ch. 7, p. 260
RT situational and developmental transition/crisis involved in adolescent giving birth, ch. 8, p. 275
RT substance abuse, ch. 8, p. 280

Parenting, alteration in
RT physical status of hemorrhaging mother, ch. 8, p. 288

Self-concept, disturbance in: role performance
RT biophysical, psychosocial, intellectual, cultural factors of adolescent pregnancy, ch. 8, p. 275
RT untimely (preterm) labor, ch. 9, p. 311
RT mother's lack of knowledge about how to meet the needs of preterm infant, ch. 9, p. 331

Social Isolation
RT adolescent pregnancy, ch. 8, p. 275

Safety

Hyperthermia
RT infection; dehydration, ch. 1, p. 24
RT prostaglandin's effect on the hypothalamus, ch. 5, p. 177

Hypothermia
(in newborn)
RT change in environment; body size; inadequate subcutaneous fat; absence of shiver response, ch. 1, p. 35

Infection, potential for
RT inadequate primary defenses, ch. 1, p. 24
RT invasive procedures, ch. 4, p. 145
RT rupture of membranes, ch. 5, p. 167
RT substance abuse, ch. 8, p. 279
RT open sinuses at placental site and/or nearness of placenta to cervix, ch. 8, p. 284

Injury, potential for: trauma
(in mother)
RT lacerations; hemorrhage; infection, ch. 1, p. 37
RT abnormal occipital posterior fetal position, larger than usual fetal diameters presenting, and possible use of forceps to assist in the delivery, ch. 2, p. 65
RT vaginal delivery of breech presentation, ch. 2, p. 67
RT vigorous uterine contractions, ch. 4, p. 135
RT prolonged labor, ch. 4, p. 146
RT injudicious administration of oxytocin, ch. 5, p. 173
RT drugs received during labor, ch. 6, p. 191
RT regional anesthesia, ch. 6, p. 204
RT paracervical anesthesia, ch. 6, p. 213
RT drug abuse and impaired mental processes, ch. 8, p. 279
RT sedation (from medications administered), eclamptic episode(s), aspiration of gastric or oral secretions, ch. 8, p. 294
RT reasons for and procedure involved in cesarean, ch. 8, p. 296

(in fetus)
RT decreased oxygenation, ch. 1, p. 25
RT longer than usual labor, precipitating fetal distress and difficult delivery, ch. 2, p. 65
RT numerous manipulations and progressive size of the fetal diameters during vaginal delivery of fetus in breech presentation, ch. 2, p. 67
RT abnormal contractions, ch. 3, p. 95
RT hypoxia, ch. 4, p. 135
RT prolonged labor, ch. 4, p. 146
RT rupture of membranes, ch. 5, p. 166
RT injudicious administration of oxytocin, ch. 5, p. 173
RT drugs received during labor, ch. 6, p. 191
RT maternal malnutrition, physiologic immaturity, and inadequate health care, ch. 8, p. 275
RT drug abuse and impaired mental processes, ch. 8, p. 279
(in fetus/newborn)
RT rapid uncontrolled delivery of the head; cord compression; inappropriate care; contamination; prematurity, ch. 1, p. 37
RT paracervical anesthesia, ch. 6, p. 213
(in newborn)
RT improper positioning, ch. 1, p. 32
RT eye prophylaxis; hemorrhage; cold stress; resuscitation, ch. 1, p. 35
RT drugs received during labor, ch. 6, p. 191
RT reasons for and the procedure involved in cesarean, ch. 8, p. 296
Skin integrity, impairment of: potential
RT uncontrolled expulsion of the fetus, ch. 1, p. 30
RT knicks in skin from shaving process, ch. 8, p. 299

Sexuality

Sexuality patterns, altered
RT labor stimulation by means of nipple stimulation, ch. 5, p. 164

Teaching/Learning

Knowledge deficit (specify)
premonitory signs of labor, ch. 1, p. 16
normal labor/delivery process, ch. 4, p. 145
in adolescent, ch. 8, p. 275
in substance abuser, ch. 8, p. 279
induction of labor, ch. 5, p. 175
implications of VBAC, ch. 7, p. 239
prepared childbirth methods, ch. 7, p. 243
cutaneous stimulation and other relaxation techniques, ch. 7, p. 256
bleeding: cause, therapy involved, ch. 8, p. 281

intrapartal hypertension, ch. 8, p. 294
cesarean delivery: reasons, procedures, methods of relaxation, pain relief, ch. 8, pp. 296–297
care of the preterm infant, ch. 9, p. 331
RT lack of information
RT inadequate preparation
RT lack of previous experience
RT lack of exposure
RT cognitive limitations
RT unfamiliarity with sources of information

Noncompliance [specify]
with instructions to inform the physician of significant decrease in fetal activity, ch. 9, p. 336
RT perceived lack of seriousness of problem, ch. 9, p. 336

Ventilation

Airway clearance, ineffective
RT aspiration of stomach contents, ch. 6, p. 218

Breathing pattern, ineffective
RT narcotic agonists, ch. 6, p. 196

Gas exchange, impaired
(in fetus)
RT head compression; decreased placental perfusion; maternal anesthesia; malpresentation, ch. 1, p. 30
RT maternal narcotic agonists received during labor, ch. 6, p. 198
RT inhalation anesthesia, ch. 6, p. 219
RT inadequate uteroplacental perfusion as evidenced by vasospasms, and/or decreased uterine relaxation, ch. 8, p. 294
RT placental abruption or oxytocin infusion as evidenced by decreased or inadequate uterine relaxation between contractions, ch. 8, p. 294
(in newborn)
RT cold stress; excess mucus; ineffective respiratory effort; intrauterine hypoxia, ch. 1, p. 35

APPENDIX C: LIST OF NURSING DIAGNOSES

According to Gordon's Functional Health Patterns Using NANDA Approved Nursing Diagnoses*

Note: "ch." refers to chapter number, and "p." refers to page reference in this book.
"RT" is the abbreviation used for "related to."

Health Perception — Health Management Pattern

Noncompliance [specify]
 with instructions to inform the physician of significant decrease in fetal activity, ch. 9, p. 336
 RT perceived lack of seriousness of problem, ch. 9, p. 336
Potential for Infection
 RT inadequate primary defenses, ch. 1, p. 24
 RT invasive procedures, ch. 4, p. 145
 RT rupture of membranes, ch. 5, p. 167
 RT substance abuse, ch. 8, p. 279
 RT open sinuses at placental site and/or nearness of placenta to cervix, ch. 8, p. 284
Potential for Injury
(in mother)
 RT lacerations; hemorrhage; infection, ch. 1, p. 37
 RT abnormal occipital posterior fetal position, larger than usual fetal diameters presenting, and possible use of forceps to assist in the delivery, ch. 2, p. 65
 RT vaginal delivery of breech presentation, ch. 2, p. 67
 RT vigorous uterine contractions, ch. 4, p. 135
 RT prolonged labor, ch. 4, p. 146

---

*Gordon, M: Manual of Nursing Diagnosis: 1986–1987. McGraw-Hill, New York, 1987.

*Gordon, M: Nursing Diagnosis: Process and Application, ed. 2. McGraw-Hill, New York, 1987.

RT injudicious administration of oxytocin, ch. 5, p. 173
RT drugs received during labor, ch. 6, p. 191
RT regional anesthesia, ch. 6, p. 204
RT paracervical anesthesia, ch. 6, p. 213
RT drug abuse and impaired mental processes, ch. 8, p. 279
RT sedation (from medications administered), eclamptic episode(s), aspiration of gastric or oral secretions, ch. 8, p. 294
RT reasons for and procedure involved in cesarean, ch. 8, p. 296

(in fetus)
RT decreased oxygenation, ch. 1, p. 25
RT longer than usual labor, precipitating fetal distress and difficult delivery, ch. 2, p. 65
RT numerous manipulations and progressive size of fetal diameters during vaginal delivery of fetus in breech presentation, ch. 2, p. 67
RT abnormal contractions, ch. 3, p. 95
RT hypoxia, ch. 4, p. 135
RT prolonged labor, ch. 4, p. 146
RT rupture of membranes, ch. 5, p. 166
RT injudicious administration of oxytocin, ch. 5, p. 173
RT drugs received during labor, ch. 6, p. 191
Rt maternal malnutrition, physiologic immaturity, and inadequate health care, ch. 8, p. 275
RT drug abuse and impaired mental processes, ch. 8, p. 279

(in fetus/newborn)
RT rapid uncontrolled delivery of the head; cord compression; inappropriate care; contamination; prematurity, ch. 1, p. 37
RT paracervical anesthesia, ch. 6, p. 213

(in newborn)
RT improper positioning, ch. 1, p. 32
RT eye prophylaxis; hemorrhage; cold stress; resuscitation, ch. 1, p. 35
RT drugs received during labor, ch. 6, p. 191
RT reasons for and procedure involved in cesarean, ch. 8, p. 296

Nutritional-Metabolic Pattern

Alteration in Nutrition: Less than Body Requirements
RT substance abuse, ch. 8, p. 279

Potential Fluid Volume Deficit
RT inadequate fluid intake, ch. 1, p. 25
RT decreased fluid intake; diaphoresis; blood loss; vomiting; hyperventilation, ch. 1, p. 30
RT bleeding from placental separation, ch. 1, p. 31
RT excess blood loss; distended bladder causing fundal relaxation, ch. 1, p. 33
RT exertion involved in abnormal labor, ch. 3, p. 95
RT excessive fluid loss, ch. 4, p. 145
RT altered blood flow at the placental site, ch. 8, p. 284

Alteration in Fluid Volume: Excess
RT decreased urine production, ch. 8, p. 294
Impaired Skin Integrity
RT uncontrolled expulsion of the fetus, ch. 1, p. 30
RT knicks in skin from shaving process, ch. 8, p. 299
Hyperthermia
RT infection; dehydration, ch. 1, p. 24
RT prostaglandin's effect on the hypothalamus, ch. 5, p. 177
Hypothermia
(in newborn)
RT change in environment; body size; inadequate subcutaneous fat; absence of shiver response, ch. 1, p. 35

Elimination Pattern

Alteration in Bowel Elimination: Constipation
RT pressure of fetal presenting part, ch. 4, p. 146; ch. 5, p. 161
Urinary Retention
RT pressure of fetal presenting part, ch. 4, p. 146
Alteration in Patterns of Urinary Elimination
RT pregnancy-induced hypertension as evidenced by diuresis and excess fluid retention, ch. 8, p. 294

Activity-Exercise Pattern

Activity Intolerance (level III or IV)
RT excessive expenditure of energy during contractions, ch. 1, p. 25
RT nonproductive labor, ch. 3, p. 95
RT inadequate rest during labor, ch. 6, p. 190
RT use of sedatives, ch. 6, p. 202
Self-Bathing-Hygiene, Dressing-Grooming, Feeding, Toileting Deficit (specify level)
RT absolute bedrest status, ch. 8, p. 294
Diversional Activity Deficit
RT prolonged labor, ch. 4, p. 145
Ineffective Airway Clearance
RT aspiration of stomach contents, ch. 6, p. 218
Ineffective Breathing Pattern
RT narcotic agonists, ch. 6, p. 196
Impaired Gas Exchange
(in fetus)
RT head compression; decreased placental perfusion; maternal anesthesia; malpresentation, ch. 1, p. 30
RT maternal narcotic agonists received during labor, ch. 6, p. 198
RT inhalation anesthesia, ch. 6, p. 219
RT inadequate uteroplacental perfusion as evidenced by vasospasms, and/or decreased uterine relaxation, ch. 8, p. 294
RT placental abruption or oxytocin infusion as evidenced by

decreased or inadequate uterine relaxation between contractions, ch. 8, p. 294

(in newborn)

RT cold stress; excess mucus; ineffective respiratory effort; intrauterine hypoxia, ch. 1, p. 35

Alteration in Cardiac Output: Decreased

RT dorsal recumbent position, ch. 1, p. 24 and p. 30

RT analgesia; anesthesia, ch. 1, p. 30

RT administration of anesthetics, ch. 6, pp. 216–217

RT excessive blood loss, positional changes, anesthetic/analgesic reactions, ch. 8, p. 298

Alteration in Tissue Perfusion (cardiopulmonary)

RT decreased placental perfusion (interruption in placental blood flow), ch. 3, p. 98

RT hypovolemia, ch. 8, p. 284

Cognitive-Perceptual Pattern

Alteration in Comfort: Pain

RT bladder distention, ch. 1, p. 25

RT contraction frequency; contraction intensity; maternal position; tension, ch. 1, p. 26

RT increased rectal pressure; strong contractions, ch. 1, p. 28

RT stretching of vagina; diaphoresis; heat production; bladder distention; strong uterine contractions, ch. 1, p. 30

RT fundal massage; perineal repair, ch. 1, p. 32

RT perineal trauma; uterine contractions; exhaustion, ch. 1, p. 33

RT fear; anxiety; hysteria; lack of medical support; rapid labor progression, ch. 1, p. 37

RT descent of occipital posterior position of fetus down maternal back bones, extended period of uterine contractions, ch. 2, p. 65

RT ineffective management of uterine contraction pain, ch. 3, p. 97

RT uterine contractions, ch. 4, p. 135

RT stripping of membranes, ch. 5, p. 160

RT full rectum, ch. 5, p. 162

RT oxytocin-induced contractions, ch. 5, p. 175

RT lack of knowledge about labor process, ch. 6, p. 190 and ch. 7, p. 243

RT inadequate use of distraction techniques, ch. 6, p. 190

RT ineffective application of cutaneous stimulation, ch. 6, p. 190

RT generalized muscle tension during labor, ch. 6, p. 191 and ch. 7, p. 256

RT inadequate support with guided imagery, ch. 6, p. 191

RT continued perception of uterine contractions, ch. 6, p. 191

RT low pain threshold during labor, ch. 8, p. 275

RT uterine contractions in the presence of anxiety, possible abruptio placenta, and oxytocin infusion, ch. 8, p. 294
RT ultrasound procedure, ch. 9, p. 314
Sensory-Perceptual Alteration: Sensory Deprivation
RT use of mixed agonists/antagonists, ch. 6, p. 200
Knowledge Deficit (specify)
premonitory signs of labor, ch. 1, p. 16
normal labor/delivery process, ch. 4, p. 145
in adolescent, ch. 8, p. 275
In substance abuser, ch. 8, p. 279
induction of labor, ch. 5, p. 175
implications of VBAC, ch. 7, p. 239
prepared childbirth methods, ch. 7, p. 243
cutaneous stimulation and other relaxation techniques, ch. 7, p. 256
bleeding: cause, therapy involved, ch. 8, p. 281
intrapartal hypertension, ch. 8, p. 294
cesarean delivery: reasons, procedures, methods of relaxation, pain relief, ch. 8. pp. 296–297
care of the preterm infant, ch. 9, p. 331
RT lack of information
RT inadequate preparation
RT lack of previous experience
RT lack of exposure
RT cognitive limitations
RT unfamiliarity with sources of information
Impaired Thought Processes
RT use of mixed agonists/antagonists, ch. 6, p. 200

Self-Perception — Self-Concept Pattern

Fear (specify)
(of pain) RT labor; delivery; examinations; needles, ch. 1, p. 22
(of long labor) RT inability to tolerate pain, ch. 1, p. 22
(of abandonment during labor) RT lack of understanding of usual routines, ch. 1, p. 22
(of internal injury or tears) RT intrusive procedures; body size, ch. 1, p. 23
(of losing self-esteem) RT doubtfulness of ability to cope; loss of control during labor, ch. 1, p. 23
(of embarrassment: nudity; urinating and defecating in bed; messiness from amniotic fluid and vaginal discharge; possibility of using foul language) RT uncertainty about acceptance of others, ch. 1, p. 23
(of helplessness) RT inability to control onset or progress of labor; inability to control what others do to her during labor and delivery, ch. 1, p. 23
(that baby might not survive labor/delivery process) RT lack of

confidence in caretaker; predictive signs (fetal distress, early gestation), ch. 1, p. 23
(that baby might be injured during delivery) RT to use of forceps/vacuum extractor; relatively large size of baby, ch. 1, p. 23
(that baby will have gross deformities) RT family history; advanced maternal age; maternal drug ingestion; unfounded myths, ch. 1, p. 23
(that baby will not come out at all) RT size of baby in relation to size of pelvis, ch. 1, p. 23
(of condition) RT self/fetus, pain, procedures, outcomes, ch. 8, p. 296

Anxiety (specify degree as Mild, Moderate, Severe)
RT uncertainty about the onset of labor, ch. 1, p. 22
RT unfamiliar surroundings, ch. 1, p. 24
RT delivery in an unplanned environment, ch. 1, p. 37
RT more painful and longer than usual labor, ch. 2, p. 65
RT unexpected, rapid labor, ch. 4, p. 135
RT changes in expected pattern of labor, ch. 4, p. 145
RT exposure during defecation, ch. 5, p. 161
RT enema procedure, ch. 5, p. 162
RT labor stimulation by means of nipple stimulation, ch. 5, p. 164
RT artificial rupture of membrane procedure, ch. 5, p. 166
RT interruption in normal labor process, ch. 5, p. 175
RT lack of exposure, ch. 7, p. 239
RT situational and maturational crises, threat to self-concept, threat of death, unmet needs, ch. 8, p. 275
RT well-being of herself and baby, ch. 8, p. 281
RT fear of unknown and lack of predictable outcomes in presence of pregnancy-induced hypertension, ch. 8, p. 294
RT cesarean procedure, ch. 8, p. 299
RT well-being of preterm baby, ch. 9, p. 311
RT amniocentesis, ch. 9, p. 315

Self-Esteem Disturbance
RT mis-(self-)diagnosed labor, ch. 5, p. 159
RT exposure during defecation, ch. 5, p. 161
RT cesarean birth implying failure in ability to birth "normally," ch. 8, p. 296
RT failure to deliver at term, ch. 9, p. 331

Role-Relationship Pattern

Anticipatory Grieving
RT loss of the "perfect" baby, potential loss of baby, ch. 9, p. 331

Disturbance in Role Performance
RT biophysical, psychosocial, intellectual, cultural factors of adolescent pregnancy, ch. 8, p. 275
RT untimely (preterm) labor, ch. 9, p. 311

RT mother's lack of knowledge about how to meet needs of preterm infant, ch. 9, p. 311
Social Isolation (Rejection)
RT adolescent pregnancy, ch. 8, p. 275
Alteration in Family Processes
RT separation of parents and newborn, ch. 1, p. 32 and p. 33
RT birth of new baby, ch. 7, p. 260
RT lack of involvement in birth process, ch. 7, p. 260
RT situational and developmental transition/crisis involved in adolescent giving birth, ch. 8, p. 275
RT substance abuse, ch. 8, p. 280
Alteration in Parenting
RT physical status of hemorrhaging mother, ch. 8, p. 288
Impaired Verbal Communication
RT withdrawal symptoms of substance abuse, ch. 8, p. 280

Sexuality-Reproductive Pattern

Altered Sexuality Pattern
RT labor stimulation by means of nipple stimulation, ch. 5, p. 164

Coping-Stress Tolerance Pattern

Coping, Ineffective (Individual)
RT rapid labor progression, ch. 1, p. 27
RT painful hypertonic contractions, ch. 3, p. 95
RT prolonged painful labor, ch. 4, p. 146
RT inadequate or ineffective support during labor, ch. 6, p. 190
RT inadequate support during labor, ch. 7, p. 260
RT situational and maturational crisis of (adolescent in) labor, ch. 8, p. 275
RT dependence and/or denial of substance abuse, ch. 8, p. 280
RT stress of pregnancy-induced hypertension, ch. 8, p. 294
RT being tired from labor or lacking sleep, ch. 8, p. 297
Ineffective Family Coping: Compromised
RT stress of pregnancy-induced hypertension, ch. 8, p. 294

APPENDIX D: RECOMMENDATIONS FOR PREVENTION OF HIV TRANSMISSION IN HEALTH-CARE SETTINGS*

INTRODUCTION

Human immunodeficiency virus (HIV), the virus that causes acquired immunodeficiency syndrome (AIDS), is transmitted through sexual contact, exposure to infected blood or blood components, and perinatally from mother to neonate. HIV has been isolated from blood, semen, vaginal secretions, saliva, tears, breast milk, cerebrospinal fluid, amniotic fluid, and urine and is likely to be isolated from other body fluids, secretions, and excretions. However, epidemiologic evidence has implicated only blood, semen, vaginal secretions, and, possibly, breast milk in transmission.

DEFINITION OF HEALTH-CARE WORKERS

Health-care workers are defined as persons, including students and trainees, whose activities involve contact with patients or with blood or other body fluids from patients in a health-care setting.

---

*From U.S. Department of Health and Human Services: Recommendations for prevention of HIV transmission in health-care settings. Morbidity and Mortality Weekly Report, *36*(2s):3s–18s, 1987, excerpted with permission.

PRECAUTIONS TO PREVENT TRANSMISSION OF HIV

Universal Precautions

Since medical history and examination cannot reliably identify all patients infected with HIV or other blood-borne pathogens, blood and body-fluid precautions should be consistently used for *all* patients. This approach, previously recommended by CDC and referred to as "universal blood and body-fluid precautions" or "universal precautions," should be used in the care of *all* patients, especially including those in emergency-care settings in which the risk of blood exposure is increased and the infection status of the patient is usually unknown.

1. All health-care workers should routinely use appropriate barrier precautions to prevent skin and mucous-membrane exposure when contact with blood or other body fluids of any patient is anticipated. Gloves should be worn for touching blood and body fluids, mucous membranes, or nonintact skin of all patients; for handling items or surfaces soiled with blood or body fluids; and for performing venipuncture and other vascular-access procedures. Gloves should be changed after contact with each patient. Masks and protective eye wear or face shields should be worn during procedures that are likely to generate droplets of blood or other body fluids to prevent exposure of mucous membranes of the mouth, nose, and eyes. Gowns or aprons should be worn during procedures that are likely to generate splashes of blood or other body fluids.
2. Hands and other skin surfaces should be washed immediately and thoroughly if contaminated with blood or other body fluids. Hands should be washed immediately after gloves are removed.
3. All health-care workers should take precautions to prevent injuries caused by needles, scalpels, and other sharp instruments or devices during procedures; when cleaning used instruments; during disposal of used needles; and when handling sharp instruments after procedures. To prevent needlestick injuries, needles should not be recapped, purposely bent or broken by hand, removed from disposable syringes, or otherwise manipulated by hand. After they are used, disposable syringes and needles, scalpel blades, and other sharp items should be placed in puncture-resistant containers for disposal; the puncture-resistant containers should be located as close as practical to the use area. Large-bore reusable needles should be placed in a puncture-resistant container for transport to the reprocessing area.
4. Although saliva has not been implicated in HIV transmission, to minimize the need for emergency mouth-to-mouth resuscitation, mouthpieces, resuscitation bags, or other ventilation devices should be available for use in areas in which the need for resuscitation is predictable.
5. Health-care workers who have exudative lesions or weeping der-

matitis should refrain from all direct patient care and from handling patient-care equipment until the condition resolves.

6. Pregnant health-care workers are not known to be at greater risk of contracting HIV infection than health-care workers who are not pregnant; however, if a health-care worker develops HIV infection during pregnancy, the infant is at risk of infection resulting from perinatal transmission. Because of this risk, pregnant health-care workers should be especially familiar with, and strictly adhere to, precautions to minimize the risk of HIV transmission.

Implementation of universal blood and body-fluid precautions for *all* patients eliminates the need for use of the isolation category of "Blood and Body Fluid Precautions" previously recommended by CDC for patients known or suspected to be infected with blood-borne pathogens. Isolation precautions (e.g., enteric, "AFB") should be used as necessary if associated conditions, such as infectious diarrhea or tuberculosis, are diagnosed or suspected.

Precautions for Invasive Procedures

In this document, an invasive procedure is defined as surgical entry into tissues, cavities, or organs, or repair of major traumatic injuries (1) in an operating or delivery room, emergency department, or outpatient setting, including both physicians' and dentists' offices; (2) cardiac catheterization and angiographic procedures; (3) a vaginal or cesarean delivery or other invasive obstetric procedure during which bleeding may occur; or (4) the manipulation, cutting, or removal of any oral or perioral tissues, including tooth structure, during which bleeding occurs or the potential for bleeding exists. The universal blood and body-fluid precautions listed above, combined with the precautions listed below, should be the minimum precautions for *all* such invasive procedures.

1. All health-care workers who participate in invasive procedures must routinely use appropriate barrier precautions to prevent skin and mucous-membrane contact with blood and other body fluids of all patients. Gloves and surgical masks must be worn for all invasive procedures. Protective eye wear or face shields should be worn for procedures that commonly result in the generation of droplets, splashing of blood or other body fluids, or the generation of bone chips. Gowns or aprons made of materials that provide an effective barrier should be worn during invasive procedures that are likely to result in the splashing of blood or other body fluids. All health-care workers who perform or assist in vaginal or cesarean deliveries should wear gloves and gowns when handling the placenta or the infant until blood and amniotic fluid have been removed from the infant's skin and should wear gloves during post-delivery care of the umbilical cord.
2. If a glove is torn or a needle stick or other injury occurs, the glove

should be removed and a new glove used as promptly as patient safety permits; the needle or instrument involved in the incident should also be removed from the sterile field.

ENVIRONMENTAL CONSIDERATIONS FOR HIV TRANSMISSION

No environmentally mediated mode of HIV transmission has been documented. Nevertheless, the precautions described below should be taken routinely in the care of *all* patients.

Sterilization and Disinfection

Standard sterilization and disinfection procedures for patient-care equipment currently recommended for use in a variety of health-care settings—including hospitals, medical and dental clinics and offices, hemodialysis centers, emergency-care facilities, and long-term nursing-care facilities—are adequate to sterilize or disinfect instruments, devices, or other items contaminated with blood or other body fluids from persons infected with blood-borne pathogens, including HIV.

Housekeeping

Environmental surfaces, such as walls, floors, and other surfaces, are not associated with transmission of infections to patients or health-care workers. Therefore, extraordinary attempts to disinfect or sterilize these environmental surfaces are not necessary. However, cleaning and removal of soil should be done routinely.

Cleaning and Decontaminating Spills of Blood or Other Body Fluids

Chemical germicides that are approved for use as "hospital disinfectants" and are tuberculocidal when used at recommended dilutions can be used to decontaminate spills of blood and other body fluids. Strategies for decontaminating spills of blood and other body fluids in a patient-care setting are different than for spills of cultures or other materials in clinical, public health, or research laboratories. In patient-care areas, visible material should first be removed and then the area should be decontaminated. With large spills of cultured or concentrated infectious agents in the laboratory, the contaminated area should be flooded with a liquid germicide before cleaning, then decontaminated with fresh germicidal chemical. In both settings, gloves should be worn during the cleaning and decontaminating procedures.

Laundry

Although soiled linen has been identified as a source of large numbers of certain pathogenic microorganisms, the risk of actual disease transmission is negligible. Rather than rigid procedures and specifications, hygienic and commonsense storage and processing of clean and soiled linen are recommended. Soiled linen should be handled as little as possible and with minimal agitation to prevent gross microbial contamination of the air and of persons handling the linen. All soiled linen should be bagged at the location where it was used; it should not be sorted or rinsed in patient-care areas. Linen soiled with blood or body fluids should be placed and transported in bags that prevent leakage. If hot water is used, linen should be washed with detergent in water at least 70°C (160°F) for 25 minutes. If low-temperature (<70°C [158°F]) laundry cycles are used, chemicals suitable for low-temperature washing at proper use concentration should be used.

Infective Waste

There is no epidemiologic evidence to suggest that most hospital waste is any more infective than residential waste. Moreover, there is no epidemiologic evidence that hospital waste has caused disease in the community as a result of improper disposal. Therefore, identifying wastes for which special precautions are indicated is largely a matter of judgment about the relative risk of disease transmission. The most practical approach to the management of infective waste is to identify those wastes with the potential for causing infection during handling and disposal and for which some special precautions appear prudent. Hospital wastes for which special precautions appear prudent include microbiology laboratory waste, pathology waste, and blood specimens or blood products. While any item that has had contact with blood, exudates, or secretions may be potentially infective, it is not usually considered practical or necessary to treat all such waste as infective. Infective waste, in general, should either be incinerated or should be autoclaved before disposal in a sanitary landfill. Bulk, blood, suctioned fluids, excretions, and secretions may be carefully poured down a drain connected to a sanitary sewer. Sanitary sewers may also be used to dispose of other infectious wastes capable of being ground and flushed into the sewer.

IMPLEMENTATION OF RECOMMENDED PRECAUTIONS

Employers of health-care workers should ensure that policies exist for:

1. Initial orientation and continuing education and training of all health-care workers—including students and trainees—on the epidemiology, modes of transmission, and prevention of HIV and other blood-borne infections and the need for routine use of universal blood and body-fluid precautions for *all* patients.
2. Provision of equipment and supplies necessary to minimize the risk of infection with HIV and other blood-borne pathogens.

3. Monitoring adherence to recommended protective measures. When monitoring reveals a failure to follow recommended precautions, counseling, education, and/or retraining should be provided, and, if necessary, appropriate disciplinary action should be considered.

Professional associations and labor organizations, through continuing education efforts, should emphasize the need for health-care workers to follow recommended precautions.

SEROLOGIC TESTING FOR HIV INFECTION

Background

A person is identified as infected with HIV when a sequence of tests, starting with repeated enzyme immunoassays (EIA) and including a Western blot or similar or specific assay, are repeatedly reactive. Persons infected with HIV usually develop antibody against the virus within 6 to 12 weeks after infection.

Testing of Patients

Previous CDC recommendations have emphasized the value of HIV serologic testing of patients for (1) management of parenteral or mucous-membrane exposures of health-care workers, (2) patient diagnosis and management, and (3) counseling and serologic testing to prevent and control HIV transmission in the community. In addition, more recent recommendations have stated that hospitals, in conjunction with state and local health departments, should periodically determine the prevalence of HIV infection among patients from age groups at highest risk of infection.

Testing programs, if developed, should include the following principles:

1. Obtaining consent for testing.
2. Informing patients of test results, and providing counseling for seropositive patients by properly trained persons.
3. Assuring that confidentiality safeguards are in place to limit knowledge of test results to those directly involved in the care of infected patients or as required by law.
4. Assuring that identification of infected patients will not result in denial of needed care or provision of suboptimal care.
5. Evaluating prospectively (a) the efficacy of the program in reducing the incidence of parenteral, mucous-membrane, or significant cutaneous exposures of health-care workers to the blood or other body fluids of HIV-infected patients, and (b) the effect of modified procedures on patients.

MANAGEMENT OF EXPOSURES

If a health-care worker has a parenteral (e.g., needlestick or cut) or mucous-membrane (e.g., splash to the eye or mouth) exposure to blood or other body fluids or has a cutaneous exposure involving large amounts of blood or prolonged contact with blood—especially when the exposed skin is chapped, abraded, or afflicted with dermatitis—the source patient should be informed of the incident and tested for serologic evidence of HIV infection after consent is obtained. Policies should be developed for testing source patients in situations in which consent cannot be obtained (e.g., an unconscious patient).

If the source patient has AIDS, is positive for HIV antibody, or refuses the test, the health-care worker should be counseled regarding the risk of infection and evaluated clinically and serologically for evidence of HIV infection as soon as possible after exposure. The health-care worker should be advised to report and seek medical evaluation for any acute febrile illness that occurs within 12 weeks after the exposure. Such an illness—particularly one characterized by fever, rash, or lymphadenopathy—may be indicative of recent HIV infection. Seronegative health-care workers should be retested 6 weeks postexposure and on a periodic basis thereafter (e.g., 12 weeks and 6 months after exposure) to determine whether transmission has occurred. During this follow-up period—especially the first 6 to 12 weeks after exposure, when most infected persons are expected to seroconvert—exposed health-care workers should follow U.S. Public Health Service (PHS) recommendations for preventing transmission of HIV.

No further follow-up of a health-care worker exposed to infection as described above is necessary if the source patient is seronegative unless the source patient is at high risk of HIV infection. In the latter case, a subsequent specimen (e.g., 12 weeks following exposure) may be obtained from the health-care worker for antibody testing. If the source patient cannot be identified, decisions regarding appropriate follow-up should be individualized. Serologic testing should be available to all health-care workers who are concerned that they may have been infected with HIV.

If a patient has a parenteral or mucous-membrane exposure to blood or other body fluid of a health-care worker, the patient should be informed of the incident, and the same procedure outlined above for management of exposures should be followed for both the source health-care worker and the exposed patient.

INDEX

A page number in *italics* indicates a figure. A "*t*" following a page number indicates a table.

AAHCC. *See* American Academy of Husband-Coached Childbirth
Abruptio placenta, 282–286
  in older woman, 276
  with vaginal bleeding, 20
Acceleration, 110
  with movement, 337
  spontaneous, 115
  uniform, 115
  variable, 115
Acme, 88
ACMN. *See* American College of Nurse Midwives
Activity, during labor, 25
Acupressure, 257
Acupuncture, 257
Admission, 20
  assessment for, 17–22
Adolescent in labor, 273–275
AIDS, precautions against, 278, 407–413
Airway clearance, 218–219
Alcohol
  abuse of, 277
  to arrest premature labor, 327–328
Alphaprodine, 198
Alternative birth centers (ABCs), 235
Ambulation, labor stimulation with, 158–160
Ambulatory monitoring, effectiveness of, 318–320
American Academy of Husband-Coached Childbirth, 245
American College of Nurse Midwives, 262
American Nurses' Association Standards of Maternal-Child Health Nursing Practice, 360
American Society for Psychoprophylaxis in Obstetrics, 147
Amniocentesis, 22, 314–315
  anxiety related to, 315
  for fetal age determination, 297
  before medical induction, 169, 171
  nursing interventions with, 318
  risks of, 315–316
Amniotic fluid
  meconium-stained, 5, 8, 342
  during rupture of membranes, 5, 8
  volume of, 337
Amniotomy, 4, 8, 138, 140, 141, 165–168
  procedure of, 166
Amphetamines, 277
Analgesia, 191–193. *See also specific agents*
  definition of, 192
  epidural blocks for, 209
  patient-controlled pump, 300
  for substance abuser, 279
Android pelvis, 57
Anemia, 273
  in preterm infants, 312
Anesthesia, 191–193. *See also specific agents*
  allergic or toxic reaction to, 217
    treatment for, 218

Anesthesia—*Continued*
complications with, emergency nursing measures for, 216–218
definition of, 192
drug-induced, 203–204
excessive, 137
abnormal fetal descent with, 143–144
general, 204
during labor and delivery, 218–222
inhalation, 219–220
injury potential with, 204–205
intravenous, 220
introduction of use of during childbirth, 235
local, 203, 328
maternal hypotension with, emergency treatment for, 217–218
neurobehavioral effects of, 204
paracervical, 212–214
protein-binding ability of, 204
regional, 203–204, 209–211, 213–216
advantages of, 205–206, 208
disadvantages of, 206–207, 208
nursing measures during, 207–208
patient position for administration of, 212
side effects of, 212
in various stages of labor/delivery, 206*t*, 212
regurgitation and aspiration of gastric contents with, 220–221
side effects of, 216–217
sites of infiltration of, *205*
Anoxia, 5, 188
Antepartal exercise, 68, *69*
Anthropoid pelvis, 57
Antihypertensive drugs, 293, 295
Anxiety
about onset of labor, 22
with amniocentesis, 315
associated with childbirth, 22–27
with emergency delivery, 37
over enema, 162
with occipital posterior position delivery, 65
pain with, 186, 243–244
with preterm infants, 331
with prolonged labor, 145, 147
with unfamiliar surroundings, 24
uterine contractions and, 97
Apgar scores
appropriate, 40
chart of, 36*t*
in emergency delivery, 39
following delivery, 35
Apresoline, 293
AquaMEPHYTON, 35, 36
Arbitration panel, 376
AROM. *See* Amniotomy; Artificially ruptured membranes
Artificially ruptured membranes, 4
Asphyxia, fetal heart rate with, 116
Aspiration, of gastric contents, 220–221
Aspirin, to arrest premature labor, 327
ASPO. *See* American Society for Psychoprophylaxis in Obstetrics
Asynclitism, 70
Atropine, 108
prior to cesarean delivery, 299
Attachment, 260. *See also* Parent-infant attachment
Augmentation, 172
Autogenic training, 258
Average length of stay (ALOS), 233, 263

Back discomfort, relief for, 70–71
Bandl ring, 86–87
Barbiturates, 202–203
abuse of, 277
for convulsion control, 217
Beats per minute, 98–99
Beta-mimetics
to arrest preterm labor, 322–326
side effects of, 323
Bethamethasone, to arrest preterm labor, 322, 327
Bi-ischial tuberosities, 63–64
Biofeedback, 258
Biophysical profile (BPP), 337, 338*t*, 340
Bi-parietal diameter, 314
Birth. *See also* Childbirth
experience of, 2
preparation for, 28, 242
Birthing centers
alternative, 235

freestanding, 261–262
Bishop score, 170–172
Bi-tuberosities, measurement of, 70
Bladder. *See also* Urinary retention
after delivery, 34-35
distention of, 25
emptying of, 72, 75
tone of, 25
Bleeding. *See also* Abruptio placenta; Hemorrhage
blood pressure and, 24
during labor, 280–282
with lacerations, 284
management of, 281
Blood pressure, elevated, 18. *See also* Hypertension
Blood replacement, 284
Bloody show, 4, 8, 28
Body alignment, to facilitate fetal descent, 71
Bonding, 260
Bony pelvis, anatomy of, 54. *See also* Pelvis
Bowels
elimination to stimulate labor, 161–162
movements before delivery, 25–26
retention in with prolonged labor, 146–147
BPM. *See* Beats per minute
Bradley, Dr. Robert, 245–246
Bradley method, 245–246
Bradycardia, 108, 110
persistent, 217
in post-term infant, 342
transient fetal, 213
Braxton Hicks contractions, 4, 6–7
Breach of duty, 358
Breast-feeding, 36
Breathing, 26
awareness of, 250
in Bradley method, 246
exhalation, 253–254
directions for, 254
for labor and birth, 249–255
modified paced, 251, 253
for pain management, 244
patterned paced, 251–253
patterns of, 250–253
pushing and, 253
rhythmic, 249
diaphragmatic patterns of, 247–248
slow paced, 250–251, 253
Breech presentation, 11, 13, 66–68
antepartal exercises for, 68, *69*
conversion of, 68
electrode placement in, 104
fetal heart rate auscutation in, 22
maternal trauma during, 67–68
mechanisms of labor in, 66–68
risks with, 67
Brethine, 326
Brow presentation, 11
Bupivacaine, 204, 209
Butorphanol tartrate, 200–201

Calcium antagonists, 326
Calcium gluconate, 293
Capaccia v. Newman, 365
Carbocaine, 204
Cardiac output, 24
Cardiff method, 336
Case law, 355–356. *See also specific cases*
examples of, 356–357, 361, 376–377
Catecholamines, 136
excessive, 139
production of, 136–137
Catheterization, after delivery, 34
Caudal block, 210
Causation, 358
Celestone, 322
Centering, 257
Cephalic presentation, 10, 13
conversion to, 68–69
Cephalopelvic disproportion (CPD), 54
Certified nurse midwives, 262
Certified Registered Nurse Anesthetist, 361
Cervical mucus, ferning of, 6, 8
Cervix, 88
changes of during labor, 4
dilatation of, 4, 8, 27, 28
abnormal patterns of, 134
assessment of rate of, 130
factors in and interventions for abnormal, 134–141
phases of S curve in, 132–133
in precipitous labor, 136
in second stage of labor, 31
edema of, 31
effacement of, 4, 8, 70, *86*
of os, 85

Cervix—*Continued*
in second stage of labor, 31
palpation of, 19
stretching of, 188
unripe, 137, 170
uterine contractions in, 85. *See also* Uterine contractions
Cesarean delivery, 295–296
with abruptio placenta or placenta previa, 286
American College of Obstetricians and gynecologists guidelines on, 237–238
anticipated sequence of events in, 299–300
candidates for, 296
confirming diagnostic procedures for, 297–298
elective, 295, 299
emotional aspects prior to, 296–297
with epidural block, 209
National Institutes of Health guidelines on, 237–238
nutrition and, 25
for occipital posterior position delivery, 65
postoperative care for, 300–301
with pregnancy-induced hypertension, 289
preparation prior to, 298–300
primary and repeat, 295
with prolonged labor, 137, 141
with transverse lie, 10
vaginal birth after, 20, 237–240
Character witness, 375
Childbirth. *See also* Birth; Delivery; Labor
emotional fears associated with, 22–27
future of, 263–265
history of, 234–235
individualized, 237
in-hospital, 235
intellectual component of, 244
introduction of medical control of, 235
maternal position during, 234, 261
methods of
alternative options in, 256–259
education for, 241–243, 263
nonpharmaceutical, 255–256
types of, 243–249
natural, 245–246
out-of-hospital options for, 261
Pavlovian conditioning for, 247
personalized environment for, 243
psychological component of, 244
psychophysical component of, 243–244
self-care concepts in, 242
support for, 260–262
Childbirth education, 243, 263
marketing of, 241–242
Childbirth Education Association, International, 244
Childbirth without Fear, 243
Chin presentation, *10*, 11
Chlamydia, prophylaxis against, 37, 40
Chloroprocaine, 204
in local perineal infiltration, 215
Chromosomal abnormalities, risk of, 275–276
Civil law, 356
Claims-made policy, 367
Clonus, 292–293
CNMs. *See* Certified nurse midwives
Cocaine, 277
Coccyx
movable, 63–64
nonmovable, 70
Cold stress, 35
Comfort, during labor, 26
Common law, 355–356
Complete breech, 11, 13
Consent, 368–372
form for, 298
Constitution, 355
Consumer advocacy, 263–264
Consumer influence, 263
Continuous caudal block, 210
Contractions. *See also* Uterine contractions
Braxton Hicks, 4, 6–7
concentration during, 27–28
in early active phase, 27
evaluation of, 28–29
hypertonic, 94–95, 96, 114, 173
hypotonic, 93–94, 96
intensity of, 26
pain with, 26
palpation of, 25
tetanic, as, 174
uterine, 4
Contraction stress test, 163, 338–339, 340–341
Contributing cause, 358

Convulsions
  control of, 217
  with pregnancy-induced hypertension, treatment of, 289–290
Cord. *See* Umbilical cord
Cortisol
  excessive, 139
  production of, 136–137
    by fetus, 3
Cost-conscious health care, 233–234
Coughing and deep breathing, following cesarean delivery, 300–301
Counterpressure, 26
Coupling contractions, 95
Creatinine levels, 316
Criminal law, 356
CRNA. *See* Certified Registered Nurse Anesthetist
Crowning, 31
Crown-rump measurement, 314
C-section. *See* Cesarean delivery
CST. *See* Contraction stress test
Cutaneous stimulation, 190

Death, of preterm infant, 333
Deceleration (FHR)
  causes of, 111
  early, 110, 114
  irreversible, 111
  late, 110–111, 114, 217
    nursing interventions for, 114–115
  reversible, 111
  with shoulders, 112, *113*, 114
  smoothing out of, 112
  variable, 111–112, *113*, 114
    nursing interventions for, 114–115
Decrement, 88
Deep tendon reflex, 292–293
  evaluation scale, 292
Deformities, fear of, 23
Dehydration, 24, 146
DeLee-Hillis stethoscopes, *100*
DeLee mucus trap, 38
Delivery, 9. *See also* Childbirth; Labor
  drug-induced anesthesia during, 203–204
  emergency, nursing responsibility for, 37–41
  general anesthesia during, 218–222
  nursing care during, 16–41
  precipitous, 135
  regional anesthesia during, 204–216
Demerol, 197–198, 200
Depositions, 375
Descent. *See* Fetal descent
Dextrostix, 342, 343
Diabetes
  fetal heart rate decelerations with, 111
  medical induction with, 169, 171
  in older women, 276
Diagnostic related groupings (DRGs), 233
Diagonal conjugate, 59, *60*, 69–70
Diaphoresis, 28
Diazepam, 217
Dick-Read, Dr. Grantly, 243–245
Direct cause, 358
Discovery process, 375
Distraction, for pain management, 190
Distress, with pain, 187
Diversion, with prolonged labor, 145
Documentation, 372–374
Doppler unit, 100–103
Down syndrome, risk of, 275–276, 277
Drugs. *See also specific agents*
  action and side effects of during labor, 195–203
  commonly used during labor, 196*t*
  considerations that influence decision to use, 193–195
  maternal/fetal effects of, 194–195
  for pain management, 185–222
    post-test for, 225–231
  potency of, 194
Dry birth, 5
Duranest, 204
Dysmature infants, 333
Dyspnea, with tocolytic agents, 323
Dystocia, 93

Eclampsia
  medical induction with, 169, 171
  with prenancy-induced hypertension, 289

ECV. *See* External cephalic version
EDC. *See* Estimated date of confinement
Effacement, 4, 8, 27, 70, *86*
  of internal os, 85
    in second phase of labor, 31
Effleurage, 26
EFM. *See* Electronic fetal monitor
EFW. *See* Estimated fetal weight
Electrical nerve stimulation, transcutaneous, 258
Electrocardiogram, baseline, 323
Electrodes
  potential for fetal infection with, 105
  scalp, 104
Electronic fetal monitor, 102
Electronic fetal monitoring, 91
  continuous, 103–107
    documentation of, 373
    with post-term labor, 342
    with pregnancy-induced hypertension, 293, 295
  external, *103*, 104, *105*, 107
  internal, 104–105, *106*, 107
    with short-term fetal heart rate variability, 120
  with pregnancy-induced hypertensions, 293–294
Elimination
  to facilitate fetal descent, 72
  during labor, 25–26
Emergency delivery, 37–39
Emotional attachment, 260. *See also* Parent-infant attachment
Emotional problems, 296, 298
Emotional tension, signs of, 70
Endogenous pain control theory, 255, *256*
Endometrium, 84
Endorphins, in pain control, 255
Enema
  contraindications to, 161–162, 163
  during labor, 25–26
  as labor stimulant, 161–163
  questioning of value of, 261
Energy, sudden burst of, 6
Enflurane, 220
Engagement, 3–4, *15*, 16, 141
  absence of, 4
  in breech presentation, 66, 67
  in multipara, 141
  in nullipara, 141–142
  in pelvic inlet, 61
  station and, 12
Environment, orientation to, 24
Epcom hand-held Doppler, *101*
Epidural blocks, lumbar, 209
Epinephrine, 136
Episiotomy, 31, 33, 35
  edema following, 33–34
  indication for, 70
  questioning of value of, 261
Erythromycin ointment, 37, 40
Estimated date of confinement, 313
Estimated fetal weight, 69
Estriol levels, 335
Ethanol, to arrest premature labor, 327–328
Ethrane, 220
Etidocaine, 204
Exhalation breathing, 263–264
  directions for, 254
Expert witnesses, 375
Expulsion, 14, 64
  in breech presentation, 66, 67
Extension, 14, *15*
  with occipital posterior position, 65, 66
  in pelvic outlet, 63, 64
External cephalic version, 68
External fetal monitoring, 91, 93, *103*, 104, *105*, 107
External os, 88
  dilatation of, 85
External rotation, 14, *15*, 63
Eye fixation, 259
Eye infection, prophylaxis against, 36–37

Face presentation, *10*, 11
False labor, 4, 137
  ambulation for, 158–160
Family-centered care
  clinical practice of, 237
  consumer influence on, 235–236
  contemporary, 236
  definition of, 236
  historical perspectives on, 234–235
  marketing and education and, 241–242
  obstetrical design trends and, 240–241
  philosophic foundation of, 236–237

with VBAC, 237–240
Fat cells, measurement of, 316
Father, 260
presence of at birth, 31
Fear. *See also* Anxiety
alleviation of, 190
associated with childbirth, 22–27
pain with, 188
Femoral calcification measurement, 314
Ferning of cervical mucus, 6, 8
Fetal activity, 335–336
nonstress test for, 336–337
Fetal activity acceleration determinations, 336–337
Fetal activity test, 336
Fetal alcohol syndrome, 277
Fetal biophysical profile, 337, 338*t*, 340
Fetal bradycardia
persistent, 217
transient, 213
Fetal descent, 14–16, 31
abnormal patterns of, 143, 144
arrest of, 143, 145
assessment of rate of, 130
decreasing resistance to, 73–74
facilitation of, 145
in multipara, 142–143
in nullipara, 142
patterns of, 141–145
in pelvic inlet, 61
pressure with, 188
progression of, 12, 14
promotion of, 71–75
protracted patterns of, 143
Fetal distress
with administration of anesthesia, 217
oxygenation for, 341
with prolonged labor, 139
testing for, 339
variable deceleration with, 111–112, 114
Fetal head
adaptation by, 54–56
descent into pelvic inlet of, 59–61
extension of, 63
external rotation of, 63
flexion of, 62
internal rotation of, 62
molding of, 70
in pelvic outlet, 63
transverse arrest of, 70
Fetal heart rate, 25
acceleration of, 110
with movement, 337
recognizing, 115–116
artifact in tracing of, *106*
assessment of, 83, 84, 121
with amniocentesis, 315
apparatus for, 99–103
continuous, 103–107
intermittent, 98–103
auscultation of, 19
baseline, 108–110
categories of in beats per minute, 108–109
decelerations in, 110–115
assessment and intervention for, 114–115
late, 217
recognizing, 110–114
electronic monitoring of, 104
first, 335
long-term, 117
monitoring of, 317
with ethanol administration, 328
in second stage of labor, 31
ultrasonic, 313
saltatory pattern of, 119–120
sinusoidal pattern of, 117, 119–120
variability in, 116–120
long-term, 120
short-term, 116–117, 120
in verlex or breech presentation, 22
Fetal monitor, external, *103*, 104. *See also* Electronic fetal monitor
Fetal monitoring. *See also* Electronic fetal monitoring
components of, 83–84
external, *105*, 107
internal, 104–105, *106*, 107
with short-term fetal heart rate variability, 120
liability potential with, 364
Fetal reserve test, 338
Fetal skull, 54, *55*
pH, 339, 341
Fetal tone, 337
Fetopelvic disproportion, 140
abnormal fetal descent with, 143–144, 144
medical induction and, 172

Fetoscope, 102–103
  in fetal heart rate assessment, 99, 100
Fetus. *See also* Fetal descent; Fetal distress; Fetal head; Fetal heart rate
  attitude of, 10, 13
    longitudinal, 71
  back of, stroking of, 75, 76
  blood sample of, 339
  breathing movements of, 337
  estimated weight of, 69
  expulsion of, 14, *15*, 63–66
  extension of, 64
  growth retardation of, 111
  infection of with electrodes, 105
  lie of, 10, 12*t*, 13
  lung maturity of, acceleration of, 327
  maneuvers of head during labor and delivery, 14, *15*. *See also* Fetal head
  movement of, resistance to, 70
  oxygenation of, 341
  position of, 11–12, 12*t*
    nursing interventions to change, 75–76
  reactivity of, 103
  relationship of to maternal pelvis, 10–14. *See also* Fetopelvic disproportion
  response of to uterine contractions, 98
  risk to with pregnancy-induced hypertension, 293–294
  rotation of, 75–76
  trauma to
    with breech presentation, 67–68
    heart rate and, 25
    with oxytocin administration, 173
    with prolonged labor, 146, 147
  well-being of
    post-mature, 335–341
    preterm, 309–334
FHR. *See* Fetal heart rate
Flexion, 14, *15*, 16, 62
  in breech presentation, 66, 67
  of fetal head, 55–56
  in occipital posterior position, 64, 66
Floating, 359
Flow sheets, 373
Fluid intake, inadequate, 25
Fluid volume deficit, 33
  with abnormal contraction patterns, 95
  with prolonged labor, 145–146
Fluothane, 220
Foam test, 316
Footling breech, 11, 13
  mechanism of labor in, 67
Forane, 220
Forceps
  fear of use of, 23
  inappropriateness of, 70
  introduction of use of, 235
  for occipital posterior position delivery, 65
Fourth Amendment, 355
Frank breech, 11, 13
Friedman's labor curves, 130, *131*
Fundal height, 313, 317, 335
Fundus, 88
  after delivery, 35
  of mother after delivery, 33
  palpation of, 90–91, 93
  uterine contractions in, 84–85
Funic souffle, 99

Gas exchange, impaired, 35, 219
Gate Control Theory, 255
Gestation, prolonged, fetal well-being with, 333–343
Gestational age, methods of determining, 313–318
Goff v. Doctor's General Hospital from San Jose, 365–366
Gonococcal infections, prophylaxis against, 36, 40
Grandparents, 260
Gravity, fetal descent and, 72, 159–160
Gray-scale imaging ultrasound, 314
Grieving
  at death of preterm infant, 333
  for potential loss of baby, 331
Gross fetal body movements, 337
Guided imagery, 191
Gynecoid pelvis, 57–58
  inlet of, *59*
  mechanisms of labor through, 54–68
  midpelvis of, 61–62

Hallucinogens, 277
Halothane, 220
Headache, postspinal, 207
Health care
individualized, non-fragmented, 237
rising costs of, 233–234
trends in, 233–234
Health care providers, attitude of, 237
Health care system, restructuring of, 232–233
Health maintenance organizations, 233
Heart rate, fetal. *See* Fetal heart rate
Heat loss, prevention of, 39
Hematomas, 287
Hemorrhage. *See also* Abruptio placenta; Bleeding
with hypertension, 280–281
intracranial, 67–68
during labor, 280–282
from placental implantation site, 33
postpartum, 286–288
in preterm infants, 312
Heroin, 277
Herpes lesions, 22
Herrup v. South Miami Hospital Foundation, Inc., 363
Hiatt v. Groce, 377
Histamine release, 196
HIV transmission, recommendations for prevention of transmission of in health-care settings, 407–413
HMOs. *See* Health maintenance organizations
Home birthing, 262
Hospital standards, 360–361
Human immunodeficiency virus (HIV) transmission, recommendations for prevention of transmission of in health-care settings, 407–413
Husband-coach, 245
Hydralazine, 293
Hydramnios, 5, 8
medical induction and, 172
Hydration, 25
Hydrotherapy, 256
Hydroxyzine, 203
Hydroxyzine pamoate, 202
Hypermagnesemia, 294
Hypertension
convulsions with, 289–290
nursing actions for, 289–290, 291
excessive bleeding with, 280–281
fetal heart rate decelerations with, 111
in older woman, 276
pregnancy-induced, 273, 288–291
delivery with, 291
fetal risk with, 293–294
treatment for, 291–295
Hyperthermia
with infection, 24
with prostaglandin gel, 177
Hypertonic contractions, 94–96, 114
with oxytocin administration, 173
Hyperventilation, fetal distress with, 187
Hypnosuggestion, 258–259
Hypocalcemia, 294
Hypotension, maternal, 114
with anesthesia, 216
emergency treatment for, 218
with regional anesthesia, 206–207
supine, 300
therapy for, 217–218
with tocolytic agents, 323
Hypothalamus, 163
prostaglandin effects on, 177
Hypothermia, of newborn, 35
Hypotonic contractions, 93–94, 96
Hypoxia, fetal, 108, 112, 136
with oxytocin administration, 173
with pain, 187
with prolonged labor, 139
testing for, 339

ICEA. *See* Childbirth Education Association, International
Iliopeclineal lines, 61
Imaging, 258
Incoordinate contractions, 95
Increment, 88
Individual practice associations (IPAs), 233
Indomethacin, 327
Induction, 165, 178

Induction—*Continued*
medical, 169–171
with oxytocin, 171–176
with prostaglandin gel, 176–177
surgical, 165–169
Infants. *See* Neonate
Infection, 24
in preterm infants, 312
with prolonged labor, 145
with rupture of membranes, 167–168
Informed Consent Form, 298
Infusion pump devices, 173
Inhalation anesthesia, 219–220
advantages and disadvantages of, 219
Injury, 358. *See also* Fetus, trauma to; Maternal trauma
Internal fetal monitor, 116–117
Internal fetal monitoring, 91–92, 104–107
advantages of, 92, 93
with short-term fetal heart rate variability, 120
Internal os, 88
effacement of, 85
Internal rotation, 14, *15*, 16, 62
in breech presentation, 66, 67
in occipital posterior position, 65–66
Interrogatories, 375
Intestinal peristalsis, 161, 163
Intracranial hemorrhage, with breech presentations, 67–68
Intrauterine growth retardation, 293
with adolescent pregnancy, 273
indication of, 313
Intrauterine pressure catheter, 91–92
Intravenous anesthesia, 220–222
complications of, 221–222
disadvantages of, 220
Ischial spines, 62, 70
Isoflurane, 220
Isoxsuprine, 108
to arrest preterm labor, 322, 326
nursing interventions with, 327
IUC. *See* Intrauterine pressure catheter
IUGR. *See* Intrauterine growth retardation

James v. Kennebec Valley Medical Center of Maine, 365
Joint Commission on Accreditation of Hospitals standard, 359–360
Jury, 376

Karmel, Marjorie, 246–247
Knee-chest position, 75
Knee-jerk reflex, 292
Kneeling breech, 67

Labor
acceleration phase of, 133
active phase of, 132–134
arrest of, 138–141
slow slope, 137–138, 140
adolescent in, 273–275
beginning of, 1–2
cause of pain in, 187–189
complicating factors in, 273–302
post-test on, 305–308
contemporary approaches to, post-test for, 266–271
deceleration phase of, 133
drug action and side effects during, 195–203
drug-induced anesthesia during, 203–204
false, 4, 137
ambulation for, 158–159, 160
first stage of, 8
active phase of, 8, 132–134
arrest of, 138–141
early active phase of, 27–28
latent phase of, 8, 22, 132
prolonged latent phase of, 134
transition phase of, 8, 28–30
fourth stage of, 9, 32–35
general anesthesia during, 218–222
graphing course of, 130
methodology of, 130–131
post-test for, 149–157
induction of
medical, 169–177
surgical, 165–169
maternal activity during, 25
maternal position during, 261
mechanisms of, 14–16, *15*, 53–54, 58
modified, 64–68

nursing implications related to, 69–76
post-test for, 79–82
through gynecoid pelvis, 54–64
nursing care during, 16–35
nursing implications for support of, 261
onset of, 130–131
ambiguous definition of, 137
recognition of, 16–17
out-of-hospital options for, 261. *See also* Birthing centers
post-test on overview of, 43–52
precipitous, 134–136
problems with, 136
premonitory signs of, 3–8
preterm, 310–333
process of in future, 263–265
prolonged, 136–140
in active phase, 140–141
care with, 145–147
in latent phase, 137–138
medical management of, 137–138, 140
supportive therapy for, 137, 139
regional anesthesia during, 204–216
second stage of, 8, 30–31
sitting and standing positions during, 75
stages of, 8–9, 30–35
standing or sitting postures during, 72–73
support for, 260–262
theories of, 2–3
third stage of, 9, 31–32
uterus anatomy and physiology of during, 84–88
Labor/delivery/recovery/postpartum room, 240
Labor-delivery-recovery room, 28, 240
Labor stimulants, 158–164
simulation of
forms of, 165–178
post-test for, 181–184
Lacerations, 284
postpartum hemorrhage with, 287
Lamaze, Dr. Fernand, 247
Lamaze method, 70, 246–249
parts of, 247
Laminaria tents, 170, 171
LDR. *See* Labor-delivery-recovery room
LDR/P. *See* Labor/delivery/recovery/postpartum room
Leffscope, 99–100
Legal considerations, 354–355
documentation and, 372–374
malpractice and, 367–368, 375–377
in nursing, 355–358
patient's rights and, 368–372
post-test for, 380–383
"reasonable nurse" standard and, 361–363
standard of care and, 360–361
Legal liability, 358–360
in each step of nursing process, 363–376
elements required to establish, 358
Leopold's maneuvers, 18–19, 21, 99
Levallorphan, 199, 200
Liability insurance, for birthing centers, 262
License sanction, 356
Lidocaine, 204
in local perineal infiltration, 215
Lightening, 3–4
Litigation, 356
strategies to discourage, 372–374
Lochia
after cesarean delivery, 300
after normal delivery, 33
Lorfan, 199, 200
L/S ratio, 316, 317
Lumbar epidural block, 209

Magnesium sulfate
to arrest preterm labor, 326
ideal level of, 293
for pregnancy-induced hypertension, 291–292, 295
toxicity of, 292
signs of, 327
Malposition, 137
abnormal fetal descent with, 143–144
Malpractice, 357, 358
insurance for, 367–368
lawsuit, components and procedures of, 375–377
Mandatory licensure law, 355
Marcaine, 204
Massage, 257
in uterine hemorrhage, 287

Maternal complications, 272–273, 301–302
of adolescent, 273–275
bleeding in, 280–288
with cesarean delivery, 295–301
of older woman, 275–277
post-test for, 305–308
with pregnancy-induced hypertension, 288–295
of substance abuser, 277–280
Maternal-fetal monitoring, 83–84. *See also* Electronic fetal monitoring; Fetal monitoring
post-test for, 124–128
Maternal fever, 108–109
Maternal pelvis. *See also* Pelvis
fetal relationship to, 10–14
quadrants of, *11*
Maternal position, 26, 261
Maternal regurgitation, 220–221
Maternal symptoms, 70
Maternal trauma
with breech presentation, 67
with prolonged labor, 146, 147
Maternity care
contemporary, pillars of, 236–242
dynamic system for, 233–234
family-centered, 234–242
marketing of, 263
Maternity units
dehumanizing routines of, 235
length of stay at, 233, 263
May v. Wm. Beaumont Hospital, 365
Meconium aspiration syndrome, 342
Meconium-stained amniotic fluid, 5, 8, 342
Medical chart, 372
relevant information on, 373–374
Medicare, DRGs of, 233
Medulla, stimulation of, 196
Membranes. *See also* Rupture of membranes
stripping of, 160–161
Mental relaxation, 246. *See also* Relaxation
Meperidine hydrochloride, 197–198, 200
Mepivocaine, 204
in local perineal infiltration, 215
Metabolic acidosis, fetal, 112
Methadone, 277
Methergine, 35
Midpelvis, 61–62
borders of, 62
contraction of, 70
diameters of, 62
Midwives, 262
Molding, 54, 56, 70
Mouth rinses, 26
Mouth-to-mouth resuscitation, of newborn, 39
Movable coccyx, 63–64
Multipara
labor curve of, 132, 133
medical induction and, 173
Multiple gestation pregnancy, 172. *See also* Twinning
Muscular relaxation, 247, 249. *See also* Relaxation
Music, in relaxation, 257–258
Myometrium, 84, 88
dysfunction of, 137

NAACOG standards, 91, 360, 362, 363
Naegele's rule, 313
Nalbuphine hydrochloride, 201
Naloxone, 198–199, 200, 201
Narcan, 198–199, 200
Narcotic agonists, 200
action and side effects of, 195–198
neonatal neurobehavior effects of, 197
Narcotic agonists/antagonists, 200–201
Narcotic antagonists, 198–200
Narcotic depression, 198–199
Natural childbirth, 245–246
Natural Childbirth, 243
Natural healing method, 256–257
Nausea, with anesthesia, 217
Negligence, 357, 358
gross, 359
Nembutal, 202
Neonate
behavioral changes of with barbiturates, 203
family-centered care of, 234–242
floppy but alert, 204
immediate care of, 35–37
neurobehavioral effects of anesthesia on, 204
nursing of, 36
placement of on maternal abdomen, 32, 38, 41
positive identification of, 33, 36

reaction to first sight of, 32
respiratory depression of, 198–199
resuscitation of, 39, 217
substance abuse effects on, 277
weighing of, 36
Nerve ganglia compression, 188
Nesacaine, 204
Nesting, 310
Nifedipine, 326
Nipple stimulation
contraction test, 338
contraindications to, 164
as labor stimulant, 163–164
Nisentil, 198
Nitrazine test tape, 5, 8
Nitrous oxide, 219–220
Nonstress test, 336–337, 340
Norepinephrine, 136
Novocaine, 204
Nubain, 201
Nuchal cord, 38, 41
Nullipara
engagement in, 141, 142
labor curve of, 133
Numorphone, 198
Nurse practice acts, 356–357
Nurses
duty of, 358
law applied to, 355–358
legal liability of, 358–360
malpractice insurance for, 367–368
malpractice suits against, 375–377
understaffing of, 359
Nursing assessment
at admission, 17–22
of laboring woman, 16–17
liability potential in, 363
of mechanisms of labor, 69–76
of mother after delivery, 33–34
during precipitous labor, 135
prior to cesarean delivery, 298
in second stage of labor, 35
Nursing care
during post-term labor, 341–342
standards of, 360–361, 362–363
Nursing diagnoses
with abnormal contraction patterns, 95–96
in emergency delivery, 37
at fourth stage of labor, 32–33
liability potential with, 365
for newborn immediately after delivery, 35
list of, 384–406
for pregnant adolescents, 275
for second stage of labor, 30
for substance abuser, 279–280
at third stage of labor, 31–32
Nursing interventions
with amniocentesis, 318
to change fetal position, 75–76
for dealing with fears associated with childbirth, 23–27
for fetal heart rate decelerations, 114–115
liability potential with, 364–365
for nonpharmacologic management of pain, 190–191
potential liability in each step of, 363–367
for pregnant adolescents, 274–275
to promote descent, 71–75
Nutrition, 25

Oblique position, 55
Obstetric care
contemporary changes in, 237
conventional vs. family-centered, 238*t*
malpractice insurance in, 367–368
trends in, 240–241
Obstetric conjugate, 59, *60*
Obstetric history, 17, 69
Occipital posterior position, 64–66
problems for mother and fetus with, 65, 66
Occipital presentation, 10
Occipitofrontal diameter, 55, *56*, 59, 61
Occiput anterior position, 11
Occiput presentations, *See* Vertex presentations
Occiput transverse position, 55
Occurrence policy, 367
Older woman, labor of, 275–277
Oligohydramnios, 5
Ophthalmia neonatorum, prophylaxis against, 36–37
Ophthalmia Neonatorum of the National Society of Prevent Blindness, Committee on, 37

Organ communication system theory, 2–3
Os, internal and external, 85, 88
Overprotectiveness, 310
Overshoots, recurrent, 115–116
Oxygen, 341–343
  decreased, 135
  for fetal heart rate decelerations, 115
  for hypotension, 217
  inadequate, 114
Oxymorphone hydrochloride, 198
Oxytocic drugs, 35
  hyperstimulation with, 111
Oxytocin
  administration of, 32, 173–175
    liability potential with, 364–365
  for augmentation, 172
  cervix response to, 288
  conditions warranting use of, 169
  contraindications to use of, 172–173
  coupling with, 95
  discontinuance of, 114, 217
  as labor stimulant, 135, 140–141, 144, 167, 169–176, 341
    in obese women, 92
  with magnesium sulfate, 293, 295
  pituitary release of, 39, 163, 172
    inhibition of, 327
  to stimulate descent, 144
Oxytocin challenge test, 338
Oxytocin stimulation theory, 2

Pain
  alternative options in control of, 256–259
  analgesia and anesthesia for, 191–193
  causes of in labor, 189
  with contractions, 26
  as distress, 187
  drugs for
    considerations in decision to use, 193–195
    post-test for, 225–231
  endogenous pain control theory of, 255
  endorphins and, 255
  fear of, 22
  gate control theory of, 255
  in labor, causes of, 187–189
  management of, 185–222
  nonpharmacologic interventions to relieve, 189–191
  physical control of, 256
  psycho-physiologic responses to, 186–187
  socially conditioned, 243–245
  as stress, 187, 189
  of uterine contractions, 97–98
Palpation, of fundus, 90–91
Panting, 31
Paracervical block, 212
  advantages and disadvantages of, 213–214
  injection sites for, *212*
  injury potential with, 213
Parental-infant attachment, 332
Parenthood, transition to, 260, 262
Parenting, effects of postpartum hemorrhage on, 288
PARU. *See* Post-anesthesia recovery unit
Patellar reflex, 292
Patel v. South Fulton Hospital, 363
Pathologic retraction ring, 86
Patient's Bill of Rights, 369, 371
Patient-controlled analgesia pump, 300
Patient's rights, 368–372
Pelvic diameter, 59
Pelvic inlet, 58–61
  boundaries of, 59, 61
  diagonal conjugate, 69–70
  diameter of, 61
  shape of, 57
Pelvic outlet, 63–64
Pelvic rock, 26, 75, 76
Pelvimetry, x-ray, 20, 22, 59
Pelvis, 10–14
  anatomy of, 54
  characteristics of, 57–58
  measurements of, 69–70
  planes of, 58
  types of, 57–58
Pentazocine hydrochloride, 201
Pentobarbital sodium, 202
Perimetrium, 84
Perineal infiltration, local, 215–216
Perineal muscles, relaxation of, 216
Perineal pads, 281
Perineal preparation, 24
Perineal stretching, 38, 41
Perineum
  assessment of after delivery, 33–34

cold compresses or ice for, 35
observation of, 40
stretching and displacement of, 188
Persistent occipitoposterior position, 65, 70–71
Phenergan, 202
Phosphatidyl glycerol, 316
Phospholipids, measurement of, 316
Physical dissociation-eye techniques, 259
Physiologic retraction ring, 85–86
Pitocin, 35, 171, 176, 300
Placenta
delivery of, 32
expulsion of, 9, 38
insufficiency, 341
interruption of blood flow of, 98
maturity, determination of, 314
progesterone production by, 2
separation of, 32, 35
Placenta previa, 282–286
with vaginal bleeding, 19–20
Placental abruption, 111
Placental grading, 315*t*
Placental stage, 9
Placental sufficiency test, 338
Plaintiff, 375
Platypelloid pelvis, 57
Pneumonitis, 342
Pneumothorax, 342
Polyhydramnios, 5, 8
Pontacaine, 204
Position, 11–12, 14
occipital posterior, 64–66
Post-anesthesia recovery unit, 300
Postmature infant, 333
appearance of, 335
characteristics of, 334–335
Postmature syndrome, 334
Postmaturity, 277
fetal heart rate decelerations with, 111
risk of, 275
Postpartum hemorrhage, 286–288
nursing actions for, 288
Postspinal headache, 207
Post-term infant
immediate care of, 342–343
physiologic disadvantages of, 343
Post-term labor
assessment for fetal well-being with, 335–341
effects of on mother and infant, 333–335
immediate care of infant with, 342–343
nursing measures for, 341–342
post-test for, 348–353
PPM. *See* Psychoprophylactic method
Predictive assessment data, 69–71
Pre-eclampsia, medical induction with, 169, 171
Preferred provider organizations (PPOs), 233
Pregnancy-induced hypertension, 288–291
convulsions with, 289–291
fetal risk with, 293–294
nursing diagnoses with, 294
treatment for, 291–295
Pregnant Patient's Bill of Rights and Responsibilities, 370, 372
Premature infant. *See* Preterm infant
Presentation, 10–11, 12*t*
breech, 11, 13, 66–68, *69*, 104
cephalic, 10, 13
conversion to, 68–69
presenting part and, 13–14
vertex, 10, 22, 54, 68
Presenting part, 12*t*, 13–14
Preterm delivery, nursing measures for, 328–329
Preterm infant
acceptance of by parents, 329–330
cardinal signs of, 330
death of, 333
parental attachment to, 332
physical features of, variations in, 329–330
physiologic hindrances of, 311–312
psychological effects of on mother, 310–311
psychological tasks for mothers of, 331
Preterm labor
ambulatory monitoring for, 318–320
determining gestational age in, 313–318
early symptoms of, 318
facilitation of parental-infant attachment in, 332
interventions to arrest, 318–328
nonpharmacological interventions for, 318–322

Preterm labor—*Continued*
nursing measures for delivery in, 328–329
pharmacological interventions for, 322–328
and physiologic hindrances of preterm infant, 311–312
post-test for, 348–353
preterm infant death and, 333
preterm infant physical features in, 329–330
psychological effects of on mother, 310–311
psychological tasks of mother in, 331
risk factors for, 318, 319*t*
Procaine, 204
Progesterone, 2
Progesterone deprivation theory, 2
Promethazine, 202–203
Prospective payment systems (PPS), 233
Prostaglandin
gel, 176–177
release of, 2
Prostaglandin synthetase inhibitors, 327
Proteinuria, 293
Pseudosinusoidal patterns, 119
Psychological support, 257–258
Psychoprophylactic method, 246–249
Pubic arch, measurement of, 70
Pudendal block, 214–215
Pushing, 31, 35
breathing and, 253
decreased effectiveness of, 207
to promote fetal descent, 74

Quickening, 313
time of, 335

Radiographic studies, 314
in pelvic measurement, 69
Read method, 243–245
Real-time scanning ultrasound, 314
"Reasonable nurse" standard, 361–363
Regulations, 355
Relaxation, 26
in Bradley method, 246
between contractions, 28
with imager/visualization, 258
in Lamaze method, 247, 249
with music, 257–258
for pain management, 243–244
for pain relief, 190–191
Respiratory depression, 201
Respiratory distress
with meconium aspiration, 342
in preterm infants, 312
Respiratory distress syndrome, 316
Respondeat superior rule, 359
Rest interval, 89–90
external and internal monitoring of, 91
Restitution, 14, *15*, 63, 64
Resuscitation, of newborn, 39
after emergency delivery, 217
Retraction rings
pathological, 86–87
physiologic, 85–86, *87*, 88
Rh sensitization, medical induction with, 169
Ritodrine, 108, 110
to arrest preterm labor, 322, 326
nursing interventions with, 327
ROM. *See* Rupture of membranes
Rotation, of fetal head, 55–56
Rupture of membranes, 4–6, 28
artificial, 4
documentation of, 373
implications of, 167–168
infection potential with, 167–168
misconception about, 130
prolonged, 169, 171
spontaneous, 4
surgical induction of labor with, 165–169
tests for, 8

Sacral pressure, 70
Sacral promontory, 59, 61
Sacrum, 61–62, 63
Saddle block, 210
Saltatory pattern, 119–120
Scalp electrodes, 104
Scultetus binder, 71–72
Secobarbital, 299
Secobarbital sodium, 202
Seconal, 202
Sedation, excessive, 137
abnormal fetal descent with, 143–144

Sedatives, 202–203. *See also*
    specific agents
Seizures. *See* Convulsions
Self-care concepts, 242
Sermchief v. Gonzales case, 356
Sexually transmitted disease, 273
Shake test, 316
Shoulder presentation, 11
Siblings, 260
Silver nitrate, 37
Sims' position, 75
Sinciput presentation, 10–11
Single-room maternity care system,
    240, 263
Sinusoidal patterns, 117, 120
  types of, 119
Sodium pentothal, 220, 221
Spinal block, 210–211
Spontaneous rupture of
    membranes, 4
Spousal abuse, 284
Squatting position, 72–73, 75
SRMC system. *See* Single-room
    maternity care system
SROM. *See* Spontaneous rupture of
    membranes
S-shaped curve in labor, 132–133
Stadol, 200–201
Station, 12, 14
Statute of limitations, 375
Statutes, 355
Statutory law, 356
Stethoscopes, *100*
  in fetal heart rate assessment, 99
Stress
  with pain, 187, 189
  reduction of with breathing
    techniques, 249
Stress hormones, 136
Stress test, 338
Stripping membranes, 160–161
Subarachnoid block, 210–211
Suboccipitobregmatic diameter, 55,
    56
Subpublic arch, 63, 64
Substance abuse, 273–274
  complications associated with,
    278*t*
Substance abuser
  complications with, 277–280
  fetal assessment in, 279
  pain threshold in, 279
Suctioning, 342
  of post-term infant, 343
Summons, 375
Supervisory nurses, 359
Support system, for pregnant
    adolescents, 273
Supportive care, 23–24
Supportive roles, 260
Surfactant, 316
Symphysis pubis, 59, 61
Syntocinon, 35, 171, 176

Tachycardia, 108—110
  fetal, 315
  with tocolytic agents, 323
Talwin, 201
TENS. *See* Transcutaneous
    electrical nerve stimulation
Terbutaline
  to arrest preterm labor, 322, 326
  nursing interventions with, 327
Tetanic contractions, 95, 174
Tetracaine, 204
Thank You, Dr. Lamaze, 246
Therapeutic touch, 256–257
Tissue perfusion, 98
Tocodynamometer, 91
Tocolytic agents
  to arrest preterm labor, 322–328
  criteria for use of, 327
  dosages of, 324–325*t*
Tocotransducer, 91
Tonus, 88, 91, 93
Torts, 356–357
Transcutaneous electrical nerve
    stimulation, 258
  with cesarean delivery, 300
Transducer, 91, 93
  ultrasound, 104
Transient fetal bradycardia, 213
Transverse arrest, 70
Transverse lie, 10
Trauma, 284
  bleeding with, 281
  with prolonged labor, 146
Trendelenburg position, 284
Trevino v. United States, 364
Trial by jury, 376
Trial decisions, 355
  examples of, 363–365
Twinning, 277
  risk of, 275–276

Ultrasonic device, 313
Ultrasonography
  at admission, 20
  gray-scale imaging, 314
  in pelvic measurement, 69
  real-time, 314, 337
Ultrasound transducer, 104
Umbilical cord
  clamping of, 32
  compromise of, 112
  cutting of, 32
  prolapse of, 4
  wrapped around fetal neck, 38, 41
Urinary bladder
  assessment of, 34
  after delivery, 34–35
  distention of, 25
  emptying of, 72, 75
  tone of, 25
Urinary retention
  after delivery, 3
  with prolonged labor, 146–147
Urine specimen, 17
Uterine contractions, 4, 6–7
  abnormal patterns of, 93–97
  ambulatory monitoring for, 318–321
  assessment of, 83–84, 121
    methods for, 90–93
    objective, 90
  coordination of, 30–31
  decelerations of, late, 341
  duration of, 89
  frequency of, 89
  fundal dominant, 84–85, 88
  hypertonic, 94–96, 114
    with oxytocin administration, 173
  hypotonic, 93–94, 96
  incoordinate, 95
  intensity of, 89
  internal monitoring of, 92
    advantages of, 92–93
  at onset of labor, 130–131
  pain of, assessment of, 97–98
  pattern of, *88*
  promotion of for maternal safety, 39
  terms used to describe, 88–90
  tetanic, 95, 174
Uterine hypoxia, 136
Uterine impulse pathway, *193*
Uterine souffle, 109
Uteroplacental circulation, 88
Uterus. *See also* Uterine contractions
  anatomy and physiology of during labor, 84–88
  atony of, 287
  bruit of, 99
  dysfunction of
    primary, 93, 96
    secondary, 93
  hemorrhage of, in older woman, 276
  muscle fibers of, 84, *85*
  musculature of, 243
    longitudinal, 88
  parts of, 84, 88
  rupture of, 284, 286
  stimulation of, for prolonged labor, 140–141
  at term, *86*

Vaginal birth after cesarean, 20, 237–240
  bleeding with, 284
  candidates for, *239*
  options for, 238–239
  prenatal instruction for, 240
  risks of, 238
  special needs in, 239–240
Vaginal bleeding, 19, 22
  characteristics of, 282
  excessive, 280, 281–282
  following cesarean delivery, 300
  with hypertension, 280–281
  from lacerations, 284
Vaginal breech delivery, mortality and morbidity with, 68
Vaginal examination, 70
  at admission, 19–20
  contraindications for, 19–20, 22
  infection potential with, 145, 147
Vaginal lacerations, 284
  examination for, 286
Valsalva maneuver, 253
Vasodilan, 326
VBAC. *See* Vaginal birth after cesarean section
Vena cava syndrome, 114
Vernix caseosa, 5
Vertex presentation, 10, 54
  conversion to, 68
  fetal heart rate ausculation in, 22
Vistaril, 202